TABLE OF CONTENTS

CHAPTER 9: TO REPORT OR NOT TO REPORT: IS THAT THE ONLY QUESTION? CHILD MALTREATMENT AND SOCIAL WORK RESPONSIBILITIES IN ACUTE HEALTHCARE SETTINGS

CHAPTER 12: THE INTERNET AND THE RISK FOR MALTREATMENT

CHAPTER 13: THE ROLE OF LAW ENFORCEMENT IN THE INVESTIGATION OF CHILD MALTREATMENT

Recognition of
Child Abuse
for the Mandated Reporter

Chapter 1

PHYSICAL ABUSE

JOHN LOISELLE, M.D.

"Physical abuse" can be defined in a surprising number of ways. Individuals, institutions, and specialties all offer differing opinions of what constitutes physical abuse of a child. Federal, state, and even local government agencies have set forth statutes with different definitions. The current federal definition of abuse is "any recent act or failure to act that results in imminent risk of serious harm, death, serious physical or emotional harm, sexual abuse or exploitation of a child (<18 years) by a parent or caretaker who is responsible for the child's welfare" (Child Abuse Prevention and Treatment Act, 1996). Individual state laws vary with respect to the age of the child subject to abuse, who may be considered a perpetrator, what degree of injury is necessary, and whether an act or omission resulting in injury constitutes abuse. Every state also specifies individuals within certain factions as mandated reporters of physical abuse. While familiarity with the legal definition for a particular region is helpful, a detailed knowledge of the law is not necessary for mandated reporters in order to report such suspicions.

The most remarkable fact about physical abuse may not be how frequently it occurs, but how long it

was unrecognized or ignored in the past. Detailed descriptions of battered children and the study of child abuse are still relatively young. The first formal descriptions of inflicted injuries as such only appeared in the medical literature in 1946 (Caffey, 1946) and the phenomenon was not considered a significant problem until the 1960s. Even today, cases are missed that in retrospect seem obvious even to an untrained person. At times our brains refuse to acknowledge what our eyes tell us because we find it inconceivable that human beings are capable of inflicting such brutal injuries on young children. We are more willing to believe fantastic stories than to accept the obvious one to explain these injuries.

The reality is that abuse is a common cause of physical injury in children. One out of every 10 injuries treated in an emergency department is the result of abuse (Holter & Friedman, 1968). In 1997 an average of two children under age 4 years were killed each day in the United States as the result of abuse (Paradise et al., 1995). Countless cases go unidentified, and numerous more go unreported. It has been well documented that victims of abuse who remain undetected and unreported frequently face

repeated episodes of abuse (American Academy of Pediatrics, 2000).

The mandated reporter faces a number of challenges in the process of identifying physical abuse apart from the differing definitions of the condition. It is not possible for a mandated reporter to identify a physically abused child unless he or she first considers abuse to be a possibility, as is illustrated by past history. The tremendous rise in the number of reports of abuse in the past 40 years does not reflect an increase in the rate at which abuse occurs, but rather an increased realization of its existence and a willingness to address the issue. Abuse injuries can and do take many forms. They can occur in any child, in any family, and in any culture. Some factors place a child in a category considered to be at greater risk of abuse, but every child is vulnerable to some degree. Some injuries are more indicative of abuse, but almost any injury may be inflicted.

Certain types of injuries fall into an ambiguous or gray area on which not even experts can agree. Where does discipline stop and abuse begin? When is it an accident, and when is it an injury due to negligent supervision?

Definitions often leave these areas open to individual interpretation. In many instances, inflicted injury cannot be distinguished from accidental injury by appearance alone. The child who sustains a bruise on the forehead when stumbling on the sidewalk is indistinguishable from the one who sustains the same injury when physically thrown to the sidewalk.

Considering these difficulties, many mandated reporters mistakenly feel their knowledge is inadequate to recognize abuse. An extensive knowledge of physiology and medicine is not necessary. Certain common childhood injuries are familiar to all of us, and we know the general, predictable mechanisms or events responsible for these injuries. They occur in expected locations with anticipated frequency and in familiar patterns. In the same way, many abuse injuries have recognizable patterns. While some injuries can result from accidental or inflicted trauma, other injuries are overrepresented in or so highly associated with abuse as to be considered distinctly characteristic. Features more suggestive of an inflicted injury may relate to the particular pattern, location, frequency, severity, or extent of the injury. This chapter will review a number of these characteristics.

Identifying abuse does not rely on physical findings alone. Discrepancies in the history or explanation for the injury in question are often crucial in detecting an abused child (Table 1-1). Features of the history that raise a suspicion of abuse include disclosure by the child or perpetrator, a significant injury without a clear history of trauma, an explanation that is inconsistent with the severity or type of the injury, a story that changes, or a delay in seeking medical care for an injury. The history or physical findings alone may raise concerns that abuse may have occurred, but many times it is a combination of information that raises concern to the threshold of reporting. In more complex cases it may require additional information acquired through laboratory testing or imaging studies.

The mandated reporter is not required to act as a detective and track down additional evidence of abuse before registering a concern, nor does this mandate encourage overzealous attempts by individuals to actively seek out abuse or find reasons to fit injuries into this category. However, all adults involved in the care of children do have the responsibility to be aware of and remain alert for such cases. The law mandates certain individuals to report a suspicion of child abuse. The operative word is "suspicion," which falls well below the level of "proof." Abuse is rarely "proven" by the individual who initially reports the case, nor is it that individual's responsibility to provide such proof.

Numerous conditions mimic abuse injuries. Although many are discussed here, it is not the obligation nor often within the abilities of the reporter to

---

Table 1-1. Features of the History that Raise a Suspicion of Abuse

- Disclosure by the child or perpetrator

- Injury without a history of trauma

- A history or explanation that is inconsistent with the severity or type of injuries found

- A history that changes

- A delay in seeking medical care for an injury

know, consider, and exclude every possible alternative explanation for a suspicious lesion. This task is often best left to a physician or other subspecialist. The rare likelihood that one of many uncommon confounding conditions might be responsible should not overshadow the concerns about abuse and paralyze the mandated reporter to inaction, but instead should encourage further investigation.

The role of the individual and the extent to which he or she is expected to investigate an abuse case will vary depending on the individual's level of training and the specific relationship with the child. There are multiple layers in the evaluation of child physical abuse. Each step provides an additional layer of knowledge and sophistication in the assessment process. Reporters comprise the foundation. The schoolteacher who reports a suspicious mark on a pupil gains the assistance of the local division of child protective services, which can then involve a physician or nurse trained in the evaluation of abuse to further assess the injury. These individuals have access to additional subspecialists or can conduct additional studies when necessary. Specially trained social workers or police can perform further interviews or investigate the home environment. The information provided here may not be applicable to many of these personnel, but instead is intended to be comprehensive enough to provide useful information so an individual can identify cases that should be referred to the next step in the evaluation.

When faced with a child who has a questionable physical injury, the reporter should ask a number of questions:

*   What about this injury makes it seem out of the ordinary?

*   Does the explanation for this injury seem plausible?

*   Does the explanation fit the physical findings, and is it within the child's developmental capacity?

*   What other psychosocial factors may place this child at increased risk for abuse?

One goal of this chapter is to assist the reporter in answering additional questions, such as:

*   Are there features of this injury that are consistent with common mechanisms of abuse?

*   Are there characteristic findings or patterns that suggest this injury was inflicted?

*   What nonabuse conditions might explain these findings?

*   What further evaluations would be helpful in distinguishing inflicted from accidental injuries?

Not all of us who care for children are experts in identifying physical abuse, but by the nature of our contact with children, we each possess a level of expertise in our knowledge of common childhood injuries and childhood development. This knowledge is critical in identifying injuries that are out of the ordinary. This gut feeling that something is not right provides the first clue that an injury may be the result of abuse. Acting on that feeling can lead

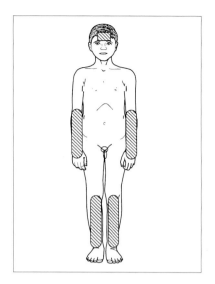

Figure 1-1. *Common distribution of bruising in a child who is walking.*

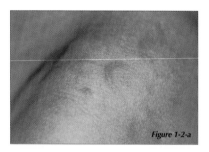

Figure 1-2-a

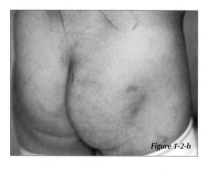

Figure 1-2-b

Figure 1-2. (a) *Loop marks from a rolled up cord. The dark coloration indicates these are old injuries.* **(b)** *Fresh loop mark above the buttock associated with scratch marks and bruising of the buttocks.*

to the appropriate identification of an abused child and to help for the child and family.

♦ SKIN

BRUISING

The skin is the most commonly injured area of the body. It can respond to a range of insults with marks that vary in shape, color, pattern, and location. Bruising is a manifestation of the rupture of small blood vessels beneath the skin's surface. In certain medical conditions bruising can occur spontaneously, but it is usually the result of trauma or pressure applied to the skin. Although bruising can occur on any region of skin, it occurs predominantly over areas with an underlying bony prominence. In the normal course of a child's play, the areas most likely to be affected include the shins, knees, forehead, forearms, and elbows. Less frequent, but not unusual, areas of bruising are the hips, cheekbones, and backbones.

To sustain a bruise, a child must first possess the mobility and developmental skills needed to generate sufficient force. A 3-month-old infant does not have the developmental capacity to roll over and cannot sustain bruises on the face from rolling off the bed. Any bruises are rare before age 8 or 9 months, when children begin to walk with support or "cruise" (Sugar, Taylor, & Feldman, 1999). At about age 2 years the toddler begins to run and climb, and bruising about the shins, forearms, and forehead becomes common. The pattern of predictable bruising is depicted in Fig. 1-1.

The most common mechanisms for accidental bruising are falls or collisions with a stationary object. Bruising from abuse occurs as the result of being slapped, punched, kicked, pinched, or struck by an object. Various objects are used to strike children, but common implements include belts, electric cords, switches, paddles, and broom handles. Each of these instruments leaves a distinctive mark on the skin. A cord that is folded over on itself will produce an elongated U shape known as a loop mark (Fig. 1-2). Switches produce two red streaks with a central linear pale streak. The resultant marks resemble train tracks (Fig. 1-3). Any bruises with a linear edge or sharp corner are consistent with trauma from a solid instrument. A belt buckle inflicts bruising in an identifiable shape corresponding to the buckle itself. A pinch or tight grasp leaves a pattern of bruising in the shape of fingerprints. Slap marks leave linear red streaks in a recognizable pattern (Fig. 1-4). As most individuals are right-handed, the majority of these wounds are inflicted on the child's left cheek. When the perpetrator is facing a child the marks are typically oriented horizontally or angled from the chin to the temple. A hand similar in size to the perpetrator's can be superimposed and matched to the site. Ligature marks on a child who has been forcibly restrained appear circumferentially around the wrists or ankles. These may be in the form of bruises or abrasions depending on the material that was used (Fig. 1-5).

Children who are abused are more likely to be struck in certain locations. Corporal punishment is customarily delivered to the buttocks. This is an area with plenty of subcutaneous tissue, and one that is normally covered with protective clothing, especially in the young child still in diapers. Thus the buttocks are relatively protected in the normal course of a child's day. Bruising here is unusual except when inflicted (Fig. 1-6). The face is also a common site to strike a child. Extensive bruising that occurs on both sides of the face is especially difficult to explain from a single fall. A child raising an arm in self-defense may sustain injuries on the outward aspect of the arms. Children reflexively break a fall with an outstretched hand and sustain bruising or abrasions on the palm. Beatings typically involve the dorsum of the hands (Fig. 1-7). The chest, thighs, and abdomen are unusual areas in which to find accidental bruising. Bilateral bruising on the upper arms suggests the child has been forcibly grasped in this area (Fig. 1-8). Bruises that occur at typical sites but in excessive numbers are also suspicious.

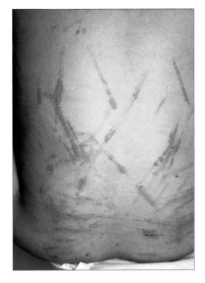

Figure 1-3. Switch marks left on the back of a young child who was disciplined for difficulty with toilet training.

Estimates of the age of a bruise based solely on color are not as precise as once thought. Previously published tables suggesting that the color of a bruise progresses over time through a predictable, orderly change are based on minimal evidence (Schwartz & Ricci, 1996). The colors in a bruise are not consistent in their time of appearance or duration. The timing of color changes varies with respect to the location and depth of the injury and the child's complexion. More recent evidence suggests the presence of yellow identifies a wound as older than 18 hours. The colors red, blue, black, or purple may occur at any point from the time the injury was incurred until complete resolution. It is still important to note the color, as well as any other details, of each bruise. Other aspects of the bruise may help in estimating the time of occurrence. The presence of a welt or raised area below the bruise suggests a recent injury.

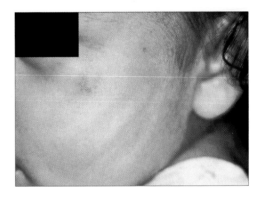

Figure 1-4. Slap marks on the left cheek of a young child. The linear dark red areas correspond to the space between fingers.

A number of medical conditions can manifest with bruising. Bleeding disorders, or coagulopathies, are generally inherited. A child who bruises frequently or extensively may have a deficiency of clotting factors, as in the case of hemophilia or von Willebrand's disease. A shortage of platelets, known as thrombocytopenia, predisposes to spontaneous or easy bruising. These disorders are easy to exclude with standard blood

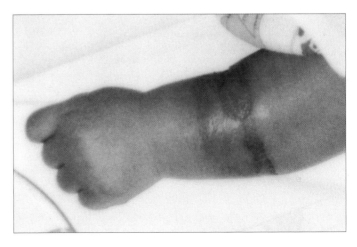

Figure 1-5. Circular bruising of wrist caused by restraints.

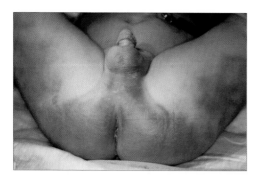

Figure 1-6. Extensive severe bruising delivered with a wooden paddle on the buttocks.

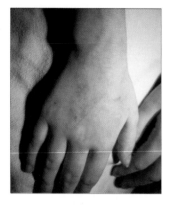

Figure 1-7. Bruising on the back of the hands from being slapped. Red linear streaks and marks on both hands are typical of slap marks. Children don't fall onto the back of both hands.

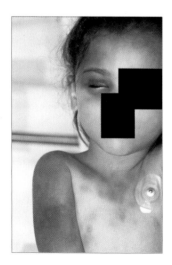

Figure 1-8. This child was violently grasped around the upper arm leaving this typical pattern of bruising. She also has bruising around the eye and chest.

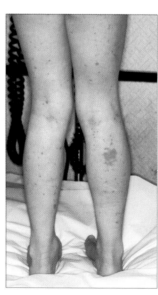

Figure 1-9. A 6-year-old girl with Henoch-Schönlein purpura. The lesions resemble bruises and occur on the back of the legs.

tests that include a platelet count, prothrombin time, and partial thromboplastin time.

Some forms of connective tissue disorders, such as Ehlers-Danlos syndrome, are associated with frequent bruising. These patients can have hyperelastic skin and fragile blood vessels that respond to minor trauma with extensive bruising. Henoch-Schönlein purpura (HSP) is an uncommon, self-limiting inflammatory condition affecting the small blood vessels. Bruising appears predominantly in the lower extremities and buttocks (Fig. 1-9). It is often associated with abdominal cramping, joint pain, and swelling of the lower extremities.

Birthmarks can have the same black and blue color as a bruise. Mongolian spots are frequent in dark-skinned individuals and occur most commonly on the lower back or buttock area but can be found almost anywhere on the body. A darkly pigmented nevus can also take on the appearance of a bruise (Fig. 1-10). These birthmarks are neither tender nor do they evolve and disappear over short periods of time like a bruise.

Coining and cupping are culturally accepted forms of treatment for some ailments. Coining is commonly practiced in areas of Southeast Asia and involves rubbing the edge of a coin vigorously against the skin leaving a symmetric pattern of bruising (Fig. 1-11). The technique of cupping involves heating the air within a small glass cup with a candle or match. The cup is then repetitively placed against the skin of the chest or back. The suction produces a circular red mark that heals in the same manner as a bruise (Fig. 1-12). These traditional folk remedies are not considered abuse.

Bruising raises suspicion of child abuse when it occurs at an unusual age, at uncommon locations, with excessive frequency or severity, or in specific patterns (Table 1-2). Alternative explanations for bruising should appropriately account for the developmental abilities of the child and the amount of force necessary to generate such injuries without the need to resort to incredible explanations.

♦ BURNS

Their naturally inquisitive nature predisposes children to accidental burns. Scalding and contact with hot surfaces constitute the majority of these injuries. By age 5 months most children can reach for and grasp objects. Older infants might tip cups of hot liquid while sitting on an adult's lap. Infants reach for hot objects such as a stove or iron but cannot crawl to them until approximately age 9 months. The depth and extent of a burn wound depend on the heat of the object, the duration of contact, and the characteristics of the body surface that comes in contact with the object. A child's sense of pain is well developed at an early age. Children and infants

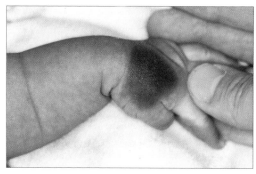

Figure 1-10. *A 4-month-old with a birthmark or nevus on the back of the hand. This can easily be mistaken for a bruise but has been present since birth and will not change color and resolve over the next week.*

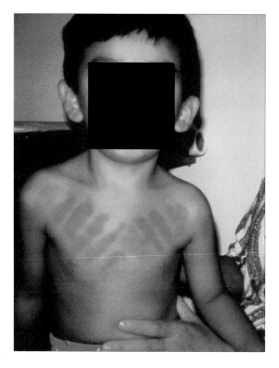

Figure 1-11. *A Southeast Asian child with typical coining lesions. Note the distribution of lesions in a Christmas tree pattern along the trunk. Also note the difference from Fig. 1-3.*

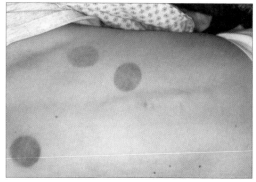

Figure 1-12. *A Russian boy with a fever and cough who has typical marks from cupping.*

rapidly withdraw a hand or attempt to escape a source of heat so that contact in accidental burns is generally brief. The American Academy of Pediatrics recommends that home hot water heaters be set to deliver water at a maximum of 120°F in order to reduce the risk of hot water burns. At this temperature it takes 5 to 10 minutes of contact to produce a second-degree burn (one that blisters) in an adult. It is unlikely that even the most curious toddler would voluntarily hold a hand in hot water for this period of time. Liquids near boiling, such as tea or coffee, cause burns within 1 second (Table 1-3). Most splash or spill burns have only a brief period of contact. Absorbent clothing may prolong this period of contact. Clothing may also protect

Table 1-2. Bruising Suggestive of Abuse

- Bruises that occur in a geometrical shape or pattern

- Bruises in the form of a handprint or fingerprints

- Circumferential bruises or abrasions of an extremity or neck

- Bruises or intra-oral injuries in preambulatory infants

- Bruising of the abdomen, chest, buttocks or genitals

- Excessive number or severity of bruises

- Bruising on multiple body sites inconsistent with single fall

- Multiple bruises of different ages

areas of the child from spilled liquids. A notable example is the child who is still in diapers. Scald burns that purportedly occur from a spill but are over the buttocks or genital area in a child in diapers should raise concerns of abuse. Hot grease or oil spills can cause deeper and more extensive burns. These fluids maintain contact longer and do not cool as rapidly as water-based liquids.

The young toddler who reaches over a countertop and pulls a cup or container of hot liquid onto himself produces a patterned burn. Large circular patches occur where the majority of the fluid falls. Smaller satellite burns surround these areas where smaller drops of liquid contact the skin. The face, chest, and abdomen are most frequently affected. A scald burn on the back is not consistent with a child pulling hot liquid onto himself.

Accidental contact burns occur when a child reaches out to touch a particularly tempting hot object. Burns consequently occur on the fingertips or palm of the hands (Fig. 1-13). The child instinctively withdraws after

Temperature (°F)	Time to Produce Scald (partial thickness) Burn in Adults (less time in children)
120°	5-10 minutes
125°	2 minutes
130°	30 seconds
135°	10 seconds
140°	5 seconds
145°	3 seconds
150°	1.5 seconds
155°	1 second or less

Table 1-3. Temperature Versus Time to Burn

Adapted from Appendix D, Scald Burn Prevention Strategy Manual, National Safe Kids Campaign, Washington, D.C., 1990.

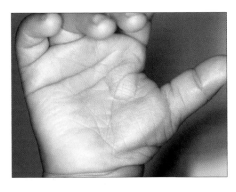

Figure 1-13. A typical second-degree burn on the palm of the hand in a toddler who reached out and touched a hot iron.

touching or grasping the surface, so such burns are rarely deeper than second-degree. Children instinctively reach for objects with the fingertips or palm of one hand. Burns on the back of the hand, deeper than second-degree, or involving both hands are indicative of abuse.

Inadvertent contact with hot objects does occur. A child may roll against a hot curling iron or fall against a heater or radiator. Although the question of adequate supervision or reasonable precautionary measures may arise, such injuries are not typically considered abusive. The child who falls against a hot object and is unable to extricate himself is at risk for sustaining much more severe burns. One example would be a child who rolls behind a bed and gets trapped against a radiator. Such episodes are rare and should, in most cases, trigger further investigation.

Burns of abuse occur from forced immersion or contact with a hot object. These actions are often intended as a form of punishment or discipline. Immersion burns occur when a body part is held in hot water. A caretaker may punish a child with dirty hands who has stained an article of clothing or furniture by holding the hands under scalding water. The perpetrator may also sustain burns on his or her hands if they contact the water during this action. The toilet training period can be a particularly trying time for parents and is a peak period for abuse. A common scenario is the toddler who repeatedly soils himself or herself and is punished by being forced into excessively hot bath water. Burns resulting from this action produce a distinctive pattern. The "glove" and "stocking" burns are circumferential burns of the hands or feet with a discrete area of demarcation marking the level of contact with the water (Fig. 1-14). When a body part is immersed, certain areas remain relatively protected, which explains the resulting burn pattern. A flexed elbow or knee will protect areas of skin that remain in contact with each other. Only skin surfaces that are exposed to the water sustain burns. Circumferential burns may occur accidentally on the hand of a curious toddler testing a hot liquid. This type of burn occurs only on the reaching hand and not bilaterally or on the lower extremities. The classic "doughnut burn" is a pattern of burn injury that occurs when a child is forced into a bathtub of hot water (Fig. 1-15). The ceramic surface of the bathtub does not conduct heat rapidly and remains cooler than the water itself. When the child is forced into a bathtub of hot water, the buttocks and heels come in contact with the ceramic surface and are

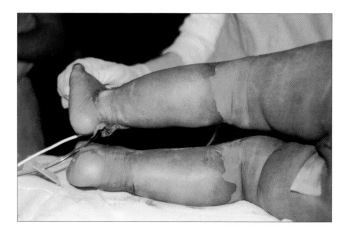

Figure 1-14. Full thickness burns of the legs occurring in a stocking distribution on a young child who was forced into a bathtub of hot water. The soles of both feet appear relatively spared because of the thickness of the skin in this area. Note the sharp upper edge of the burn marking the high level mark of the water.

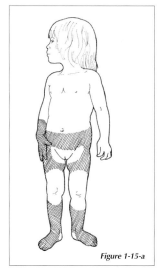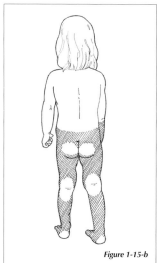

Figure 1-15-a *Figure 1-15-b*

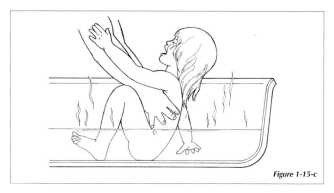

Figure 1-15-c

Figure 1-15. (a) and (b) "Doughnut burn" pattern of immersion burns on a child forced into a bathtub of hot water. (c) How the doughnut pattern of immersion burns is produced.

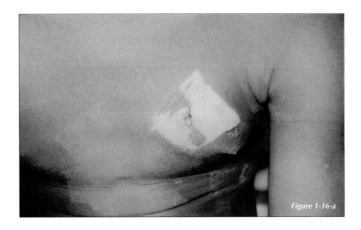

Figure 1-16-a

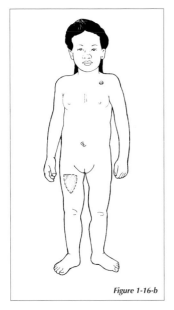

Figure 1-16-b

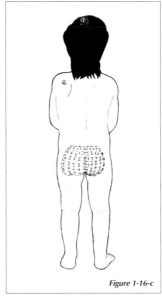

Figure 1-16-c

Figure 1-16. (a) *This contact burn with a geometric pattern was not consistent with the reported story that the child had spilled a cup of hot tea on himself.* **(b)** *and* **(c)** *Examples of geometrically-patterned contact burns.*

spared. The skin surfaces surrounding the buttocks come in contact with hot water and are burned, leaving a doughnut-shaped pattern. The palm and sole often appear relatively uninjured and blister less readily than the surrounding skin surfaces despite similar exposure, due to the thickness of the skin covering these areas. Abusive scald burns are frequently attributed to the child climbing into a bathtub and turning on the hot water. It is important to remember that a child does not have the ability to climb into a bathtub and turn a circular hot-water handle until approximately age 2 years.

Abusive contact burns are also a means of punishment and their location often reflects this. A child's hands may be held against a hot object such as a stovetop or iron as punishment or in a misguided effort to teach the child not to touch these items. The backs of the hands or buttocks are other areas where inflicted burns are found. These burns characteristically imprint the shape or form of the object used to inflict the burn (Fig. 1-16). A geometric pattern or straight edge differentiates these lesions from a standard scald burn. A scald burn forms sharp edges only where it borders an area protected by clothing. A cigarette pressed forcefully against the skin leaves a small (1 cm) circular lesion, which is often second- or third-degree in depth. Accidentally brushing against a lit cigarette is more likely to produce a first- or second-degree burn in a comet-tail configuration. Glancing blows, as when a hot object falls against a child, produce burns with a less distinct edge (Table 1-4).

Several dermatological conditions produce lesions that resemble burns. Blistering of the skin can occur with severe allergic responses to drugs as in the case of Stevens-Johnson syndrome or toxic epidermal necrolysis. These children generally appear ill and the lesions progress over time. Impetigo is frequently mistaken for a cigarette burn because of the similar shape and size of the lesion (Fig. 1-17). It can be differentiated by its more superficial involvement. Impetigo is a mildly contagious condition and matching lesions can be found on opposing areas of the body that are likely to be in physical contact. Staphylococcal scalded skin syndrome is an infectious condition caused by the bacteria *Staphylococcus aureus*. It occurs predominantly in infants or preschool children and results in a diffuse blistering and sloughing of the superficial layers of skin that can mimic burn injuries. Cultures of the skin grow the offending organism. The diagnosis can also be made with a skin biopsy.

Several other blistering disorders, both inherited and acquired, can occur in children. Most of these conditions are diagnosed at an early age or can be readily distinguished from burn injuries by a general pediatrician or dermatologist. A previously well child with an unusual or questionable lesion requires further evaluation or consultation.

◆ BITES

From the time their teeth first erupt, children are testing them out, and other children are frequently the targets of this attention. Toddlers bite misplaced hands or the face as part of an attempted kiss. Any body part within reach is at risk. A bite from a toddler will leave a circular ring of teeth marks. (Fig. 1-18) Most bites are superficial, but they can occasionally draw blood. In addition, dogs and various other animals commonly inflict bite wounds. Dogs tend to bite the face and lower extremities of children. The long canine teeth in dogs produce puncture wounds and tearing lacerations.

Adult bites inflicted on children are often a form of punishment or sexual stimulation. Certain characteristics help differentiate these bites from animal or toddler bites. A suck mark may be present that appears as a bruise in the center of the bite. Bites that appear on the back, buttocks, or genitalia are suspicious. Human bites tend to be more circular than animal bites. The distance between the canines in an adult human bite is greater than 3 cm, while children with primary teeth (less than 8 years old) leave wounds with canine teeth less than 3 cm apart. Careful measurements are useful in confusing cases. Referral and evaluation by a forensic dentist can provide detailed information regarding the perpetrator.

◆ HAIR LOSS

Young children, especially young girls with long hair, may habitually twirl or chew on hair.

Table 1-4. Burn Features Suggestive of Abuse

- Glove or stocking burns
- Doughnut burns
- Burns in a geometrical shape
- Scald burns on the back
- Burns on the buttocks or genital areas
- Burns on the back of the hands
- Contact burns involving both palms
- Cigarette burns
- Burns in multiple locations
- Burns on areas typically protected by clothing

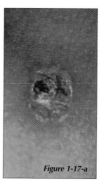
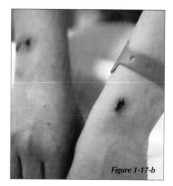

Figure 1-17-a   *Figure 1-17-b*

***Figure 1-17. (a)** and **(b)** Impetigo compared to a child with multiple cigarette burns on the back of the wrists. The cigarette burns are deeper and are present in areas where impetigo is uncommon.*

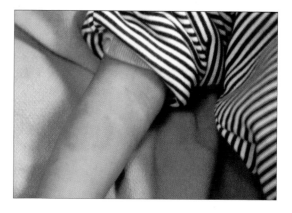

***Figure 1-18.** This child has a toddler bite on the forearm. The circular pattern is typical of a human bite and the small size is consistent with a wound from a young child.*

Frequent pulling in this manner can result in patches of hair loss, a condition known as trichotillomania. Tight hair wraps or braiding may also result in the loss of hair in a predictable pattern. Infants who lie on their backs may develop areas of hair loss from this persistent pressure.

Adults can pull out clumps of a child's hair when grabbing or pulling the child. This typically leaves broken hairs and an area of redness and tenderness on the scalp; it can even produce a hematoma or bleeding beneath the scalp. Alopecia areata is an autoimmune disorder in which hair follicles are attacked and hair falls out, leaving smooth, circular patches of hair loss in the scalp. Fungal infections of the scalp, like ringworm, result in hair loss in circular patches. Bald patches produced by fungal infections can usually be distinguished from traumatic hair loss by the circular shape and presence of scaling.

Table 1-5. Fractures Suggestive of Abuse

- Rib fractures

- Metaphyseal chip or corner fractures

- Long bone fractures in a pre-ambulatory child

- Scapular, sternal, or spinous process fractures without a history of severe trauma

- Multiple fractures in different stages of healing

- Multiple skull fractures

- Healing fractures without a consistent time of injury

◆ BONES

The adult bone has many of the properties of a large stick or branch. It possesses intrinsic strength but little flexibility. When sufficient force is applied, it eventually breaks or fractures. Childhood bones more closely resemble a sapling, with greater malleability, tending to bend or fold before breaking. Growth plates are a part of actively growing long bones. These are relative weak sites and are commonly involved in injuries to childhood bones. Because of these unique properties, young bones are not as limited in their response to different forces. The damage sustained by a child's bone provides information about the force that was applied, how it was applied, and when it was applied.

The incidence of broken bones in young children parallels that of bruises. Fractured bones in pre-ambulatory children are rare, and when they do occur they are often associated with motor vehicle accidents or a serious fall while in the arms of a caretaker. As the child's mobility increases, so does the frequency of broken bones. Stepwise increases are seen as the child graduates from walking to running to bicycle riding. The peak incidence of fractures in childhood occurs with the onset of participation in competitive sports.

Injuries reflect the mechanism involved. An experienced orthopedic surgeon, emergency physician, or sports trainer can accurately predict the likelihood and type of fracture simply by listening to the details of the incident. The history of a fall from a bed or couch is inconsistent with a femur fracture. Such a fall rarely exceeds 2 feet, and even when the underlying surface is hard, the force is not adequate to fracture such a large bone. The associated history behind the injury is therefore critical in determining the level of concern for abuse. Most fractures have a clear, consistent story, and many are witnessed.

In moments of extreme rage or loss of control, an adult may handle a child in a manner that can injure the bones. Broken bones that result from abuse

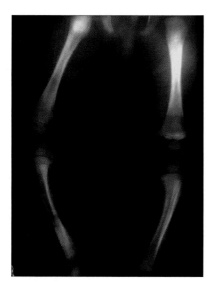

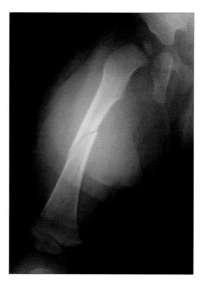

Figure 1-19. *This x-ray of a physically abused 18-month-old boy shows the presence of corner fractures at the ends of both femurs.*

Figure 1-20. *This spiral fracture of the femur in a 5-month-old infant required a great deal of force in a twisting motion and was inconsistent with the explanation that the child "rolled over on the leg funny."*

mechanisms may have predictable findings (Table 1-5). These mechanisms include vigorous shaking, twisting, squeezing, or pulling of one or more extremities. A direct blow with a solid object like a baseball bat is another common mechanism of abuse fractures.

Although any type of fracture may be inflicted, certain injuries are so highly linked with abuse as to mandate a report whenever found. Specific categories of fractures can only be determined by x-rays. The interpretation of these fractures as suggestive of abuse is therefore relevant primarily to those mandated reporters who are physicians. Metaphyseal chip or "corner" fractures are one such characteristic abuse fracture. These appear radiographically as triangular shaped fragments of bone at the end of long bones (Fig. 1-19). Chip fractures are found mainly on the femur or tibia, but can also occur in the elbow or shoulder joints. When an infant is held by the lower extremities and vigorously shaken, the relatively strong ligaments pull at their attachments to the bone and avulse or tear away these small fragments of bone. The so-called "bucket handle" fracture extends across the entire end of the bone and occurs from the same shaking mechanism. It may represent a different radiographic view of the chip fractures. A young bone that is violently twisted can fracture in a spiral pattern like a cardboard paper towel roll. Rotary force or torque is a common occurrence in a skier who has the foot immobilized by a ski under a twisting body. The pre-ambulatory infant is unlikely to encounter these same forces (Fig. 1-20).

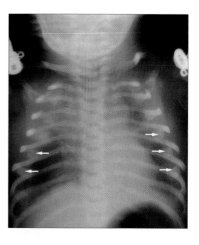

Figure 1-21. *This child has multiple rib fractures as depicted by the arrows. Also note the broken clavicle on the left.*

Rib fractures in young infants are seen so rarely in any other context that they are considered essentially indicative of physical abuse. Studies that have attempted to attribute rib fractures to cardiopulmonary resuscitation (CPR) or high falls have been largely unsuccessful. An adult can squeeze the rib cage of a child with enough force to fracture several ribs. These may be detected as acute fractures, or as healing fractures with callus formation (Fig. 1-21). Other specific fractures are indicative of abuse. Scapular fractures, sternal fractures, and spinous process fractures do not occur without a significant history of trauma.

Multiple fractures in the same child are always a cause for concern. Clearly there are children who tend to be highly active and more prone to risk-taking ventures, but, with extremely few exceptions, children do not have "weak" or easily broken bones. Explanations of frequent fractures resulting from minor falls and attributed to brittle bones should be seriously questioned.

Broken bones not only occur in a predictable fashion, but they also heal over a predictable time period and with certain radiographic findings. Serial x-rays of healing bones have provided a great deal of information regarding changes in the bone during the healing process. Healing begins immediately after the fracture occurs. An early radiographic finding of this healing is the formation of a bony callus over the area of disruption. The callus becomes visible on an x-ray between 7 and 10 days after the injury, helping to date the time of the fracture. Experienced radiologists can provide detailed estimates of the age of the injury based on the location and type of fracture, the amount of callus, and the age and general health of the child. Explanations of injuries should be consistent with these estimates of age. A history of a recent fall is inconsistent with the finding of a fracture with associated callus formation on an x-ray (Fig. 1-22). This finding suggests a delay in seeking medical care. Children with multiple fractures in different stages of healing have most likely been subjected to repetitive abuse.

To hear some defense attorneys argue in the case of an abused child, one would think that inherited and acquired bone disease is rampant among children. The

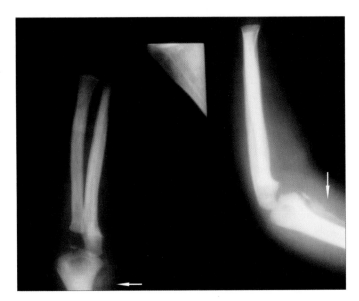

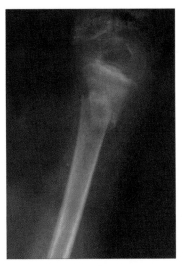

Figure 1-23. This femur fracture occurred during vigorous exercising of the muscles in this wheelchair-bound child. The bones are weak and noticeably thin from lack of use.

Figure 1-22. X-rays of the elbow in this young child who reportedly fell off his bicycle the same morning, shows vigorous callus formation (arrows) which is not consistent with a recent injury.

fact is that these conditions are extremely rare. Most can easily be ruled out by a detailed family history, radiographic evaluation of the bones, or a few simple blood tests.

Osteogenesis imperfecta is an inherited disorder of collagen synthesis. Collagen is a crucial component in the formation of bone. Afflicted patients have multiple fractures from minor trauma beginning soon after birth. These patients most often have diagnostic findings on radiographs as well as additional physical disorders such as short stature, abnormal dental development, and blue sclera. In the subtlest cases, a biochemical analysis of skin fibroblast culture can diagnose the abnormality. The incidence of type IV osteogenesis imperfecta, the mildest variant, is less than 1 per 1,000,000 children. The average pediatrician would be extraordinarily unlikely to see even a single case in a lifetime of practice.

Normal bone growth and development depend upon stimulation of bone deposition and turnover through regular use. This process does not occur in the child who is wheelchair-bound or otherwise non-ambulatory. Children with conditions such as cerebral palsy, spina bifida, or other neuromuscular diseases suffer from disuse osteopenia, or thinning of the bones, which predisposes their bones to fractures with minor forces. Fractures in these children are known to occur during the course of routine physical therapy (Fig. 1-23). The child with profound developmental delay or sensory deficits may not be able to communicate or sense these injuries in a timely fashion. They may exhibit fractures without an obvious history of trauma or with healing already present. This must be taken into account when evaluating such a child for the possibility of abuse.

A young child who limps or refuses to bear weight on one leg may have a spiral or oblique fracture at the far end of the tibia. In many cases the preceding mechanism was a fall off a step or from a slide. The child may have no clear history of trauma at all. Although the diagnosis of abuse should always be considered, in the absence of other findings this injury is consistent with what is frequently termed a "toddler's fracture" and is not considered the result of abuse.

Several metabolic conditions may predispose bones to fractures. Abnormal calcium utilization or deficiency produces rickets. Copper deficiency can be inherited or the result of nutritional deficiency. A severe deficiency of vitamin C, which is necessary for collagen synthesis, results in scurvy, a condition associated with easy bruising and bony changes. Inherited metabolic disorders are rare. Acquired vitamin or mineral deficiencies are also extremely uncommon, as commercially prepared formulas are supplemented with sufficient quantities to prevent such conditions. Specific associated physical abnormalities and features on the x-ray help to differentiate patients with an underlying metabolic disorder from children with normal bones and traumatic injuries.

Many times fractures are not a presenting complaint or not evident on the physical examination. After a short period of healing, they may not be tender and external signs may be minimal. A skeletal survey is a standardized series of x-rays that images the entire pediatric skeleton and focuses on those areas most likely to show bony injuries from abuse. The skeletal survey can be used as a screening tool to detect these silent injuries and provide evidence of a pattern of abusive injuries. The skeletal survey is indicated as a routine part of the abuse evaluation in children less than age 2 years with other conditions or findings that have raised a concern of physical abuse (American Academy of Pediatrics, 2000). Between the ages of 2 and 5 years, the utility of the skeletal survey as a screening device is less evident and the decision to perform a skeletal survey is determined on an individual case basis. In children beyond 5 years of age, it is generally not considered useful as a screening tool.

A bone scan can detect areas of bony injury or healing that may not be apparent on a simple x-ray. It should be considered when there is a high suspicion of bony injury in the presence of an apparently normal x-ray. Metabolic studies are not indicated for every case of abuse involving fractures. These should be performed only when there is sufficient suspicion based on the history, physical findings, and x-rays to suggest such conditions are a possibility.

In the evaluation of the young child with a fractured bone, it is important to consider the proposed history of injury, including an estimation of the direction and degree of force involved, as well as the specific radiographic findings. Conditions that predispose to fractures in young children are rare and in most cases can be ruled out with simple testing.

◆ BRAIN INJURIES

The leading causes of traumatic brain injury in children under age 2 years are motor vehicle accidents, falls from great heights, and child abuse. Substantial force is necessary to produce these injuries. It is important to know not only what forces or scenarios result in serious intracranial injuries, but also which mechanisms do not. Forces associated with common injuries from falls and childhood play cannot produce the same pattern or severity of injury seen in inflicted head trauma. Studies that have reviewed childhood injuries resulting from a fall down the stairs or off a bed have found predictable patterns of bruising and occasional fractures (Joffe & Ludwig, 1988). Intracranial injuries are noticeably absent from these findings.

Shaking is the mechanism most commonly attributed to abusive head injury in infants. The brain is subjected to severe rotational forces when a child is held by the trunk and shaken vigorously back and forth. The injuries sustained from this action comprise what is known as the "shaken-baby syndrome." Some discussion exists as to whether the injuries incurred in this syndrome require an actual impact of the head at the end of the shaking thus giving rise to the term "shaking-impact syndrome." Violent rotational forces stretch and break blood vessels around the brain and can bruise or even tear portions of the brain. Recent evidence suggests that a sudden deceleration resulting from the impact of the head produces many characteristic features seen in cases of inflicted head trauma. In this scenario, the injury to the brain and surrounding blood vessels results from the internal forces generated by the rapid deceleration and not from the impact itself. A hard surface is therefore not required to produce the necessary deceleration, and infants with internal injuries may have minimal or no external signs of trauma despite such an impact (Duhaime et al., 1998).

The "shaken-baby syndrome" includes a series of physical injuries that are frequently found together. Subdural hemorrhages from internal bleeding are the principal intracranial injury found in cases of shaken babies. External scalp injuries, including bruising, swelling, or lacerations, may accompany the internal injuries but, as mentioned previously, are not always present. Retinal hemorrhages are areas of bleeding within the back of the eye. Although they have been found in rare instances associated with other mechanisms, their presence is considered almost diagnostic of child abuse. Bruising and other associated cutaneous injuries are common. A high proportion of shaken babies have fractures. The most characteristic types are metaphyseal fractures and rib fractures. Many of these infants have no visible signs of injury. They may exhibit breathing abnormalities, seizures, unexplained vomiting, depressed level of consciousness or tone, or full cardiac arrest. In contrast to other episodes of severe head injury, there is no clear history that explains the brain injuries in these cases.

Skull fractures do occur among young infants as the result of accidental injuries. Common mechanisms include falls from the arms of a caretaker, from a car seat left on a table, or from a bed onto a hard surface. Skull fractures resulting from these accidental mechanisms are usually linear and not associated with significant intracranial injuries or retinal hemorrhages. Multiple skull fractures, "eggshell" or complex fractures of the skull, and skull fractures associated with other injuries are highly suggestive of abuse.

A more detailed investigation of head trauma and its relationship to abuse is the responsibility of the evaluating physician. A head CT and skeletal survey are recommended in the acute evaluation of any child with suspected brain injury as the result of abuse. Follow-up MRI studies may be useful to identify the full extent of the injury and provide further information regarding the age of the injury. An infant with intracranial hemorrhages should have an ophthalmologic examination as a routine part of the evaluation to inspect for the presence of retinal hemorrhages.

Seemingly trivial trauma may produce intracranial bleeding in infants with an underlying bleeding disorder. Bleeding tests are generally diagnostic of these cases. The most common cause is vitamin K deficiency. Newborn infants routinely receive an injection of vitamin K at the time of delivery to compensate for this deficiency. Children at risk are those who are born at home, in an ambulance, or where deliveries are not routinely performed.

♦ Intra-Abdominal Injuries

Intra-abdominal injuries in children are rare and require an impact of significant energy. It is not surprising that most intra-abdominal injuries in children occur as the result of being struck by a car or falling from a height greater than 10 feet. These accidental injuries are frequently witnessed, leave confirmatory evidence at the scene, or are associated with additional injuries typical of such massive trauma. While the initial signs of abdominal injury may be subtle, the mechanism is not. A number of abdominal injuries have been reported from bicycle accidents in which the handlebar strikes the child below the ribcage. In this case the end of the handlebar leaves a telltale circular bruise on the surface of the abdomen.

The mechanism of intra-abdominal injuries in the case of child abuse is generally blunt trauma from a closed fist or punch. The force generated from such a blow thrown by an adult is capable of causing tremendous internal damage. Bruises or tears of the spleen or liver are common. The presence of air in the intestines at the time of a violent impact can rupture the intestines in a manner similar to bursting a paper bag. The pancreas and duodenum are compressed against the thoracic vertebrae and can sustain internal bleeding. Internal abdominal injuries may or may not be associated with bruising of the skin surface. Serious intra-abdominal wounds may also be inflicted as the result of sexual abuse. The physician evaluating a child with unexplained intra-abdominal injury must carefully examine the genital and rectal areas for evidence of sexual abuse.

The history is unhelpful and often intentionally misleading in cases of abdominal injuries resulting from abuse. As opposed to accidental abdominal injuries, a history of trauma in inflicted injuries is frequently absent or attributed to common, low energy accidents such as a fall down the stairs, a fall from a couch, or rough-housing with another young child. These incidents do not produce life-threatening intra-abdominal injuries in children (Huntimer, Muret-Wagstaff, & Leland, 2000; Joffe & Ludwig, 1988; Lyons & Oates, 1993). Because of the confusing history, most cases of abuse-related intra-abdominal injury are detected based on the physical examination findings. The initial clinical signs of intra-abdominal injury in the young child are often subtle and may consist of irritability, tenderness, vomiting, grunting, pallor, tachycardia, or abdominal distention. A child who is suspected of being battered should have a careful examination of the abdomen as part of a complete abuse evaluation. Screening tests that may show evidence of abdominal injury include liver function tests, pancreatic enzyme levels, and urine tests for blood. A CT scan of the abdomen provides more specific information and is indicated in any case in which the possibility of intra-abdominal injury is being seriously considered.

Mononucleosis is one condition in which the spleen may rupture with little or no significant intra-abdominal trauma. The swelling in the spleen from the underlying infection predisposes this organ to rupture. Serology tests for the causative virus are positive in these children.

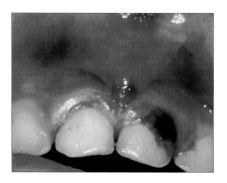

Figure 1-24. Subluxated permanent central incisor, contusions of the vestibule and laceration of the labial frenum from an open-handed slap to the mouth.

◆ MOUTH INJURIES

The mouth is a common area for both accidental and inflicted injuries. The vast majority of accidental injuries to the face, mouth, and teeth occur once the child is capable of taking steps. The relatively large head size and poor balance predispose to frequent episodes of falling forward at this age. Bruising of the forehead, nasal abrasions, bloody lips, and dental injuries are all considered part of the normal costs of learning to walk. Parents constantly reprimand children for running with an object such as a straw, lollipop, or pencil in their mouths. The predictable end result of a fall when carrying one of these implements in this fashion is a tear or puncture wound deep within the mouth or throat. The teeth, especially the frontal incisors, are prime targets for injury resulting from a forward fall. In the process of striking his or her chin, a child often lacerates the area of the tongue that is protruding beyond the incisors. As the child becomes older and more involved in organized sporting activities, the mouth is at risk from wayward elbows or balls. Children also sustain a large proportion of facial-oral injuries as the result of bicycle mishaps.

Abuse injuries involving the mouth are often the result of a frustrated caretaker forcing a bottle, spoon, or pacifier into the mouth of a crying infant. The infant sustains bruises on the lips and cheeks in a circular pattern that matches the pacifier or bottle lid. Repeated thrusts with these objects can inflict bruises or cuts on the hard or soft palate. The frenulum of the upper lip is a thin band of skin connecting the upper gums with the upper lip. The frenulum of the tongue connects the underside of the tongue with the floor of the mouth. While the upper frenulum is commonly injured in simple falls, it is unusual to find accidental tears of the frenulum of the tongue. Neither structure is likely to be injured accidentally in a child who is not yet walking (Fig. 1-24). Direct blows to the face or mouth inflict injuries that are difficult to distinguish from those sustained in a fall. Accidental or inflicted trauma can fracture or dislodge a tooth. In both instances the frontal incisors are most often affected because of their location. Injuries that are considered suspicious include those with associated slap marks on the face, or facial and oral injuries out of proportion to a simple fall. Jaw fractures, for example, are rare in young children and require a degree of force not typically encountered in a short fall. A perpetrator wearing a ring may inflict telltale lacerations when punching or slapping the child in the face. Alternatively, a suspected abuser may show injuries to a hand or fist that has come in contact with the child's teeth. Children who have been gagged or had tape applied over the mouth may show patterned bruising in the corners of the mouth or abrasions in areas where the tape has been forcefully removed. Tiny burst capillaries, or petechiae, may appear on the face of a child who has been gagged or choked. Oral injuries in the pre-ambulatory child, and injuries that occur deep within the mouth and are attributed to a simple fall are signs of probable abuse.

Several oral lesions of childhood resemble traumatic injuries. Children with bleeding disorders may incur frequent bruising within the mouth area from relatively minor or unknown trauma. A ranula is a large cyst or bulla with a purple appearance that occurs beneath the tongue on the floor of the mouth. It may appear as a large hematoma, but is not tender, has no associated injuries, and results from the buildup of fluid behind a blocked salivary gland duct. Certain strains of virus produce an irritation of the mouth referred to as stomatitis. The infection produces multiple ulcerations that are painful and may bleed. Fat tissue in the cheeks of a young infant is more susceptible to cold injury by virtue of its high proportion of saturated fat. Prolonged exposure to cold air, or contact with a piece of ice or a popsicle will produce a red swollen area on the cheek that resembles a bruise. The lesion, termed panniculitis, resolves without passing through the more typical color changes of a bruise. Children who habitually lick their lips develop a dry, irritated rash surrounding the mouth. This skin condition is known as "lip-lickers dermatitis." There is no bruising associated with the rash and it resolves with cessation of the activity and application of moisturizers or petroleum-based ointments. A dentist or physician readily recognizes many of these conditions. Simple bleeding tests can resolve questions of coagulopathies. Panniculitis and lip-lickers dermatitis have a history, appearance, and recovery that are consistent with the diagnosis.

◆ DOCUMENTATION

The sight of an abused child is an image that we expect to remain burned into our memories forever. Surprisingly, this is not the case. Over time, we forget some details and become less clear about others. The criminal justice and social service systems do not solve complicated child abuse issues overnight. Investigations and prosecutions can take several months, if not

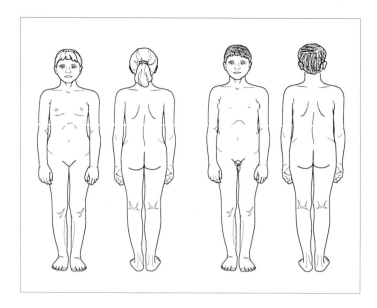

Figure 1-25. Anatomic drawings for documentation of physical abuse injuries.

years. It is crucial for the reporter to keep accurate detailed notes of the case. Most injuries resolve over time, and the reporter's account may be the only description available to police or physicians from that particular point in time. In the event the case results in legal proceedings, the reporter must rely on a carefully recorded description of any physical injuries to recall specifics. Key areas to address in cases of physical abuse include the location of injuries, accurate measurements, and descriptions of shape, color, and swelling. A drawing is extremely helpful in clarifying these details. Specific patterns should be duplicated. Most physicians who deal with abuse use a standardized form so that no pertinent information is overlooked. These forms include anatomic drawings on which detailed representations of injuries can be included (Fig. 1-25).

Photography is an exceptionally useful and accurate form of documentation. Instant-processing cameras provide immediate pictures that can be labeled at the time they are taken. A good quality 35-mm camera that is easy to use can accurately portray injuries with better color reproduction than an instant camera. Special lenses are available for close-up pictures of skin or mouth lesions. Taking multiple photographs of each injury at different angles improves the likelihood of getting at least one good photo. A whole body picture identifies the child and provides better perspective for the area of interest. A label including the patient's name and the date can be included in the photograph for additional verification that the injury belongs to the child in question. A measuring tape or recognizable object such as a coin provides the viewer with a better sense of the actual size of the lesion. Photographs are not only a useful means of recall, but are accepted as evidence in most courts (Ricci, 1991).

◆ SUMMARY

This chapter describes many abuse injuries in isolation. In reality, the physically abused child often exhibits many injuries. A single suspicious finding calls for a more detailed examination for additional physical injuries. While it is not necessarily the obligation of the reporter to perform this evaluation, it is often the combination of physical findings that raises suspicion to the level of certainty in abuse. As important as the physical findings are, they also should not be considered in isolation. As pointed out here and in later chapters, the underlying history, general attitude of the child, observed interactions with caretakers, and, at times, the results of laboratory and radiologic studies all contribute to making a final diagnosis of child abuse.

To recognize what is abnormal, one must first know what is normal. The law designates certain groups to be mandated reporters of child abuse not only because of their close interactions with children, but because of their unique knowledge of normal childhood abilities, behavior, and injuries. This chapter is intended to pull these normal findings into greater focus for the mandated reporter and to point out characteristic physical injuries that result from child abuse.

There is overwhelming evidence that unless abuse is brought to the attention of the appropriate authorities and some intervention occurs, the pattern of inflicted injuries continues. Most child homicide victims have a previous history of suspicious injuries (Jenny et al., 1999). By recognizing and reporting physical abuse, the reporter can stop the cycle of abuse and ensure the future safety of that child. A report of suspected child abuse can lead to the provision of appropriate medical care for the child and needed services and support for the family. The mandated reporter performs the crucial first step in this process.

◆ REFERENCES

American Academy of Pediatrics; Section on Radiology. (2000). Diagnostic imaging of child abuse. Pediatrics, 106(6), 1345-1348.

Caffey, J. (1946). Multiple fractures in the long bones of infants suffering from chronic subdural hematomas. American Journal of Roentgenology, 56, 163.

Child Abuse Prevention and Treatment Act (CAPTA). (1996). 42 U.S.C.A. §5106g

Duhaime, A., Christian, C. W., Rorke, L. B., et al. (1998). Nonaccidental head injury in infants—the "shaken-baby syndrome." The New England Journal of Medicine, 338(25), 1822-1829.

Holter, J. C., & Friedman, S. B. (1968). Child abuse: Early case finding in the emergency department. Pediatrics, 42, 128-138.

Huntimer, C. M., Muret-Wagstaff, S., & Leland, N. L. (2000). Can falls on stairs result in small intestine perforations? Pediatrics, 106, 301-305.

Jenny, C., Hymel, K. P., Ritzen, A., et al. (1999). Analysis of missed cases of abusive head trauma. JAMA, 281, 621-626.

Joffe, M., & Ludwig, S. (1988). Stairway injuries in children. Pediatrics, 82(3), 457-461.

Lyons, T. J., & Oates, R. K. (1993). Falling out of bed: A relatively benign occurrence. Pediatrics, 92, 125-127.

Paradise, J. E., Bass, J., Forman, S. D., et al. (1995). Minimum criteria for reporting child abuse from health care settings. Pediatric Emergency Care, 11, 335-339.

Ricci, L. R. (1991). Photographing the physically abused child: Principles and practice. AJDC, 145, 275-281.

Schwartz, A. J., & Ricci, L. R. (1996). How accurately can bruises be aged in abused children? Literature review and synthesis. Pediatrics, 97(2), 254-257.

Sugar, N. F., Taylor, J. A., & Feldman, K. W. (1999). Bruises in infants and toddlers. Archives of Pediatrics and Adolescent Medicine, 153(4), 399-403.

Chapter 2

SEXUAL ABUSE

CINDY W. CHRISTIAN, M.D.
DAVID M. RUBIN, M.D.

Sexual abuse in children is defined as the engaging of a child in sexual acts that the child does not understand, to which the child cannot give informed consent, or which violate the taboos of our society (Kempe, 1978). Sexual abuse may involve direct acts perpetrated against children as well as other nontouching abuses, which include exhibitionism, voyeurism, or the use of children for pornographic purposes.

Although precise incidence data are lacking, sexual abuse of children occurs commonly in our country and throughout the world. It has been estimated that as many as one in four girls and one in 10 boys will be victims of sexual abuse by the time they become adults (Finkelhor, 1993; Leventhal, 1988). While boys are reported as victims less often than girls, recent studies have suggested that the

number of male victims may in fact be higher as a result of a reluctance to report cases of sexual abuse among boys (Holmes & Slap, 1998).

The purpose of this chapter is to assist the mandated reporter and other professionals in their investigations of child sexual abuse by exploring the following topics in detail:

- *Presenting complaints for child sexual abuse*

- *Interviewing the child victim*

- *Medical referrals and examination*

- *Screening for sexually transmitted diseases*

- *Reporting child sexual abuse*

- *Pitfalls of investigations*

- *Mental health referrals*

- *Case examples*

A common theme throughout this chapter is that the medical examination of suspected victims of sexual abuse is usually normal. We will explore the multiple reasons why the examination is normal later in the chapter. As a result, the most important determinants for indicating whether sexual abuse has occurred involve the child's disclosure and how the child interfaces with the child welfare system and law enforcement once a report is made. Ultimately, it is in the early stages of the investigation, when police officers and child protective services (CPS) workers are most involved, that the greatest potential exists for securing the most important evidence—the history from the child.

◆THE PRESENTATION OF CHILD SEXUAL ABUSE

Although each case that is reported to the child welfare system is unique in its origins, the majority of children reach attention in one of three ways:

- The child discloses a history of sexual abuse to a third party (e.g., parent), who then seeks advice from professionals who care for children.

- The child presents with nonspecific behavioral or medical symptoms which are manifestations of underlying sexual abuse.

- The child has unexplained injury or medical findings which are suspicious for sexual abuse.

A child's disclosure to a third party is the most common presentation for child sexual abuse. The child often discloses a history of abuse to a caregiver, friend, or teacher. A caregiver is alerted, who then brings the child to an appropriate authority for evaluation.

Children also come for evaluation of behaviors that are thought to be sexually inappropriate, but without a verbal history of abuse. An evaluation is then needed to determine if the behaviors are inappropriate and, if so, what their etiology is.

To determine what behaviors are normal or abnormal sexual exploration in young children, Friedrich and colleagues distributed surveys about childhood sexual behavior to parents of healthy, nonabused children (Freidrich, Grambsch, Broughton, Kuiper, & Beilke, 1991). In general, pre-school children engage in more sexual exploration than school-age children. While children commonly engage in self-masturbatory touching or ask sexually-related questions, they infrequently simulate sexual acts with other children or their parents.

Sexualized behavior should be of concern to the mandated reporter, but is not diagnostic of sexual abuse. It is important to ask the family specific questions about the home situation, namely, whether the child has witnessed public nudity, adult sexual activity, or pornography. Frequently, the roots of such behavior remain unanswered, and a referral to a psychologist for further evaluation and counseling may be indicated.

Occasionally, the child victim who is coerced or threatened into secrecy may develop nonspecific physical or psychiatric symptoms of illness that mask an underlying history of sexual abuse. Therefore, some children come to medical and childcare professionals with nonspecific psychiatric or medical disorders as primary manifestations of sexual abuse. Mandated reporters should remain alert for the child with signs of unexplained anxiety, depression, self-abusive behavior, and multiple somatic complaints (e.g., headaches, abdominal pain) (Krugman, 1986). School officials should be wary of the child whose school performance drastically worsens during the school year. An overlooked victim may be the older child who perpetrates sexual abuse against younger children; the child perpetrator often has a history of being a victim as well (Krugman, 1986).

The child who comes to a medical professional with a physical complaint that involves the genital region of the body (i.e., vaginal discharge, vaginal bleeding) may be a victim of sexual abuse. The physician, however, must determine whether or not the problem is related to sexual abuse. Although sexually abused children are occasionally identified because of isolated physical injury, it is far more likely that there will also be behavioral indications of sexual abuse (e.g., disclosure or behavioral change) in conjunction with the injury. As a result, the child with physical findings that are of concern, but no disclosure or other parental suspicion of sexual abuse, may leave a clinician in a quandary as to how to interpret the physical findings. This situation will be discussed further later in this chapter.

♦ INTERVIEWING CHILDREN DURING SEXUAL ABUSE EVALUATIONS

Once a concern is identified, the most important aspect of the sexual abuse evaluation becomes the interview with the child (when developmentally possible) (Reed, 1996; Saywitz & Goodman, 1996). Interviewing children is challenging because children may go through several emotional stages during the disclosure process. The sexual abuse accommodation syndrome describes the emotional stages a child victim may encounter, which include helplessness, secrecy, entrapment and accommodation, spontaneous disclosure, and recantation (Summit, 1983). The interviewer must be aware of these stages and must be prepared for the possibility that a single interview may not uncover the full details of the abuse that has occurred.

Understanding the dynamics of a disclosure and the relationship of the perpetrator to the child may help predict the difficulty in obtaining a consistent and full disclosure during the interview process. In some cases a child is accidentally overheard revealing a suspicious event to a friend and may be reluctant to discuss the abuse with the interviewer (i.e., "accidental disclosure"). In most cases, the perpetrator is well-known to the child and has engaged in escalating sexual behavior with the child over time. It is not uncommon for the perpetrator to threaten or coerce the child into secrecy. If the perpetrator has gained the child's trust, the child may be reluctant to incriminate the perpetrator and may also wish to protect him or her.

Depending on the emotional conflict a child may feel for revealing sexual abuse, an interviewer must realize that a child may not be prepared to talk at length about the allegation. Pushing the distressed child does not aid the investigation and may endanger any trust development between the interviewer and the child. The interviewer may need multiple sessions to complete the child's evaluation. The interviewer may also choose to continue the evaluation via a referral for psychological counseling and therapy.

Although every interviewer has an individual style, several techniques are commonly employed to enhance the success of the interview with young children:

- *Develop rapport before initiating the interview:* Interviews take time, particularly with young children, whose shyness may interfere with the ability to perform an interview. Often, engaging in activities with children at eye level (e.g., coloring or block building) helps break the ice and encourage conversation with the child before initiating the interview.

- *Avoid too many distractions:* The interviewer should not overwhelm and distract the child with multiple toys or dolls. Interruptions should be avoided.

- *Establish from the outset that you don't want the child to guess an answer to a question:* The interviewer should encourage the child to tell the interviewer when the interviewer makes an incorrect statement. The interviewer should encourage the child not to guess an answer to a question.

- *Use age-specific language:* The interviewer should find out from the parents or child what words the child uses to describe his or her anatomy. The interviewer should avoid long questions or words that confuse the child.

- *Avoid leading questions; if necessary, balance the interview with directed and open-ended questions:* The interviewer should avoid directed questions such as, "Did he touch you there?" or "Did he touch you with his pee-pee?" The interviewer should instead use open-ended questions to help the child disclose spontaneously. Occasionally, a directed question may be necessary to help clarify an issue. For instance, the interviewer may ask, "Do you know what good touch and bad touch is?" If the child answers yes, the interviewer may respond, "Tell me about that." If the child responds appropriately, the interviewer may follow with the question, "Has anyone ever touched you bad or where you didn't want to be touched?" If the child answers "yes," the interviewer may respond, "Tell me what happened" or "Could you tell me about that?"

- *Document accurately the information provided during the interview:* It is important that the interview be documented in a detailed fashion to adequately convey how the interview was conducted. Some locales have employed the use of routine videotaping to accurately record child interviews. While there has been considerable debate regarding the use of videotaped testimony, many proponents believe that when properly done, videotaping reduces the trauma to which the child is exposed. Subject to the scrutiny of attorneys at trial, routine videotaping also raises the standards of interviewing practices over time (Van Dokkum, 1994). If investigators wish to explore the use of videotaped testimony, they should consult their local district attorney's office for further guidance.

◆REFERRALS FOR MEDICAL EXAMINATION OF CHILD VICTIMS

Suspected victims of sexual abuse reach medical attention in many ways. Parents may choose to visit their child's pediatrician in search of help when a sexual abuse allegation is made, prompting the physician to complete a thorough medical examination. Mandated reporters, police officers, or social service workers also refer families to physicians for evaluation. Some children may be referred to the emergency department, others to their family doctor, and others to a child abuse specialist at a referral pediatric institution.

Given the anxiety that a sexual abuse allegation provokes in a family, children are commonly referred or brought by a family to the emergency department of a local hospital. Despite the best intentions, a referral to an emergency department is often not the ideal setting in which to provide a comprehensive medical evaluation of a sexually abused child. The emergency department may be a frightening setting for a young child. The lack of privacy also makes the emergency department an ill-equipped setting for interviewing the child, which may be necessary if a report has not yet been made. For a child who is frightened about the consequences of a disclosure, the emergency room experience may be further traumatizing and may impede the likelihood of obtaining a consistent disclosure. Finally, in contrast to pediatric physicians who regularly examine children, some emergency physicians may have little training in sexual abuse evaluations of children.

Although the emergency department is not an ideal setting for the medical evaluation of a young, sexually abused child, there are specific circumstances that demand referral for immediate evaluation. Indications for immediate referral to the emergency department include the following:

1. The need for collection of forensic evidence

2. The presence of acute symptoms that cannot wait for evaluation by the patient's primary physician (e.g., acute vaginal discharge, genital trauma/bleeding)

3. The unavailability of the physician when the family is in crisis

The best example of immediate referral to an emergency department is for the collection of forensic evidence from the child's body to link the alleged perpetrator to the child. Physicians may obtain a "rape kit," which consists of swabs of the mouth, vagina/penis, and rectum. The swabs and occasionally other collected specimens (pieces of hair or skin under the fingernails) are then sent to a crime laboratory for analysis.

Unlike adult rape, the likelihood of obtaining forensic evidence directly from the prepubertal child's body diminishes greatly after the first 24 hours following an assault (Christian et al., 2000). After 24 hours, there may still be a possibility of recovering forensic evidence, but the evidence usually comes from the analysis of bed linens, the child's clothing, or the child's underwear present at the time of the assault. The likelihood of recovering any physical evidence diminishes greatly after the first 72 hours.

While most children need not be seen in the emergency room setting for forensic evidence collection, all children who report an acute sexual assault within the past 72 hours should still be seen as soon as possible for the detection of injury (American Academy of Pediatrics, 1999). Understanding the improbability of recovering physical evidence from prepubertal children after 24 hours should help mandated reporters opt instead to refer a younger child to a pediatrician for the sexual abuse evaluation within the 72-hour time frame, if possible. For children who have reached puberty, an emergency room referral is still appropriate over the entire 72-hour window after an assault. Regardless of age, if a child reports a recent assault, the reporter should request that the family recover any clothing or sheets present during the assault and place them into a paper bag. The family should then provide the specimens to the police officers or other investigators assigned to the case.

Although children may not need to be seen in the emergency department after an alleged sexual assault, a timely medical examination should still occur because the likelihood of finding an injury decreases with the time elapsed since the assault (Finkel, 1989; McCann & Voris, 1993). Many pediatricians are comfortable providing this evaluation, and if they are not, the child can often be referred for a semi-urgent evaluation at a local child abuse center. Although the medical examination in most cases of alleged sexual abuse is normal (see below), the likelihood of detecting injury (particularly in a girl) increases when the examination is performed acutely and the child reports both pain and bleeding at the time of a sexual assault (Christian et al., 2000). If a family tells a mandated reporter that both pain and bleeding were noted, the reporter should communicate this information to the referring physician so that the child can be seen as soon as possible for the medical examination.

♦ THE MEDICAL EXAMINATION OF SUSPECTED SEXUAL ABUSE VICTIMS

In most cases of child sexual abuse, the medical examination of the child is normal (Berenson et al., 2000; Adams, Harper, Knudson, & Revilla, 1994). Understanding the relationship of a child victim to a perpetrator helps explain why the examination is normal in most cases. A perpetrator who is known to a child and who victimizes the child over a considerable period of time usually pursues a pattern of escalating behavior to prevent detection. The known perpetrator may wish to avoid physical injury to the child, opting instead to engage in repeated events of fondling or genital to genital contact without full penetration past the hymenal opening (vulvar coitus). This may accomplish the goal of gratifying the perpetrator without physically injuring the child. As one might expect, the physical examination of such a child would reveal normal genital anatomy.

Although a detailed discussion of medical anatomy is beyond the scope of this text, mandated reporters and investigators should have some familiarity with the medical documentation of sexual abuse examinations.

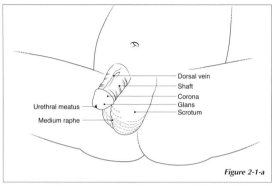

Figure 2-1-a

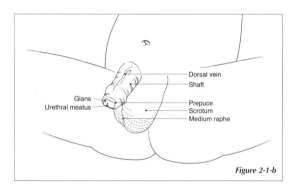

Figure 2-1-b

Figure 2-1. Male genital anatomy: **(a)** circumcised, **(b)** uncircumcised.

While the medical examination of a boy's genitals may be easy to interpret, the medical examination of a girl's genitals is more complex. (Note: Compare Figures 2-1a and b with Figure 2-2). For a boy, the central issue regards the presence of swelling, bruising, or abrasions over the genital region (anal exam discussed below). For a girl, however, the vaginal anatomy is more complex. There are multiple layers of anatomy before the vaginal opening is encountered (Fig. 2-2).

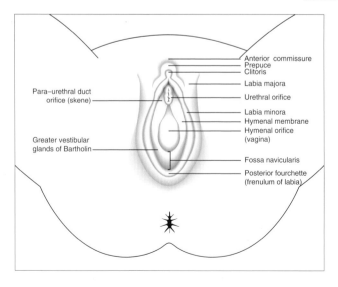

Figure 2-2. Female vaginal anatomy.

A girl is typically examined while lying on her back in the "frog-legged position." The physician separates the labia majora and often applies traction, revealing the hymen and the vaginal opening. The child is examined for injuries to the vulva, the hymen, and the surrounding tissue. Penetrating genital injury most often occurs to the posterior vulva and hymenal rim, so these areas require careful inspection. In most cases, the hymen appears very smooth and can have different configurations, most commonly annular or crescentic. Physicians should carefully note the appearance of the hymen, particularly the lower half (commonly described as 3:00 to 9:00), for evidence of transections or clefts which extend to the vaginal wall. In acute sexual assaults, abrasions, bruising, and bleeding transections may be directly visualized and then documented by diagram or photograph. Physicians should culture any vaginal discharge, if noted, to determine if there is a sexually transmitted disease.

Most commonly, though, the hymenal examination (Fig. 2-3) reveals normal anatomy or nonspecific changes that can be seen in normal children as well as healing trauma. Such variants include bumps, incomplete clefts, hymenal asymmetry, and rolled hymenal edges. Contrary to popular myth, the size of the hymenal opening is not predictive of the likelihood of sexual abuse.

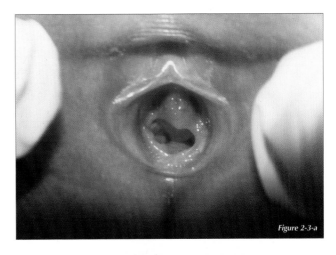

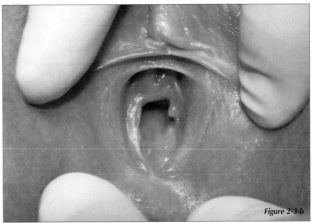

Figure 2-3. The vaginal examination. *(a)* A three-year-old girl with a history of fondling by a male caregiver. Exam reveals a normal crescentic hymen, with no evidence of injury. *(b)* An eight-year-old girl with a history of recurrent vaginal penetration. Exam reveals a significant loss of hymenal tissue with a deep, wide cleft extending to the vaginal wall. The exam is diagnostic of penetrating injury.

In performing an anal examination (Fig. 2-4) in children, a physician carefully notes the symmetry and tone of the anus when the buttocks are separated. In addition to symmetry, the physician should note the presence of extra tags, fissures, or scars. With the exception of a bleeding laceration after a report of sodomy, the presence of tags, bumps, and scars may be nonspecific findings that do not confirm whether a child has been sexually abused. Furthermore, documented anal injury after a child sexual assault is distinctively uncommon (Adams et al., 1994).

Ultimately, in most cases of suspected sexual abuse, a physician will encounter an examination with normal or nonspecific anatomical features of the genitals. The reasons for a relatively normal examination and forensic evaluation in suspected victims of sexual abuse include the following:

1. The anal and hymenal tissues heal extremely quickly, and findings may disappear within days of an assault (Finkel, 1989; McCann & Voris, 1993).

2. Most sexual abuse involves behaviors that gratify the perpetrator but do not physically injure the child (e.g., fondling, rubbing genitals against a child's genitals without penetration).

3. There are relatively few findings diagnostic of sexual abuse without a corresponding disclosure (Adams, 2001).

4. Sexually transmitted diseases are uncommonly identified in sexually abused children (see below) (Ingram et al., 1997).

5. Recovery of semen from a child's body is unlikely after the first 12-24 hours following an assault (Christian et al., 2000).

6. Although a child may state that a perpetrator "put his pee-pee in me," the child may be unable to distinguish full anal or hymenal penetration from a perpetrator rubbing his genitals against a child's vulva (vulvar coitus) or buttocks (gluteal coitus). The latter would be expected to leave no injury.

7. There can be significant labial penetration to the hymenal orifice without full hymenal penetration.

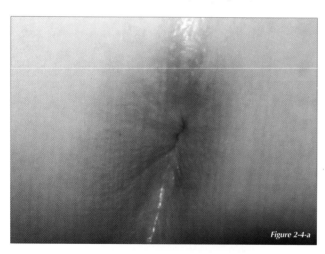

Figure 2-4-a

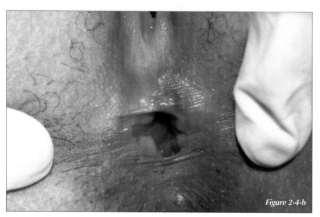

Figure 2-4-b

Figure 2-4. *The anal examination.* **(a)** *Normal exam with normal tone and symmetric appearance.* **(b)** *An eight-year-old girl with a history of sodomy by her father. Exam reveals poor anal tone and significant perianal scarring.*

8. The vaginal and anal mucosa is elastic, allowing for significant distension without disruption of tissue (Bays & Chadwick, 1993).

9. Pubertal, adolescent girls develop thick, estrogenized, redundant hymenal tissue which is more elastic and difficult to examine for evidence of penetrating trauma.

Of the above considerations, perhaps the most important are whether injury would occur based on the history and, if so, how rapid and complete healing can be. Children with significant acute penetrating injuries have been serially examined to document that rapid healing occurs (Finkel, 1989; McCann & Voris, 1993). Since most children disclose a history of sexual assault long after it has occurred, the likelihood of detecting a remote injury is very low (Adams et al., 1994). As already mentioned, the probability of detecting a physical injury is highest when an assault has occurred with the last 72 hours, or when the child reports a history of both pain and bleeding.

♦ **LABORATORY EVALUATION**

Universal screening for sexually

transmitted diseases (STDs) is not necessary for victims of sexual abuse (American Academy of Pediatrics, 1999). Most children without symptoms of an STD (vaginal or penile discharge or pain) are unlikely to have a sexually transmitted disease (Ingram et al., 1997). According to Seigel, Schubert, Meyers, and Shapiro (1995), a recognized protocol for testing for STDs would include the following:

- Any symptomatic child with discharge
- Any child found to have another sexually transmitted disease
- Any child with a sibling found to have a sexually transmitted disease
- Any child who is post-menarchal (having regular menstrual periods)

Finding an STD in a child who discloses a history of sexual abuse or exhibits behavior worrisome for sexual abuse can supplement an investigation. However, the likelihood of an STD representing evidence of sexual abuse is made more difficult when there is no other evidence of sexual abuse in the child (parental concern, behavioral change, child's disclosure). Many sexually transmitted diseases can be vertically passed to a child during routine childbirth. Some pathogens, most notably human papillomavirus (genital warts) and chlamydia, may have long incubation periods before overt symptoms (warts or discharge) appear. The outside limit of incubation for perinatally acquired genital warts and chlamydia is unknown, but is generally regarded to be less than 3 years. Other pathogens like herpes simplex virus and *Trichomonas vaginalis* can be spread by autoinoculation or innocent transmission by close household contacts. Although all sexually transmitted diseases raise suspicion of sexual abuse, acquired gonorrhea and syphilis are most suspicious for sexual abuse without other corroborating concerns (Hammerschlag, 1998).

◆ MANDATED REPORTING

Mandated reporters are required to report children with suspected sexual abuse to the child welfare system and law enforcement for investigation. Reporters make critical judgments with an understanding of the implications that making a report may have on the family. Additionally, professionals who care for children and families also are aware that false accusations of sexual abuse can have significant consequences to the accused parties. In a field where the majority of reports center more around a child's disclosure than a physical examination finding, each mandated reporter is forced to define a personal threshold that, when reached, will compel them to make a report. Discussed here are some common dilemmas when the decision to report may not be self-evident.

THE THIRD-PARTY REPORT

When a child discloses a history of sexual abuse to a mandated reporter, the reporter has an obligation to contact the local authorities for an investigation. However, in some cases, a third party, usually a parent, provides a history of a disclosure by the child, which cannot be reproduced by interviewing the child. If the physical examination of the child is normal, the mandated reporter must then decide if his threshold to report the case has been reached.

This decision can be especially challenging if the concern arises around custody issues (in a divorce proceeding, for example). To remain consistent and objective, the following unbiased approach may be helpful in evaluating a child who makes a disclosure to a parent, but who is unable to make a disclosure to the mandated reporter:

1. Ensure that the caregiver and child are interviewed separately employing proper child interviewing technique (see below).

2. Ask the caregiver about sexual expression within the home, including nudity, pornography, and public displays of affection or sexual activity in front of the child. The child who witnesses sexual activity or pornography in the home may imitate what he sees, leading others to suspect that sexual abuse has occurred.

3. State your concern for what the third party is reporting, but let the caregiver know that you were unable to elicit the same information from the child.

4. Assist the caregiver or third party as they make an anonymous report to the proper authorities (child welfare or law enforcement).

5. Consider a referral to a psychologist or therapist to further explore statements the child has made to a caregiver.

This approach allows the mandated reporter to assist concerned caregivers who report a child's disclosure without questioning the caregiver's motivation. Most families are very understanding of the difficult position a mandated reporter is in when the reporter has no direct information from the child to support a sexual abuse allegation. These families most need the proper counseling on how to proceed with an investigation. Taking the time in the office to explain to a family how child sexual abuse reports are made and walking the family through those steps while in the office ensures that the children are reported for a proper investigation. However, since the caregiver is assisted in making a report, the mandated reporter is removed from making a report when he or she has no direct information provided by the child.

THE CHILD WITH AN ISOLATED PHYSICAL COMPLAINT

As mentioned earlier in this chapter, the child who presents to a mandated reporter with a genital complaint (e.g., vaginal discharge or bleeding) may prompt suspicion for sexual abuse. It is not surprising that children who present with isolated physical complaints, without a disclosure or abnormal behavior, are frequently reported to social services for an investigation without involving a medical subspecialist who is experienced in child sexual abuse evaluations. However, most large pediatric institutions now provide referral services for medical consultations in cases of suspected sexual abuse. Although up to two-thirds of children with isolated physical complaints are reported to social services before medical subspecialty referral, only 15% of these children will have findings suspicious for sexual abuse when they are examined by an experienced clinician (Kellogg, Parra, & Menard, 1998). This should alert the mandated reporter to consider a referral for the child with isolated physical complaints to a pediatric child abuse specialist for a second opinion before determining whether a child protective report is necessary.

THE CHILD WITH AN STD AND NO DISCLOSURE

Because of the potential for autoinoculation and a prolonged carrier state following perinatal transmission, a mandated reporter may be confused as to when to report a child with an STD who has not disclosed a history of sexual abuse. The likelihood of an STD representing evidence of sexual abuse is reviewed in Table 2-1. Although some children with an STD may not have

Table 2-1. When Sexually Transmitted Diseases in Children Compel a Report

STD Confirmed	Likelihood of Sexual Abuse	Suggested Action
Gonorrhea	Diagnostic*	Report
Syphilis	Diagnostic*	Report
HIV	Probable**	Report**
Chlamydia	<1-3 years of age:. Possible$^\alpha$	Report
	>3 years of age: Probable	Report
Trichomonas Vaginalis	<1 year of age: Possible$^\alpha$	Consider Report
	>1 year of age: Probable	Report
Herpes (genital)	<3 years of age: Possible$^\beta$	Report$^\beta$
	>3 years of age: Probable	Report
***Condyloma Accuminata* (Anogenital Warts)**	<3 years of age: Possible$^\psi$	Consider Report
	>3 years of age: Probable	Report
Bacterial Vaginosis	Nonspecific	No Report

* *If not perinatally acquired*

** *Must exclude perinatal and transfusion-related transmission*

α *Outer limits of incubation from perinatal transmission unknown*

β *Must exclude autoinoculation (more likely HSV1) from caregiver or child. If clear evidence of autoinoculation, may opt not to report.*

ψ *Long incubation from perinatal transmission; most cases under 3 years of age likely to be from perinatal transmission; consider other risk factors from history in making decision to report*

been abused, a report is generally recommended to investigate all children with a sexually transmitted disease. The only exception to make is for young children with no behavioral indicators of abuse who have genital warts, which are most often innocuously transmitted at birth. If a mandated reporter is unsure whether to report a child whose only concern is a sexually transmitted disease, the reporter should contact the local child abuse specialist or forensic pediatrician for assistance with the case.

♦ Pitfalls of the Ensuing Investigation

Once a report is made, the most common problem faced during an investigation may be the multiple interviews to which a child is subjected. Because of this, the mandated reporter has a responsibility to advocate for reducing unnecessary interviews of the child. Multiple interviews by parents, physicians, police officers, and child welfare workers are often the most damaging aspect of child sexual abuse investigations. Children, particularly when they are toddlers, are susceptible to suggestibility (Reed, 1996). Multiple interviews, often by personnel not fully trained to interview children, may elicit partial disclosures and changing statements that, when viewed in hindsight by the legal justice system, taint the most important evidence in the case. The result may be a case being deemed unfounded or unsubstantiated by child welfare or the legal justice system, despite a mandated reporter's original inclination that inappropriate sexual contact may have occurred. Furthermore, an unsubstantiated report may result in a child and potentially other children still being at risk from the alleged perpetrator.

The best way to avoid tainting a child's disclosure is to recognize the role a mandated reporter assumes during the course of a sexual abuse investigation. A useful guideline is that, when a family is being seen for a sexual abuse complaint, the mandated reporter must determine if the complaint has already been reported to the proper authorities. If a report has not been made, the mandated reporter is obligated to interview the child to establish whether suspicion for sexual abuse exists. This does not necessarily mean an exhaustive interview, but one to gather enough information to satisfy a reporting threshold. If a report has already been made, the child may have been referred only for consultation, as occurs with physicians who perform the physical examination. In such a case, it is rarely useful to interview the child again.

Community-wide efforts may also reduce the number of interviews to which a child is exposed (Jaudes & Martone, 1992). Many states and counties have multidisciplinary centers (e.g., child advocacy centers) established to promote collaboration among child welfare and law enforcement investigators through co-housing of agencies. When a report is made, a single investigator interviews the child while other investigators watch by closed-circuit television or through a one-way mirror. In areas where no multidisciplinary teams exist, the mandated reporter can still discuss the issues of suggestibility and multiple interviews with the family before the investigation begins. Families can be instructed to advocate for a single collaborative interview with both law enforcement and child welfare officers present.

◆ MENTAL HEALTH REFERRALS

Regardless of the decision to report or the results of an ensuing investigation, victims of sexual abuse benefit from some form of ongoing counseling or therapy. While most referrals for mental health services follow an investigation, a mental health referral may preempt a decision to report, particularly when a mandated reporter is unable to obtain a disclosure of sexual abuse from a child at risk. For instance, if a child makes disjointed, sexually explicit statements that parents find confusing, but the child does not disclose a history of sexual abuse during the interview process, the mandated reporter may refer the child for counseling or therapy. Over time, the therapist can explore the root of the child's statements. If the therapist elicits more information over time to substantiate a child sexual abuse complaint, then the therapist, as a mandated reporter, will be compelled to report the case to the proper authorities.

◆ SUMMARY

A review of the medical literature regarding childhood sexual abuse reveals that in the majority of sexual abuse cases, the physical examination is normal. Given that the examination is often normal, statements provided by the child and other witnesses become the most important evidence in these cases. While a normal examination cannot prove whether sexual abuse has occurred, one must avoid discrediting the child who makes a cogent disclosure, but whose examination is normal. The duty of a mandated reporter is not to provide proof that an abusive situation exists, but to report suspicion of abuse to the proper authorities.

◆ APPENDIX: CASE EXAMPLES

Case One: A 3-year-old girl is brought to daycare, at which time the mother tells the daycare worker that the child told her that "pop-pop (paternal grandfather) has been putting his pee-pee in me." The daycare worker talks with the child alone, but the child does not disclose any information about anyone touching her. The mother asks the daycare worker what she should do.

Questions: What other questions should the daycare worker ask?

Should the daycare worker report the case to child welfare?

Should the daycare worker recommend the child be seen for a medical exam?

Discussion: This case is a classic example of a third party report when a parent tells a mandated reporter that a child has disclosed that another family member is sexually abusing him or her. In spite of this report, the daycare worker is unable to confirm the information with the child. The daycare worker should talk to the parent separately to elicit whether there have been previous concerns of sexual abuse, how often the child spends time with the grandfather, and whether the child has had any change in behavior or has made any other statements in the past. While many professionals who work with children may opt to file a report when a parent states this history, an alternative in this case would be for the daycare worker to assist the parent in filing a report to child welfare, since it was the parent who heard the disclosure. The child should be referred for a medical examination, but unless the child's contact with the perpetrator was within the last 24 hours, the child should be referred to his or her pediatrician or to a pediatric child abuse specialist in the area. The daycare worker should confirm with the parent that the child will be safe and have no further contact with the alleged perpetrator while the investigation is in progress.

Case Two: A school counselor is approached by the mother of a 5-year-old girl with concerns that the girl has been fearful of spending time at her father's home the last two months (parents are divorced). Mother has also noted that the child has not been acting her usual self, and that her school performance has declined. When the mother has asked the child what is wrong, the child has at times cried, but has refused to talk to her. The mother states that she is concerned the child may have been sexually abused, although she has no evidence of it. The mother asks the counselor what she should do.

Questions: What should the counselor instruct the parent to do?

Should the counselor file a report to child welfare?

What other options does the counselor have?

Discussion: This case exemplifies the subtleties in diagnosing sexual abuse when the sexually abused child manifests with only psychological symptoms. Although the temptation is to be extremely concerned when a parent tells such a story, we would caution against reaching a premature conclusion regarding the diagnosis of sexual abuse. A report at this time may in fact be premature, as there is insufficient evidence to warrant a report. This, however, does not mean there is not cause for concern. A reasonable plan of action in this case would be to refer the family to a therapist who can work with the girl over time to explore her behavioral changes. At the same time, a referral to the child's pediatrician would allow for medical screening in the remote chance there is suspicious genital anatomy to warrant a report to child welfare.

Case Three: A 6-year-old girl tells her school teacher that she is having bleeding from her "private area." The girl denies that anyone has touched her. The teacher calls the parents, who state that she has had some intermittent bleeding for the last week. The parents report no concern for sexual abuse, but state they had planned to discuss the problem with their doctor.

> *Questions:* Should the school teacher file a report to child welfare?
>
> What other options does the teacher have?

Discussion: This case is a good example of a child who has a physical finding in the genital region without a corresponding history of parental concern, disclosure, or unusual behavior. While sexual abuse should be considered whenever a child has an abnormal genital finding, only about 15% of such children will be found to have findings suspicious for sexual abuse when they are examined by a child abuse specialist. Therefore the proper course of management in this case is not to report (unless other concerns are elicited) and to recommend the family see their pediatrician or a child abuse specialist in their area who is familiar with pediatric gynecology.

♦ REFERENCES

Adams, J. A. (2001). Evolution of a classification scale: Medical evaluation of suspected child sexual abuse. Child Maltreatment, 6(1), 31-36.

Adams, J. A., Harper, K., Knudson, S., & Revilla, J. (1994). Examination findings in legally confirmed child sexual abuse: It's normal to be normal. Pediatrics, 94(3), 310-317.

American Academy of Pediatrics. (1999). Guidelines for the evaluation of sexual abuse of children. Pediatrics, 103, 186-191.

Bays, J., & Chadwick, D. (1993). Medical diagnosis of the sexually abused child. Child Abuse and Neglect, 17, 91-110.

Berenson, A. B., Chacko, M. R., Wiemann, C. M., Mishaw, C. O., Friedrich, W. N., & Grady, J. J. (2000). A case-control study of anatomic changes resulting from sexual abuse. American Journal of Obstetrics and Gynecology, 182, 820-834.

Christian, C. W., Lavelle, J. M., De Jong, A. R., Loiselle, J., Brenner, L., & Joffe, M. (2000). Forensic evidence findings in prepubertal victims of sexual assault. Pediatrics, 106, 100-104.

Finkel, M. A. (1989). Anogenital trauma in sexually abused children. Pediatrics, 84, 317-322.

Finkelhor, D. (1993). Epidemiological factors in the clinical identification of child sexual abuse. Child Abuse and Neglect, 17, 67-70.

Freidrich, W. N., Grambsch, P., Broughton, D., Kuiper, J., & Beilke, R. L. (1991). Normative sexual behavior in children. Pediatrics, 88, 456-464.

Hammerschlag, M. R. (1998). The transmissibility of sexually transmitted diseases in sexually abused children. Child Abuse and Neglect, 22, 623-635.

Holmes, W. C., & Slap, G. B. (1998). Sexual abuse of boys: Definition, prevalence, correlates, sequelae, and management. JAMA, 280, 1855-1862.

Ingram, D. L., Everett, V. D., Flick, L. A., et al. (1997). Vaginal gonococcal cultures in sexual abuse evaluations: Evaluation of selective criteria for preteenaged girls. Pediatrics, 99, e8-11.

Jaudes, P. K., & Martone, M. (1992). Interdisciplinary evaluations of alleged sexual abuse cases. Pediatrics, 89, 1164-1168.

Kellogg, N. D., Parra J. M., & Menard, S. (1998). Children with anogenital symptoms and signs referred for sexual abuse evaluations. Archives of Pediatrics and Adolescent Medicine, 152, 634-641.

Kempe, C. H. (1978). Sexual abuse, another hidden pediatric problem: The 1977 C. Anderson Aldrich lecture. Pediatrics, 62(3), 382-389.

Krugman, R. D. (1986). Recognition of sexual abuse in children. Pediatrics in Review, 8, 25-30.

Leventhal, J. M. (1988). Have there been changes in the epidemiology of sexual abuse during the 20th century? Pediatrics, 82, 766-773.

McCann, J., & Voris, J. (1993). Perianal injuries resulting from sexual abuse: A longitudinal study. Pediatrics, 91, 390-397.

Reed, L. D. (1996). Findings from research on children's suggestibility and implications for conducting child interviews. Child Maltreatment, 1, 105-120.

Saywitz, K., & Goodman, G. (1996). Interviewing children in and out of court: Current research and practical implications. In J. Briere, L. Berliner, J. Bulkley, C. Jenny, & T. Reid (Eds.), The APSAC handbook on child maltreatment (pp. 297-318). Thousand Oaks, CA: Sage Publications.

Seigel, R. M., Schubert, C. J., Meyers, P. A., & Shapiro, R. A. (1995). Prevalence of sexually transmitted diseases in children and adolescents evaluated for sexual abuse in Cincinnati: Rationale for limited STD testing in prepubertal girls. Pediatrics, 96, 1090-1094.

Summit, R. (1983). The child sexual abuse accommodation syndrome. Child Abuse and Neglect, 7, 177-193.

Van Dokkum, N. (1994). Preparing a child witness in sex abuse cases: The destruction and re-creation of testimony. Medicine and Law, 13(5-6), 473-488.

Chapter 3

CHILD NEGLECT AND ABANDONMENT

MARK D. JOFFE, M.D.

The full spectrum of child neglect is difficult to capture in a single chapter. Examining the various ways that children's basic needs are not met in the most affluent society in history is as bewildering as it is disconcerting. Child neglect is antithetical to the evolutionary imperative to nurture our young and see our genes enter the next generation. Medical professionals who seek to understand and successfully intervene in cases of child neglect must have an appreciation for the complexity of this problem. Simplistic or overly politicized arguments about whether responsibility for child neglect should fall upon parents or society at large are neither enlightening nor constructive. Child neglect exposes deficiencies in individuals, families, communities, and culture that need to be addressed at every level.

We pay a dear price for child neglect, the magnitude of which is impossible to estimate. Child neglect adversely impacts both the biological and environmental factors necessary for a child to develop into a healthy, happy, and productive adult.

The size and cultural diversity of our country make it difficult for many people to see the shared benefit of improving the lot of all children. A toxic cynicism asserts that attempts at intervention are futile, despite anecdotal and some experimental evidence to the contrary. Child advocates proclaim that "children are our future," a mantra that is not as altruistic as it may seem. It focuses on the future value of today's children to the adult community. Underlying this assertion is the investment model that the resources we devote to children today will offer a return to us in the future. Even if this were not true, children have "the equal and inalienable rights of all members of the human family" (United Nations Convention, 1990). We have an obligation as human beings to ensure a nurturing environment for them, regardless of whether or not it pays off for us in the future.

♦ DEFINITION OF NEGLECT

Neglect may seem like a concept that is easy to define. In reality, we know it when we see it, but a definition does not always come easily. Children require food, shelter, clothing, health care, education, and emotional nurturance. Neglect occurs when a child's basic needs are not met, usually through caregiver omissions. The concept of "demonstrable harm" is important in defining neglect, although placing a child in a dangerous environment or situation constitutes a form of neglect despite the absence of harm. Certainly in the most egregious forms of neglect there is little argument about whether a line has been crossed. Every parent, however, occasionally makes errors of omission or commission in the rearing of children. Neglect ranges from poor parenting to criminal negligence, with no clear boundary line to simplify the task of mandated reporters. The age of the child is also a factor. As independence grows in adolescence, the responsibilities of the parent become more difficult to define.

A child suffers from neglect when his or her basic needs are not met, regardless of the circumstances leading to the inadequacy of care. Some legal definitions associate neglect with culpability, however, arguing that poverty and caregiver disability are exemptions from neglect. A child is labeled "dependent" if his or her needs are not met through no fault of the caregiver. This awkward, legalistic terminology defines neglect based on a judgment of parental behavior. Certainly an understanding of contributing factors is important in designing effective interventions, but neglect is perhaps better defined from the child's perspective, for it results in suffering and harm regardless of circumstances.

♦ INCIDENCE

Data are available on reports of child neglect, but an accurate estimation of the incidence is quite difficult to derive. Child maltreatment in all of its forms is often not observed, much less reported. The Third National Incidence Study (NIS-3) used sampling and statistical methods to estimate the incidence of child abuse and neglect (Sedlak & Broadhurst, 1996). It used definitions of neglect that included an Endangerment Standard and a more stringent Harm Standard. The estimation of neglect using the Harm Standard was 879,002 cases in the United States per year, or 13.1 per 1,000 children (Table 3-1). Neglect is the most prevalent form of child maltreatment. One third of all child maltreatment fatalities are the result of neglect. This life-threatening condition is as much a public health problem as it is a social services issue.

DYNAMICS OF NEGLECT

Professionals working with neglected children have identified many factors that are frequently present in the lives of neglected children. This body of knowledge in no way undermines the importance of individual assessments. Obviously each case is unique and can best be managed by understanding the particular problems each caregiver must face. Most of the emphasis in describing child neglect has focused on the child's mother, who is the primary caretaker in a majority of cases. Neglect has been identified, however, in children in foster care, in children in the custody of fathers or other relatives, and in children reared in institutional settings.

SOCIAL FACTORS

Poverty is strongly associated with child neglect (Daro & McCurdy, 1992; National Center for Children in Poverty, 1991). It is more powerfully

Table 3-1. Incidence of Child Abuse and Neglect (NIS-3, 1996)*

Category	Number of Children	Rate per 1,000 Children
Neglect		
Physical	338,888	5.0
Emotional	212,843	3.2
Educational	397,323	5.9
Neglect Total	879,002	13.1
Abuse		
Physical	381,675	5.7
Sexual	217,654	3.2
Emotional	204,485	3.0
Abuse Total	743,238	11.1
Maltreated Total	**1,553,786**	**23.1**

* Data based on "Harm Standard." Numbers and rates using "Endangerment Standard" are higher.

associated with neglect than with physical or sexual abuse (Drake & Pandey, 1996). Unquestionably, some circumstances make child rearing extremely difficult, but the majority of impoverished children are not neglected. Using resourcefulness, energy, and community supports, low-income parents in the United States are generally able to provide for their children's basic needs. A safety net for children exists in this country, but it is a complex, confusing, cumbersome web with many holes so that parents are often unable to access the food, clothing, and shelter available for their children. Material deprivation may be the major factor in many cases of child neglect, but usually other problems are essential contributors (Fig. 3-1).

Humans evolved in clans of extended family, where kinship relationships

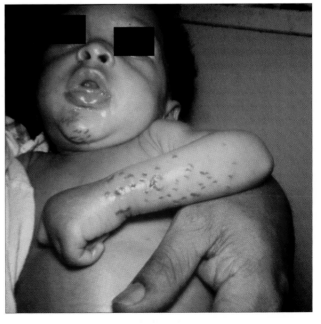

Figure 3-1. *This infant, left unsupervised in dilapidated housing, suffered multiple rat bites. Poverty is more closely correlated with neglect than child abuse.*

invested the entire group in the nurturance of its children. One theory to explain the prevalence of neglect in our affluent society links it to social isolation. The family unit in our culture is smaller and more independent than at any time in human history. Greater mobility has separated parents and children from grandparents and other extended family members. Studies have documented an association between network supports, single parenthood, and estrangement from relatives with the incidence of neglect (Coohey, 1995; Coohey, 1996). Social isolation may be a symptom of family dysfunction, but it also appears to be an important contributing factor in the dynamics of child neglect. Social support can prevent child neglect in a variety of ways. Children may be insulated from the effects of a temporary loss of income through the material assistance of family and close friends. Family members may confront a parent with negligent behavior more readily than neighbors or other strangers. Ignorance often contributes to neglect. Extended family members with experience in child rearing may provide information or a reality check that an isolated, inexperienced mother may lack. Maternal disabilities may be identified and the mothers brought for treatment by caring family members and friends before they impact on the children's well-being. Loneliness often contributes to depression, which undermines a parent's ability to properly care for children. The social structure of modern America, with small, isolated families surrounded by unrelated strangers, does not provide the support to dysfunctional families that protects children.

MATERNAL/PATERNAL FACTORS

Neglectful parents often lack basic problem solving skills and social competence (Daro, 1988). They may be young, inexperienced, and ignorant of the nutritional, developmental, and safety needs of their children. Mothers with mental retardation or other developmental disabilities may need extra support to prevent neglect of their children.

The prevalence of major affective disorders, especially depression in women, appears to be increasing. Symptoms often include lethargy, apathy, sleep disturbance, irritability, and inability to make decisions and think clearly. A depressed parent usually cannot meet the daily demands of parenting. Postpartum depression has been linked to failure to thrive in young infants. The array of effective treatments for depression has never been wider, but poor, depressed mothers are less likely to receive care than their wealthier counterparts.

Alcoholism or drug abuse or both are noted in over one quarter of negligent families (Kelleher, Chaffin, Hollenberg, & Fischer, 1994). With the exception of alcohol, effects of in-utero drug exposure are poorly understood. The consequences of drug abusing parents, however, are clear. Parents addicted to alcohol or other drugs have a compulsion that may be stronger than their motivation to care for their children. Intoxication leads to a variety of neglectful situations. Clearly an intoxicated parent cannot provide the guidance and emotional support children need. When not intoxicated, addicted parents devote their time and material resources to procuring more drugs. Children may be left alone in unsafe environments for prolonged periods of time. In addition, access to drugs and alcohol can put young children at risk for intoxication.

CHILD FACTORS

Child factors generally do not play an important causative role in neglect. Some authors have tried to describe children at particular risk for neglect. Passive, quiet children may be less demanding and therefore less likely to have their needs met. There may be a poor fit between the personality of the parent and the temperament of the child. These descriptions may misleadingly suggest that the child is responsible for the neglect.

Children with special needs, a population that has increased dramatically in recent years, are at greater risk for neglect. Medical neglect is especially likely when medical needs are great. The daily administration of multiple medications to children with chronic illnesses may exceed the capabilities of any family. The stress of prematurity or other medical illness on families, as well as abnormalities in attachment to a baby who spent his or her early life in the hospital, increases the likelihood that these children will suffer from neglect. Health insurance for children is not universal, making provision for their medical needs quite costly for parents. The responsibility of parents to make sure the basic needs of their children are met can be quite challenging (Fig. 3-2).

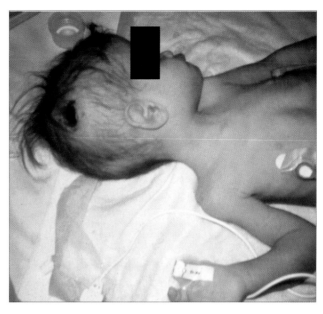

Figure 3-2. *This blind child was ignored for prolonged periods of time. A decubitus ulcer has developed on her head. Children with disabilities are more likely to suffer from neglect.*

◆ TYPES OF NEGLECT (TABLE 3-2)

FAILURE TO THRIVE

Inadequate growth of infants and young children is one of the most common presentations of neglect, but failure to thrive is not one disease, nor is it synonymous with neglect. A multitude of biological and psychosocial problems can lead to inadequate growth. The traditional categorization of failure to thrive as organic versus non-organic is being replaced with a more sophisticated interactional model. Children with increased caloric requirements or problems with intake due to medical conditions may also have dysfunctional families who are unable to meet their special needs. Organic and non-organic causes of failure to thrive may coexist in patients.

Table 3-2. Types of Neglect
Physical neglect
Failure to thrive
Inadequate supervision
Abandonment/expulsion
Custody issues
Other physical neglect
Medical neglect
Refusal of health care
Delay in health care
Educational neglect

In general, weight gain reflects the balance between caloric intake and metabolic expenditure, but humans are much more complex than simple input-output machines. Organic causes of failure to thrive may diminish a child's ability to take in and retain adequate nourishment, decrease absorption of ingested nutrients, impair utilization of absorbed molecules, or increase overall metabolic requirements. Occasionally patients do not gain weight despite receiving adequate calories, but inaccurate dietary history, unrecognized malabsorption, medical illness that increases caloric needs, or a combination of the above factors is usually responsible.

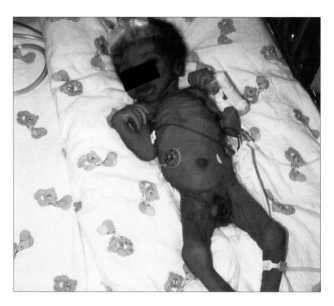

Figure 3-3. *Failure to thrive is usually related to non-organic, psychosocial factors.*

"Non-organic" or "psychosocial" failure to thrive, which describes the majority of cases, applies to normal children, usually infants, who are receiving inadequate calories. Nutritional neglect may occur because the mother is uninformed about proper nutritional requirements, distracted by other demands, disturbed by psychiatric problems, mentally impaired, or abusing alcohol or other drugs. Emotional deprivation almost invariably accompanies the nutritional deprivation. In the majority of cases, poverty is the context in which maternal and family problems lead to failure to thrive (Fig. 3-3).

First, a clinician needs to determine if failure to thrive is in fact a problem. Despite our culture that idealizes thinness in adults, many parents are worried that their properly nourished children are not as fat as they would like. Conversely, negligent parents often express no nutritional concerns in children with obvious nutritional deficits. The child's weight, length/height, and head circumference should be measured and plotted on an appropriate growth chart. Growth velocity is a more useful parameter than a single weight measurement in detecting failure to thrive. A child who has crossed two major percentiles on the growth chart in a downward direction may be identified as failing to thrive before he or she drops below the 5th percentile. A single measurement of weight below the 5th percentile will, by definition, suggest failure to thrive in the 5% of normal children who happen to be small. Calculating a growth velocity requires more than one measurement, which illustrates the importance of continuity of medical care in a home for children whose growth is of concern.

Caloric deprivation causes a decrease in weight percentile before length/height is affected. The head circumference is usually spared in all but the most severe cases of starvation. Children with poor weight gain who have relatively normal axial growth are said to have "asymmetric" failure to thrive, which suggests caloric deprivation. Those with "symmetric" failure to thrive, in whom percentiles for weight, length/height, and head circumference are all equally low, are more likely to suffer from an organic condition such as fetal alcohol syndrome, congenital infection, or dwarfism. Measurement of skin fold thickness is a useful tool in assessing nutritional status. A child with small parents who has normal growth velocity and normal skin fold thickness, but is below the 5th percentile, is likely to be achieving his genetic potential for growth.

Once poor growth has been identified, clinicians must complete a comprehensive evaluation to understand all of the factors that contribute to an individual child's failure to thrive. Assessments include the child's physical, nutritional, and developmental status, the diet, and the family structure and dynamics. Obtaining a quality history is usually the key to diagnosing the cause of failure to thrive. The prenatal history is especially important to detect in-utero exposures (alcohol) or congenital infections that can cause persistent growth retardation. Clinicians with strong prior relationships with families and excellent interviewing skills are better able to obtain information, such as alcohol and drug use in pregnancy, that parents may be reluctant to disclose. Fetal alcohol syndrome (Table 3-3) is an important cause of failure to thrive that must be considered by clinicians, especially when a child remains short and microcephalic despite inter-

Table 3-3. Fetal Alcohol Syndrome	
Persistent growth deficiency (weight, length, head circumference)	
Mental retardation	
Face	short palpebral fissures
	epicanthal folds
	thin upper lip
	maxillary hypoplasia
	micrognathia
Cardiac	septal defects
Limb/joint abnormalities	

ventions. Controlling for prematurity and other factors, in-utero exposure to marijuana, cocaine, or narcotics alone does not appear to cause significant post-natal growth retardation. A human immunodeficiency virus infection may first manifest itself with slow growth. Since failure to thrive may result from chronic problems with any body system, clinicians must ask about symptoms of respiratory, cardiac, and neurologic problems in addition to the obvious questions about gastrointestinal function. A detailed dietary history, including questions about types of foods, formula/food preparation, and amount and frequency of intake, is essential. Information from babysitters, day care workers, and other caretakers can reveal problems that are not known or not reported by the parent. The inability to obtain a detailed and non-idealized dietary history suggests non-organic failure to thrive.

Failure to thrive usually reflects dysfunction in the parent-child dyad, so evaluation of the caregiver, often the mother, is as important as assessment of the child. Questions about the caregiver should be asked in a supportive way to avoid defensiveness. Uncovering maternal depression, substance abuse, and other causes of parental disability may be the solution to the child's future weight gain. Knowledge of family stressors (e.g., finances, separation, divorce, family illnesses, relocation) that are temporally associated with the onset of the failure to thrive may be diagnostic. The family's strengths as well as weaknesses are important in planning an effective intervention.

A careful and thorough physical examination is aimed at assessing the child's current clinical state, as well as uncovering the cause of the failure to thrive. Many neglected infants and children with failure to thrive appear apathetic, with dull eyes, poor eye contact, and involvement in self-stimulatory behaviors. The cardiorespiratory, abdominal, and neurologic examinations are particularly important in excluding an organic cause of failure to thrive. Children with failure to thrive have thin extremities, prominent ribs, and wasted buttocks. Flattening of the occiput with hair loss is a less specific finding now that the supine position is recommended for infants. Poor general hygiene, with diaper rash, impetigo, dirty, unclipped fingernails, and unwashed skin and clothing often accompany nutritional neglect. The clinician should observe a feeding in the office. A professional eye may detect oral-motor problems or improper feeding techniques that limit the child's intake. Observation of the mother is as important as observation of the child. Bonding and physical contact between mother and child can be assessed while feeding. Poor bonding, no response to separation from the child and a lack of perception of child's needs suggest an attachment disorder, which often underlies psychosocial failure to thrive. Signs of maternal depression can alert the clinician that the parent needs to seek treatment.

The cause of failure to thrive is seldom determined at a single visit. Weekly visits can more accurately determine growth velocity. A more exact calculation of caloric intake is possible with a food diary. First-line interventions for poor weight gain can be assessed with frequent follow-up. Numerous medical conditions can cause failure to thrive (Table 3-4). If basic nutritional counseling does not result in improved weight gain at the 1- or 2-week follow-up visit, laboratory testing should be undertaken to rule out many of the conditions that cannot always be diagnosed based on history and physical examination alone (Table 3-5). Early identification and intervention with close follow-up may eliminate the need for more in-depth medical and psychosocial evaluation.

A state-of-the-art evaluation and treatment plan for a child with significant failure to thrive entails more than most medical offices can provide. The expertise of nutritionists, developmental specialists, and social workers can add to the physician's resources in dealing with the complex mix of medical and social issues. They can provide home assessments and ongoing monitoring of the child and family through the intervention phase. Multidisciplinary teams are available in some regions, and clinicians should be informed about resources available in their communities.

Intervention depends on the cause and severity of failure to thrive and the family and community resources that are available. Failure to thrive is a chronic condition that benefits from long-term, multidisciplinary follow-up. Intervention starts with access to quality medical care. Significant non-organic failure to thrive should be reported to Child Protective Services (CPS). In collaboration with CPS, family support should be organized, a treatment plan developed and instituted, and follow-up arranged and monitored.

Initially, acute medical problems such as dehydration, hypoglycemia, and hyponatremia must be stabilized. Some children with severe failure to thrive should be hospitalized (Table 3-6). When provided with >150 calories/kg/day, most infants with non-organic failure to thrive feed avidly and gain 1-2 ounces per day. Behavioral changes, with increased interactivity and positive affect, are often noted by nurturing hospital staff.

During the hospital stay, social workers can assist families with enrollment in food programs such as the Special Supplemental Food Program for Women, Infants, and Children (WIC) and put them in contact with resources to deal with problems with housing, heat, health insurance, and family issues. Education and treatment of negligent mothers begins immediately, but will need to be continued after discharge. Enlisting the support of extended family members often plays an important role in maintaining the progress made after returning to the home environment. Approximately three-quarters of patients with non-organic failure to thrive return to their homes with supplemental

Table 3-4. Organic Causes of Failure to Thrive	
Gastrointestinal	*Vomiting*
	Gastroesophageal reflux
	Pyloric stenosis
	Reduced intake
	Cleft palate/lip
	Inflammatory bowel disease
	Malabsorption
	Cystic fibrosis/pancreatic insufficiency
	Celiac disease (gluten-sensitive enteropathy)
	Parasites
	Liver/biliary disease
	Lactose intolerance
Neurologic	Static encephalopathy
	Degenerative disorders
Renal	Urinary tract infection
	Renal tubular acidosis
	Chronic renal failure
Cardiopulmonary	Congestive heart failure
	Bronchopulmonary dysplasia
	Chronic asthma
	Recurrent/chronic pulmonary infections
	Severe adenotonsillar hypertrophy
Endocrine/metabolic	Diabetes mellitus
	Hypothyroidism
	Inborn errors of metabolism
Congenital	Genetic/chromosomal disorders
	Fetal alcohol syndrome
	Congenital infections (HIV, CMV, syphilis)

services. Clinicians should not be overly optimistic, however, that a short-term intervention will change the child's home in the long run. Weekly office visits, home visitation, and close monitoring must continue to prevent recurrences.

Table 3-5. Laboratory Testing for Failure to Thrive (as indicated)

- Complete blood count
- Free erythrocyte protoporphyrin
- Lead level
- Erythrocyte sedimentation rate
- Urinalysis and urine culture
- Electrolytes, blood urea nitrogen, creatinine
- Alkaline phosphatase, calcium, phosphorus
- Liver function tests
- Albumen
- HIV, syphilis serology
- Tuberculin skin test
- Skeletal survey
- Sweat test

Table 3-6. Indications for Admission in Failure to Thrive

- Severe malnutrition
    - Below birth weight at 6 wks
- Dehydration
- Head circumference crossing 2 or more percentiles downward
- Organic cause requiring admission is suspected
- Failure of outpatient intervention
- Physical abuse or gross neglect
- Unsafe home
- Caregiver disability/inadequacy

MEDICAL NEGLECT

When failure to meet healthcare needs causes demonstrable harm, the child has clearly suffered medical neglect. Medical neglect includes failure or delay in seeking care as well as noncompliance with treatment plans. Extreme noncompliance, especially with chronically ill children, can also be called medical neglect because of the imminent risk of serious consequences. For instance, failure to administer anticonvulsant medication to a child with a seizure disorder may be medical neglect, especially if breakthrough seizures have occurred. Failure to complete an antibiotic prescription is simple noncompliance. Missed appointments for health maintenance visits and failure to fully immunize are frequent problems that warrant the involvement of a social worker, but generally do not constitute medical neglect.

Physicians often share some of the responsibility for medical neglect. While parents are expected to make reasonable medical decisions for their children, expectations must take into consideration both the medical knowledge and judgment of parents and the available family resources to comply with treatments. Physicians can prevent medical neglect by ensuring that parents understand the importance of medical treatments and follow-up care. Families without health insurance and transportation may not be able to comply with expensive treatments or frequent visits to distant offices. Knowledge of the family's resources can help the physician anticipate noncompliance before it becomes medical neglect. Clinicians who are frustrated and angry about noncompliance should not use a report to CPS to punish parents when the definition of medical neglect has not been met.

Religious-based medical neglect is a controversial subject. Some jurisdictions provide exemptions to adherents of "well-recognized" religions who provide spiritual treatments. Most courts, however, will override parental religious practices when certain criteria are met. The refused treatment must be clearly superior to alternatives, significant complications of therapy must be unlikely, and failure to treat must be expected to result in serious harm or death. The child must be likely to enjoy a relatively normal life in the future, a provision that gives parents the right to refuse aggressive treatment for severely handicapped or terminally ill children. If the child is old enough, he or she must also consent to the therapy (Bross, 1982). Healthcare providers who report medical neglect in families who refuse treatment based on religious reasons need not worry about legal retribution, even if the court later upholds the religious exemption. Our legal system is increasingly recognizing that religious preference is an adult decision. While the parents are not considered neglectful, minor children cannot be denied the medical care that they need.

EDUCATIONAL NEGLECT

Truancy that is endorsed or tolerated by parents is a common form of educational neglect. Many adolescents who skip school come from dysfunctional families, but this type of truancy often is not supported by the family and therefore is not educational neglect. Conduct disorders are common in adolescent truants. School refusal or school phobia, which are disorders commonly associated with anxiety or depression, can appear to be educational neglect to teachers and school administrators who are unaware of the underlying problem. Educational neglect also applies to families who never enroll their children in school despite the children reaching the age of compulsory education. Children may not receive the expected support from their families in preparation for school or in completing homework assignments, but these issues generally do not comprise neglect. CPS can work with the school's personnel to design a plan to reduce educational neglect. Physicians and other healthcare providers have numerous opportunities to emphasize the importance of education to the long-term welfare of children when instructing parents about school absence and return to school after illness. The consequences of educational neglect include academic underachievement, compromised employment potential, and social problems.

ABANDONMENT

Abandonment is perhaps the most extreme act of neglect. All child neglect reflects a degree of emotional abandonment, but occasionally physical abandonment also occurs. Abandonment rates in the United States are not systematically measured, but they vary widely from 0.4% in San Francisco to almost 2% in Washington, D.C. (Abedin, Young, & Beeram, 1993; Takayama, Wolfe, & Coulter, 1998). In the 1990s, the abandonment rate in Romania exceeded 4%. One hospital in Hungary placed incubators in their lobby so abandoned infants would not become hypothermic before they were found. In poorer countries there is a clear relationship between economic trends and the rate of abandonment, but the vast majority of even the poorest parents would not consider abandoning their children. A study in St. Petersburg, Russia, demonstrated that hospital efforts to promote early attachment between mothers and newborns could dramatically reduce the rate of abandonment, despite worsening economic conditions and a rising rate of abandonment in the general population (Lvoff, Lvoff, & Klaus, 2000). The dynamics of abandonment in the United States are comparable. Similar to all child neglect, attachment problems in the context of poverty are the basis of most cases of child abandonment.

Physical abandonment includes a variety of circumstances, such as infants left out of doors with intent to kill, infants left where they are likely to be found, children left with others who will meet their needs, and older children who are thrown out of their homes. Some cases of abandonment result from a decision not unlike the decision to have one's child adopted. A child safely abandoned at a hospital may have better prospects for a happy and productive life than one who remains with his or her biological parents. Children who are left in places where they are likely to be found are put at risk, however, especially if left out of doors. When an infant is left out of doors with no expectation of being found, child abuse or attempted infanticide is a better description than child neglect.

Premature infants and other newborns who require prolonged hospitalization are at risk of abandonment. Parents do not have the opportunity to bond normally with these children. The neonatal intensive care environment may be so unnerving for some parents that they do not visit regularly. The realistic expectation of significant ongoing medical problems after discharge can overwhelm some parents, leading to withdrawal. Procedures that encourage early involvement of parents in the care of their hospitalized newborn can have important effects on attachment. Older children with chronic illnesses and prolonged hospitalization may also be abandoned when parents do not show up at the time of discharge. Most hospitals and municipalities will notify CPS of abandonment 48 hours after a child's scheduled discharge, assuming no lack of notification or extenuating circumstances.

◆ OUTCOME OF NEGLECT

Child neglect has profound consequences on both the physical and psychological development of children. There is a clear association between infant malnutrition and persistent deficits in growth. Malnutrition compromises immune function and puts the child at risk for a variety of infectious diseases. Medical neglect is often defined by the preventable illness that occurs.

The neuropsychological consequences of child neglect are difficult to clearly define, as quality longitudinal studies that control for other factors are few. Numerous adverse neuropsychological and behavioral outcomes have been associated with child neglect, including cognitive deficits, academic underachievement, depressed affect, behavior problems, and poor peer relations (Erikson, Egeland, & Pianta, 1989). Neglect has been associated with subsequent alcoholism, drug abuse, criminal convictions, and premature death (McCord, 1983). Some children, however, show remarkable resilience to the effects of child neglect when placed in a stimulating, supportive environment. Providing food supplementation and emotional support to mothers and children results in improved affect, better peer relations, and improved problem-solving skills (Barrett & Frank, 1987). Positive long-term outcomes may be more affected by developmental stimulation than nutritional assistance. The societal burden created by neglected children who never reach their full potential as adults is enormous. In addition to being the right thing to do, intervention and prevention of child neglect can have substantial, tangible, and enduring benefits.

NEGLECT VERSUS ABUSE

Neglect and child abuse are often lumped together as child maltreatment, suggesting that the risk factors, dynamics, and outcomes are similar. Child abuse has gotten more publicity than neglect in recent years, prompting several authors to discuss the "neglect of neglect." Recent evidence suggests neglect is different from child abuse in many ways. Negligent parents are more disengaged from their children and have more negative interactions with their children than abusive parents (Bousha & Twentyman, 1984). Negligent mothers have lower perception of personal and social adequacy and lower self-esteem than physically abusive mothers (Christensen et al., 1994). Several studies provide evidence that neglect is more damaging to a child's development than child abuse. Neglect and emotional abuse have a more profound negative long-term effect on academic performance, psychological distress, and psychopathology than abuse alone (Brunner, Parzer, & Schuld, 2000; Kendall-Tackett & Eckenrode, 1996; Melchert, 2000; Widom, 1999). The persistence and pervasiveness of neglect in the life of a child seem to be especially harmful to cognitive and psychological development.

INTERVENTIONS

The spectrum of child neglect necessitates a variety of interventions based on the type of neglect, the condition of the child, and the dynamics of the family. Child neglect is usually identified after the child has suffered for a prolonged period of time. Interventions for complex and chronic conditions necessarily require considerable time, often 12 to 18 months or longer (Dubowitz & Black, 1994). Some cases of neglect can be managed by a physician and local CPS workers. In more complex cases, particularly when the child's medical condition is poor, involvement of an established team of physicians, nutritionists, social workers, therapists, and specialists in child development is advisable. Experienced multidisciplinary teams can perform a more comprehensive assessment, access a wider variety of resources for families, coordinate a multifaceted intervention, and monitor follow-up in consultation with the primary care provider. Physicians should know where and how to access these services in their communities.

Once neglect has been identified, the first step is to stabilize any acute medical problems, such as dehydration. This may require hospitalization. Once the acute problems are controlled, careful assessment is necessary to understand the circumstances that led to neglect and to identify family strengths that will be essential to the long-term intervention. Interviews with multiple family members and friends will give a more accurate picture of the family. Home visitation is often instructive.

Many cases of neglect are related to inadequate food, housing, heat, or health insurance. Social workers can access programs to supplement the resources in the home. Enrollment in WIC, specialized feeding programs, Medicaid, Supplemental Security Income, and other support programs can be the first step in overcoming many cases of neglect. It is generally easier to improve nutrition, heat the home, and access health insurance coverage than change family members and family dynamics.

Head Start and other early intervention programs provide for the child's developmental and psychological needs and are successful at fostering rapid developmental progress in neglected children. As respite for parents, adult needs can be addressed during the time children are in programs. Older children may benefit from group therapy.

The problems of neglected children often pale in comparison to the problems of the negligent parent. Detailed assessment and understanding of the parent can direct the intervention. The intervention should be structured and goal-directed, modeling the organization that many negligent parents lack. Treatment of depression, addiction, family conflicts, and other personal problems is perhaps the most important intervention in the long run. Parent training is important, especially for young, inexperienced parents and parents of children with special needs. Parenting skills, stress reduction, impulse control, money management, job placement, and marital counseling are components of successful programs (Lutzker & Rice, 1984). Family therapy that includes extended family members may be more effective than individual therapy because it can create a more supportive network for parents who are isolated socially. Unfortunately, a significant number of neglected children suffer subsequent neglect despite attempts at intervention. Some circumstances involving severe neglect, significant physical injury, unremitting parental disability, or extreme family dysfunction require placement of the child with either a relative or a foster family.

Clinicians should recognize how difficult it is to overcome many of the problems that lead to child neglect. Ongoing monitoring of neglected children and their families is crucial to prevent these vulnerable children from future neglect. Physicians and other healthcare providers cannot monitor these families by themselves. Scheduled health maintenance visits, however, are both an important monitor of the child's health status and a useful marker of improved family functioning. Continued communication between the physicians and CPS can help ensure a successful intervention.

Prevention is obviously the preferred intervention. Astute clinicians who detect maternal inexperience, depression, drug addiction, mental illness, or extreme poverty should make every effort to intervene before the children are neglected. The expertise of a social worker should be one of the services clinicians can obtain for their patients and families. Early intervention programs that have proven successful for neglected children are available for at-risk children. Programs for home visitation in high-risk cases are currently being studied and offer hope for primary prevention in the future.

◆ SUMMARY

Child neglect, the failure to meet a child's basic needs, is a complex and multifaceted problem that is more prevalent than the better-publicized problem of child abuse. Its long-term impact on physical and cognitive development can be severe. Social factors, such as poverty and lack of social supports, and parental disabilities, such as depression and substance abuse, play important roles in many cases of child neglect. Interventions must be individualized and long-term to be successful in creating a more nurturing environment for neglected children.

◆ REFERENCES

Abedin, M., Young, M., & Beeram, M. R. (1993). Infant abandonment: prevalence, risk factors, and cost analysis. AJDC, 147, 714-715.

Barrett, D. E., & Frank, D. A. (1987). The effects of undernutrition on children's behavior. New York: Gordon and Breach.

Bousha, D. M., & Twentyman, C. T. (1984). Mother-child interactional style in abuse, neglect and control groups: Naturalistic observations in the home. Journal of Abnormal Psychology, 93, 106-110.

Bross, D. C. (1982). Medical care neglect. Child Abuse and Neglect, 6, 375.

Brunner, R., Parzer, P., & Schuld, V. (2000). Dissociative symptomatology and traumatogenic factors in adolescent psychiatric patients. Journal of Nervous and Mental Disease, 188, 71-77.

Christensen, M. J., Brayden, R. M., Dietrich, M. S., et al. (1994). The prospective assessment of self-concept in neglectful and physically abusive low income mothers. Child Abuse and Neglect, 18, 225-232.

Coohey, C. (1995). Neglectful mothers, their mothers, and partners: The significance of mutual aid. Child Abuse and Neglect, 19, 885-895.

Coohey, C. (1996). Child maltreatment: Testing the social isolation hypothesis. Child Abuse and Neglect, 20, 241-254.

Daro, D. (1988). Confronting child abuse: Research for effective program design. New York: The Free Press.

Daro, D., & McCurdy, K. (1992). Current trends in child abuse fatalities and reporting: The results of the 1991 50-state survey. Chicago: National Center for the Prevention of Child Abuse.

Drake, B., & Pandey, S. (1996). Understanding the relationship between neighborhood poverty and specific types of child maltreatment. Child Abuse and Neglect, 20, 1003-1018.

Dubowitz, H., & Black, M. (1994). Child neglect. In R. Reece (Ed.), Child abuse: Medical diagnosis and management. Philadelphia: Lea and Febinger.

Erikson, M. F., Egeland, B., & Pianta, R. (1989). The effects of maltreatment on the development of young children. In D. Cicchetti and V. K. Carlson (Eds.), Child maltreatment: Theory and research on the causes and consequences of child abuse and neglect. Cambridge: Cambridge University Press.

Kelleher, K., Chaffin, M., Hollenberg, J., & Fischer, E. (1994). Alcohol and drug disorders among physically abusive and neglectful parents in a community-based sample. American Journal of Public Health, 84, 1586-1590.

Kendall-Tackett, K. A., & Eckenrode, J. (1996). The effects of neglect on academic achievement and disciplinary problems: A developmental perspective. Child Abuse and Neglect, 20, 161-169.

Lutzker, J. R., & Rice, J. N. (1984). Project 12 ways: Measuring outcome of a large in-home service for treatment and prevention of child abuse. Child Abuse and Neglect, 8, 519.

Lvoff, N. M., Lvoff, V., & Klaus, M. H. (2000). Effect of the baby-friendly initiative on infant abandonment in a Russian hospital. Archives of Pediatrics and Adolescent Medicine, 154, 474-477.

McCord, J. (1983). A forty-year perspective on effects of child abuse and neglect. Child Abuse and Neglect, 7, 265.

Melchert, T. P. (2000). Clarifying the effects of parental substance abuse, child sexual abuse, and parental caregiving on adult adjustment. Professional Psychology—Research and Practice, 31, 64-69.

National Center for Children in Poverty. (1991). Alive and well? A research and policy review of health programs for poor young children. New York: Columbia University School of Public Health.

Sedlak, A. J., & Broadhurst, D. D. (1996). <u>The third national incidence study of child abuse and neglect (NIS-3 final report).</u> Washington, DC: US Department of Health and Human Services; US Government Printing Office (Contract #105-94-1840).

Takayama, J. I., Wolfe, E., & Coulter, K. P. (1998). Relationship between reason for placement and medical findings among children in foster care. <u>Pediatrics, 101,</u> 201-207.

United Nations Convention on the Rights of the Child. (1990).

Widom, C. S. (1999). Childhood victimization and the development of personality disorders: Unanswered questions remain. <u>Archives of General Psychiatry, 56,</u> 607-608.

Chapter 4

EDUCATIONAL NEGLECT

PEGGY S. PEARL, ED.D.

Neglect is failure by the caregiver to provide for the basic needs of a child. The basic needs are usually defined by state statutes to include food, clothing, shelter, and medical and dental care. Supervision and education appropriate to the age and developmental level of the child are also usually included as part of the definition. States assist parents in their responsibility to educate their children by providing free public education for all children.

The Third National Incidence Study of Child Maltreatment (NIS-3) identified educational neglect in approximately 14% of maltreatment cases. It defined educational neglect as follows (Sedlak & Broadhurst, 1996):

Permitted chronic truancy

Habitual truancy averaging at least 5 days a month if the parent or guardian has been informed of the problem and has not attempted to intervene.

Failure to enroll/other truancy

Failure to register or enroll a child of mandatory school age, causing the child to miss at least 1 month of school, establishing a pattern of keeping a school-age child home for non-legitimate reasons (e.g., to work, to care for siblings, etc.) an average of at least 3 days a month.

Inattention to special education need

Refusal to allow or failure to obtain recommended remedial education services, or neglect in obtaining or following through with treatment for a child's diagnosed learning disorder or other special education need without reasonable cause.

All states allow parents to choose public, private, religious, or home education for their children. States are very zealous in the protection of this parental right to choose the type or means of fulfilling the responsibility to educate their children. Most states require that parents declare their decision in writing to a local governmental agency, usually the public schools. Some states require that parents demonstrate that the child is making educational progress and achieves a minimum level of proficiency. Proficiency is usually measured periodically for all children regardless of methods of schooling chosen. For example, all children in the geographic area of a school district may be required to complete and pass periodic skills tests, especially at grades 8 and 12.

The U.S. Constitution gives states domain over education. However, both state and federal court cases have formed the case law that guides a parent's right to select his or her child's form of education. The *Meyer v. Nebraska* (1925) decision ruled that parents had the right to teach their own children. *Pierce v. Society of Sisters of the Holy Name* (1925) ruled that Oregon could not require children to attend public schools. Parents could choose private, parochial, secular, or public schools. The parental right to follow religious beliefs in educating their children was the basis of the 1972 *Wisconsin v. Yoder* Supreme Court decision that exempted Amish children from the requirement that students attend school until the age of 16. Very different from the Amish religious beliefs, public secondary school systems are based on competitiveness, self-achievement, and success. These court cases reinforced both the parents' rights and responsibilities in educating their children.

During the early years of our nation, children were educated by parents or other adults in their own homes, or in the homes of neighbors or extended family. This changed in the last half of the 19th century. Universal public schooling then became the common means of educating children from age 6 to 16. Not until the last 20 years of the 20th century did this begin to change significantly. In addition to the increase in private and parochial education, growing numbers of parents were choosing to home school their children. Home schooling is "instruction and learning, at least some of which is through planned activity, taking place primarily at home in a family setting with a parent acting as teacher or supervisor of the activity" (Lines, 1991). In the 1970s it was estimated that between 1,000 and 15,000 children were home schooled. By the 1999-2000 school year in the United States, the number had increased to between 1,300,000 and 1,700,000 children (National Home Educational Research Institute [NHERI], 1999).

In response to this trend, state legislatures passed laws or regulations to guide the home schooling process. These laws and regulations vary significantly from state to state. Some states don't require that parents file a curriculum or list a particular person as responsible for the teaching, while three states require a certified teacher. In states where "outcomes testing" is required, the results are comparable to the public schools. Most states offer some support to parents and require periodic academic testing. Some states allow public dollars to be used for curriculum materials and allow children to participate in extracurricular activities, summer programs, teams, and large group activities (Berger, 1998).

♦ CAUSES OF EDUCATIONAL NEGLECT

Most parents want their children to get an education. They use their resources to help them achieve that goal. Other parents fail to provide an appropriate education for their children, which is defined as educational neglect in many states. This is when child protective agencies and/or law enforcement becomes involved. This neglect may be seen in both overt, confrontational ways, as well as subtle, almost invisible ways. Table 4-1 contains a list of possible indicators of educational neglect. For example, parents may fail to enroll children in school following a move or may not allow older adolescents to return to school in the fall *(see Example 1)*. This non-enrollment often goes unnoticed by the school system and instead is noticed by someone who realizes that the child is of school age and not in school during the usual school hours *(see Example 2)*.

Although enrolled, other children fail to attend on a regular basis, resulting in failure to progress at the expected rate. This truancy may be with or without parental knowledge, consent, or concern. Parents who had poor experiences in formal education may pass their own negative attitudes about school and school attendance on to their children. The parents and other adults in the child's life may also fail to model the routine or discipline necessary for learning. The child's role models may also devalue formal education, books, homework, class projects, and responsible behavior, all of which are necessary for school success. Some children enter kindergarten or first grade with the attitude that school is a place where bad things happen and they should do

---

Table 4-1. Indicators of Educational Neglect

Objective Indicators

Excessive absences for no apparent reason.

Excessive absence that parent fails to correct, i.e., head lice, school immunizations.

Failure to follow through with needed referrals for special services and therapy, especially as part of an individualized educational plan (IEP).

Parental Behavior

Fails to correspond with school without reasonable justification. For example, does not return phone calls, attend parent-teacher conferences, or return notes from teacher.

At parent-teacher conference, parent focuses only on self or others, never on the child under discussion.

During discussions and conferences, blames child for all of parent's problems.

Degrades child in presence of child and others.

Fails to recognize child's strengths.

Fails to participate in child's school activities when child desires and there is no apparent reason not to attend.

Child Behaviors

Consistently performs below ability level when at school.

Has poor self-esteem.

Reports disinterest of parents in education and general lack of interest in the child's interests and activities.

Reports parental agreement that child can drop out of school prior to legal age or completion of high school.

Describes staying home to care for siblings or other family members with parental approval.

anything to get out of it. Parents often support the child's efforts to stay home with notes saying they are sick or had to go to the doctor/dentist when in fact the child just did not want to go to school. There is a high correlation between poor school attendance and later status offenses, criminal behavior, and unemployment.

Failure to attend school regularly is also an indicator of other problems within the family *(see Example 3)*. Parents can be so overwhelmed with issues such as poverty, substance abuse, unemployment, mental illness, domestic violence, and/or poor housing that they cannot focus on the child's needs, including educational needs. If the child has special educational needs, the parent may be even more overwhelmed and immobilized by the challenges in his or her life. These families need help with all their problems and frequently do not know where to begin in problem solving. These families commonly have so few resources that they feel "helpless and hopeless" to make positive changes. The child's lack of clothing and/or school supplies may have been more than the parent could handle. These parents need a parent aide or family support worker to assist them in daily living tasks and resource management, including someone to assist them with their possible mental health, job skills, or substance abuse problems. Children may in fact be staying home to care for the parent or siblings. Homes where educational neglect occurs are frequently homes where there are other types of neglect, i.e., medical, nutritional, emotional, or poor housing and sanitation. Occasionally, there is physical abuse, and the child is kept home to hide the signs of the physical abuse from the outside community. When there is substance abuse in families, there is frequently a combination of neglect and physical abuse along with psychological abuse.

Dubowitz, Giardino, and Gustavson (2000) call for health providers to screen all children with the simple question, "How are things going at school?" The professional can follow up with questions about behavior, learning, and peer relations. Other follow-up that might be part of the screening assessment includes:

- If truant or not enrolled, why? How much school has been missed? What has the parent done about it? What has the school done?

- If problems have been identified, what assessment has been done? What has been recommended? What has been implemented? Have there been any results?

- Request permission to talk to a teacher to help clarify the situation.

Management of the child and family relies on impressing upon the family the importance of a sound educational foundation for life. Dubowitz, Giardino, and Gustavason (2000) suggest the following:

1. Strategize around ensuring school attendance.

2. Demand appropriate educational evaluation and services.

3. Support the family in seeking out the necessary services.

The causes of educational neglect are many and diverse. Common in neglectful families is the failure of the caregiver to appropriately bond with the child. The parent fails to consistently recognize and respond to the child's basic needs right from birth. This early pattern of parent-child interaction may have established a relationship where the child's needs are secondary, at best, to the parent's needs. This results in children who not only fail to trust their primary caregivers, but who also fail to trust their own feelings and abilities. They may lack a sense of initiative, self-confidence, and empathy for others, all of which are necessary social skills for appropriately constructing knowledge of the world around them. The lack of bonding may be caused by environmental factors such as repeated losses, poverty, and/or community and domestic violence, as well as organic problems such as mental illness or substance abuse. Whatever the causes of the educational neglect, it rarely corrects without some type of external intervention. Like other types of child maltreatment, each added abuse tends to become more serious as the instances become more frequent. Families in which there is educational neglect need help to resolve some of the family issues and allow the adults to more appropriately meet the educational needs of their children.

◆ NEGLECTING THE CHILD WITH SPECIAL NEEDS

Children with special needs are at significantly higher risk for educational neglect than their siblings and age-mates without special needs. Two general forms of educational neglect situations may occur. In one form, the parent may fail to accept that the child has special educational needs and may stay in the stage of denial to the point that the child's special needs are never met. The parent's denial results in the child being denied the therapy, assistive device, special tutoring, medication, or medical attention necessary for his or her appropriate educational needs to be met. An example may be failing to purchase hearing aids for a hearing-impaired child to facilitate learning and language development because the parent refuses to believe the child's hearing is impaired and doesn't want people thinking the child is "deformed." Other parents may deny physical therapy for a physically-challenged child, refusing to accept that it would make any difference and saying "it would just be a waste of time and money."

In another form of educational neglect, parents may burn out on parenting a child with special needs. Parents give up or give out on the challenging job of meeting the child's educational needs. Their time and energy resources become depleted. Some parents are unable to sufficiently renew their resources. They give up and stop providing for the child's special educational needs—resulting in educational neglect and often physical and/or psychological abuse through physical and verbal attacks. When one parent never accepts the child's ability level (or disability level), all of the care can become the responsibility of the other parent, and this parent is often unable to sustain the level of effort necessary to meet the special educational needs of the child.

Providing appropriate educational adaptations for children with special needs is difficult. For some children, appropriate education means learning the life skills necessary to live in an environment separate from their parents in a group home, assisted living facility, or supportive living environment. Some overly protective parents do not permit their children with developmental delays or multiple impairments to gain appropriate independence. These cases require sensitive handling by case managers to ensure that each individual is given the opportunity to perform at his or her optimal level.

♦ Consequences of Educational Neglect

Educational neglect is more than a young child missing school. It may be a total lack of concern by parents for the educational needs of their child. There is a considerable body of educational research indicating that when parents are not actively involved in the lives of their children, the children are less likely to experience academic success and more likely to drop out before age 16. The level of parental interest in and support of children is the primary factor affecting whether or not children succeed in school (Boyer, 1991). When children do not have this interest and support, they do not reach their potential, they fail in the classroom, and they fail in life. They fail to feel the joy of learning. They feel left out of their peer groups. Overall, they often see themselves as failures and worthless. Many children who fail in the early years of school due to educational neglect continue to experience failure in the educational system until they drop out, turn to drugs or anti-social behaviors, and often prey on others.

♦ Summary

Educational neglect is a tangible indicator that caregivers are failing to provide one of the necessities of life for children. Educational neglect does not generally occur in isolation from other child maltreatment and family violence. When educational neglect is present in a family, closer observation usually reveals many other family problems. These problems may include poverty, substance abuse, unemployment and underemployment, mental illness, domestic violence, and animal abuse. Children with special needs are at higher risk for educational neglect than their peers, as parents may burn out from the stress of providing for those needs, or they may deny the special needs exist. Appropriate external intervention is needed to assist the family with meeting basic needs and improving family functioning, or the situation will grow worse, with more negative consequences for the children. The family dynamics that cause educational neglect are most often long-term, chronic problems that require both short-term and long-term assistance and support. The consequences are not just educational delays but also diminished self-worth, social problems, and poor peer relationships, including victimizing others. Educational neglect teaches children anti-social behaviors that require multi-disciplinary intervention or the behaviors will grow more damaging. When schools report educational neglect and social service agencies get involved, they often discuss medical neglect, lack of supervision, and psychological and physical abuse. As part of the child's wellness team, healthcare providers should ask general questions about how school is going at regular visits, in the emergency room, or in the urgent care facility to open dialogues about school and screen for possible educational neglect.

Example 1: The Peters family moves to a nearby city in June. Mrs. Peters and Maria, her 14-year-old daughter, find jobs fairly quickly. By mid-July, the second daughter, Samantha, is very fortunate to find a job with a major bank that will allow her to continue working full-time while she takes the classes needed for graduation. Mr. Peters is still searching for a day job that pays as well as he was making before he was laid off. By August, he finds a job and the family is finally comfortable and everyone likes his or her job. When the time for school registration rolls around, Samantha registers and begins classes. Maria likes her job and does not want to go to school. She persuades her parents to let her quit school and go to night school and get her G.E.D.

Since neither Mr. nor Mrs. Peters finished high school, they feel they can do little to make Maria go to school against her wishes. At least she does have a job.

Example 2: It is a warm Monday in late October in a middle-class, suburban neighborhood. Mrs. Jones is home ill from work and notices Sam, the neighbor boy, is also home and outdoors riding his bike. The next day, as she returns home from her appointment with the doctor, she notices him outside again. This continues for the remainder of the week. On Friday she is so curious she goes outside to talk to Sam. In the conversation, she asks where he attends school. Sam shrugs his shoulders and goes back into the house. Confused, Mrs. Jones calls the neighborhood elementary school and tells them her concerns. She is told that due to rights of confidentiality, they cannot tell her whether Sam is enrolled, and that parents have the right to choose alternatives to public schools for their children.

Example 3: Carlos, a shy third grader, is absent again. The teacher notes that this is the second time this week, the 8th time this month, and the 15th time in the 2 months since school began. He works hard when he is at school, but he is barely making passing grades because he is absent so much. Most days he comes back with a note from his mother that just reads "Carlos was sick yesterday." When he returns to school, he appears healthy but not always clean. The teacher shares her concern with Ms. Santos, the school nurse. Ms. Santos tries to call Carlos' home. The phone has been disconnected. She drives to his home. No one answers the door. She has come before and no one ever answers the door. As she leaves school around 4 p.m. the next day, she once again drives to Carlos' home. This time Carlos is playing on the steps with a toddler. Ms. Santos sits down on the steps to visit with Carlos. He says, "I didn't go to school 'cause my mom's sick and I got to take care of my baby sister." Ms. Santos asks Carlos if she could talk to his mother. Carlos says she is sleeping and does not want to be bothered. Ms. Santos asks when Carlos' father will be home. Carlos says, "I don't know, just later. I'm to keep my sister outside and be quiet so Mom can sleep." Ms. Santos talks with Carlos for about 30 minutes, then feels she must leave. Carlos is not at school the next day. Carlos' teacher and the school nurse confer and decide to call child protective services.

◆ REFERENCES

Berger, E. H. (1998). Rights, responsibilities and advocacy. In <u>Parents as partners in education.</u> Englewood Cliffs, NJ: Merrill.

Dubowitz, H., Giardino, A. P., & Gustavason, E. (2000). Child neglect: Guidance for pediatricians. <u>Pediatrics in Review, 21</u>(4), 111-116.

Lines, P. (1991). Home instruction: The size and growth of the movement. In H. Van Galen and M. A. Pitman (Eds.), <u>Home schooling: Political, historical, and pedagogical perspective</u> (pp. 9-42). Norwood, NJ: Ablex Publishing.

National Home Education Research Institute (NHERI). (1999). <u>Facts on home schooling.</u> Retrieved September 11, 2001 from the World Wide Web: http://www.nheri.org/98/research/general.html

Sedlak, A. J., & Broadhurst, D. D. (1996). <u>Third national incidence study of child abuse and neglect (NIS-3 final report).</u> Washington, DC: US Department of Health and Human Services; US Government Printing Office (Contract #105-94-1840).

Chapter 5

PSYCHOLOGICAL ABUSE

PEGGY S. PEARL, ED.D.

Psychological maltreatment of children and youth consists of acts of commission (such as repeatedly telling the child that she is stupid) and omission (such as ignoring the child), both of which are psychologically damaging. Psychological abuse involves the presence of hostile behavior as well as the absence of positive parenting techniques. Such acts immediately or ultimately damage the behavioral, cognitive, affective, or physical functioning of the child. Psychological abuse is a concerted attack on a child's development of self and social competence. It may or may not be a conscious act by the parents or other caregivers. Psychological abuse damages the child's psychological development and emerging personal identity. Since emotions are primary to cognition and precede the development of cognitive processing skills, the assessment of cognition can yield evidence of psychological abuse. (Claussen & Crittenden, 1991; Garbarino, Guttman, & Seeley, 1987; McGee & Wolfe, 1991).

Psychological abuse is the most elusive diagnosis in child maltreatment. It interrupts the process of attachment, affective development, and the evolution of empathetic capacities. As a result of the failure to develop empathy, the child is impaired in his or her

ability to appropriately receive and transmit emotional information. Some researchers feel that the lack of attachment, continual attack on the child's sense of worth, and failure to provide emotional nurturance found in psychological abuse, when coupled with neglect and perhaps early physical abuse, can impair the child's total capacity to respond emotionally. Alexithymia, an inability to consciously experience and communicate feelings, appears to be linked to human maternal deprivation. Because affective development precedes cognitive and physical development, early diagnosis and treatment are needed to minimize damage to the child's development and maturation. This will hopefully reduce the societal costs of psychological abuse and increase the likelihood that the victim will live a full and productive life (Barnett, Miller-Perrin, & Perrin, 1997; Belsky, 1991; Miller-Perrin & Perrin, 1999; O'Hagan, 1995; Wolfe, 1991).

♦ FORMS OF PSYCHOLOGICAL ABUSE

Psychological abuse can take many forms. It is a repeated pattern of caregiver behaviors or extreme incidents that convey to children that they are worthless, flawed, unloved, endangered, or of value only in meeting another's needs. It is always involved in the adult's struggle for absolute control of the child. The younger the child and the less developed the child's sense of self and identity, the more serious the physical, social, and emotional consequences. Emotional abuse of older children with a well-established sense of self may have less impact than the same action on a younger child or a previously maltreated child.

When a child experiences the emotion of fear or feels distress, a parent normally responds with compassion and love as well as physical comforting. Such emotionally interactive responses are appropriate and form a core component of "attachment." When parents do not respond in this way, but repeatedly respond with anger and rejection, attachment does not develop and the child experiences psychological maltreatment. (Garbarino, Guttman & Seeley, 1987; Wolfe, 1991).

Psychological abuse varies in intensity from occasional to mild to extreme over a sustained period of time. Categories of psychological abuse are listed in Table 5-1.

Table 5-1. Categories of Psychological Abuse

1. Ignoring or degrading the child and failing to provide necessary stimulation, responsiveness, and validation of the child's worth in normal family routine

2. Rejecting the child's value, needs, and requests for adult validation and nurturance

3   Isolating the child from the family and community; denying the child normal human contact

4. Terrorizing or threatening the child with continual verbal assaults; creating a climate of fear, hostility, and anxiety, thus preventing the child from gaining feelings of safety and security

5. Corrupting or exploiting the child by encouraging and reinforcing destructive, antisocial behavior until the child is so impaired in socioemotional development that interaction in normal social environments is not possible

6. Verbally assaulting the child with constant name-calling, harsh threats, and sarcastic put-downs that continually beat down the child's self-esteem with humiliation

7. Overpressuring the child with subtle but consistent pressure to grow up quickly and to achieve too early in the areas of academics, physical/motor skills, and social interaction, leaving the child feeling he or she is never quite good enough

8. Overexposing children to domestic and community violence and other behaviors that prevent children's personal safety

---

In most dysfunctional families, children experience many types of maltreatment. In some families, all children are treated or mistreated similarly, while in others each child is treated uniquely and affected individually. The child's developmental stage influences both the parent-child interaction and the impact of the interaction on the child. The more nurtured the child has been before the maltreatment and the more secure the child's attachment to his or her caregiver(s) early in life, the less impact the maltreatment will have on the child.

IGNORING

A parent or other caregiver exhibiting ignoring behavior fails to acknowledge the child's presence or needs (Table 5-2). The ignoring parent is physically and psychologically unavailable for the child, either consistently or on an unpredictable basis. Ignoring is often part of serious physical neglect in which the child is not fed, clothed, sheltered, bathed, supervised, or acknowledged as being in need of these basics.

CASE EXAMPLE

Martha seldom, if ever, calls any of her children by name. She neither talks to them nor looks at them. Martha's house is spotlessly clean but meals are rarely prepared and seldom is there food that the children can readily prepare for themselves. Following a visit with her daughter, Martha's mother brought the youngest child to the emergency room, concerned about the child's lack of appetite. He was diagnosed as having nonorganic failure to thrive. On examination of the other children, each child was found to be in the lowest percentile on growth charts, with abnormally short limbs, poor skin coloring, and extreme delays in muscle development. A visit to the school found that the oldest child was barely passing, had poor social skills, and was withdrawn and passive. Discussion with Martha revealed that her husband, Tom, is a workaholic, a very successful lawyer who spends long hours at the office. His income is one of the highest in the community, from which he generously provides for his family. However, he spends little time at home and little of that time with his children. Even from cursory observation of Martha, she appears depressed and merely says that she misses her husband's company.

CASE EXAMPLE

Jane is a 21-year-old single mother of three children. She had normal pregnancies, and each child was observed as normal at birth. However, each

Table 5-2. Parental Ignoring Behaviors
• Not responding to child's needs
• Failing to stimulate child in an appropriate manner
• Failing to look at child or call child by name
• Not attaching or bonding to child
• Failing to recognize child's presence
• Showing no affection for child
• Being psychologically unavailable for child on consistent basis

child now appears developmentally delayed and malnourished. Their skin is dry with little resiliency and a pale color. Their hair is dull, dry, and brittle. Their scalps are very dry. The children appear lethargic, as if drugged. The oldest child, at 3 years, 6 months of age, lacks language. In the doctor's waiting room, nurses observed the eldest child feeding the 6-month-old infant. The mother sat nearby, ignoring the children and their activities.

RESULTING CHARACTERISTICS

Studies of ignored children in institutions describe socioemotional deprivation so severe as to cause infant mortality of more than 33%. Most maternal deprivation cases involving infants do not result in death because of medical intervention. However, each year the number of failure-to-thrive cases is growing (Crittenden, 1992).

In addition to the physical harm, the ignored child learns to live under the absolute control of adults who cannot be trusted. Children of depressed mothers, who were emotionally unavailable to their children on a consistent basis, show both emotional and cognitive developmental delay. The parent with schizophrenia or a character disorder also is in such need emotionally that she or he is consistently unavailable to the child. Ignoring is an act of omission—passive and neglectful. Rejecting, however, is an act of commission—active and abusive (O'Hagan, 1995; Portwood, 1999; Wright, 1994).

REJECTING

Parents exhibiting rejecting behavior refuse to touch or show affection to their child and do not acknowledge the child's presence or accomplishments, as well as constantly rejecting and demeaning age-appropriate behaviors. Table 5-3 lists parental rejecting behaviors.

With an infant, the parent exhibiting rejecting behavior refuses to form an attachment. The parent does not respond to the child's requests to have basic needs met, such as when the child cries for food or with a wet diaper. The parent also does not respond to the child's smiles and vocalizations of pleasure. As the child grows, the parent does not talk with the child or become involved in the preschooler's activities. The child is not included in family activities. The child may spend long periods of time in solitary play, often in another room with the door closed. As the child develops, the parent consistently communicates a negative definition of self to the child. The parent belittles the child and his or her accomplishments, both privately and publicly calling the child "dummy," "clumsy," "dunce," "nerd," "freak," or other such names. The parent has very low expectations of the child in school, telling the child that he or she can't expect to pass or do well in school because he or she is not smart enough to succeed. The school-aged child or adolescent is treated like a small child and not allowed to act in age-appropriate ways. The parent does not acknowledge, or openly rejects, the changes associated with adolescence, including social roles, physical size, sexual development, or increased cognitive ability. The child is told of his failures and seldom if ever included as a valued individual within the family. The parent commonly fails to have empathy for the child's needs (O'Hagan, 1995; Romeo, 2000).

Rejecting parents generally appear overwhelmed by the convergence of social and economic hardships. Commonly, rejecting parents are reacting to large families, limited material resources, limited education and job skills, and few emotional and social supports, all of which stress the parents and limit their ability to nurture their children (Table 5-4). These parents feel materially and psychologically unable to move beyond concern for themselves to concern about their roles as caregivers, teachers, and providers of emotional support for their children.

Table 5-3. Parental Rejecting Behaviors

- Refusing to allow child to get needed psychological or medical treatment or educational services
- Belittling and ridiculing child
- Purposefully and continually embarrassing child
- Singling child out for criticism and punishment
- Failing to allow child to develop autonomy or independence
- Undermining child's attachment with others
- Routinely rejecting child's ideas
- Ridiculing or punishing age-appropriate behaviors as too immature
- Routinely calling child negative names, e.g., dumb, stupid, freak, nerd
- Routinely putting child down, publicly and privately
- Inappropriately attributing undesirable characteristics to child
- Continuing to treat adolescent as young child
- Denying child's needs and making child meet adult needs

CASE EXAMPLE

Jane feeds her son on schedule but seldom, if ever, holds him while she gives him his bottle. She lays him on the sofa and props the bottle, telling him and others how much of her time he takes and what better things she could be doing than taking care of him. When she feeds him baby food, she fails to make eye contact or talk to him. When she changes his diaper the only comments she makes are in disgust at how terrible it smells and what a mess he has made that she must clean up. She is seldom in the same room as the child and does not talk to him or play with him when they are physically near each other. She describes him as a "troublesome baby." However, other family members comment that he is a good baby since they never hear him cry.

RESULTING CHARACTERISTICS

Children who have been psychologically and/or physically rejected by parents or other primary caregivers are hostile and aggressive, have impaired self-esteem, and show either excessive dependency on parents and/or other adults or "defensive independence." These children and teens appear emotionally unstable and unresponsive, eventually perceiving the world in negativistic terms. They see themselves as having few strengths and skills. They view the world as being hostile and unwilling to assist them. They feel isolated and in turn may reject others, including their own children.

Table 5-4. Family Circumstances Associated with Increased Risk for Rejection

- Unwanted pregnancies

- No opportunity for caregiver to spend time alone

- Lack of involvement by father in child rearing

- Marital discord

- Social and instrumental isolation of family from the community

- Parental mental illness

ISOLATING

Isolation of children can come from a variety of parental motivations, but the resulting behavior prevents children from having normal opportunities for social relations with both adults and peers. Table 5-5 lists parental isolating behaviors. Some isolating parents are themselves fearful of the outside world and may attempt to protect their children from the dangers they believe exist from contact with others. These families usually have a very limited amount of social contact, which deprives the children of learning social skills with a variety of individuals.

Table 5-5. Parental Isolating Behaviors

- Not allowing child to participate in normal family routine

- Not allowing child normal contact with peers

- Physically separating child from family unit

- Not allowing child to participate in the social aspects of school

- Routinely teaching child to avoid and distrust peers

- Locking child in room, basement, attic

- Punishing requests for interaction with family or others

- Binding or gagging child to prevent interaction

- Refusing, without justifiable reason, to allow child contact with noncustodial parent, grandparent, or siblings

- Hiding child from outside world

Isolation is also present in sexually abusive families and in families in which ritualistic abuse occurs. The isolation is to keep what happens in the family a secret and to keep the children from learning that there is any other way of life. Other isolating parents are themselves without social skills. They merely lack their own social contacts or supports, and do not provide the opportunity for their children to acquire these.

CASE EXAMPLE

Neither Maria, 14, nor Christine, 10, are allowed to have friends over to play or go to other homes to play. Their mother believes that other children will introduce her girls to drugs and other "evils of the world." The girls were taught at home until recently, when their mother had to go to work to help pay off some medical and home repair bills. Since entering the public schools, the girls have not made friends. Christine has had problems doing group assignments in social studies and language arts. Both girls are excessively anxious about trying new experiences at school. Their peers tease them because they worry about someone taking advantage of them.

RESULTING CHARACTERISTICS

Isolating families often directly teach their children that contact outside the family is undesirable. School-aged children are not allowed to participate in co-curricular school activities, youth activities, or neighborhood play groups. Adolescent children are given home responsibilities and are prohibited from participation in school activities. Some families even remove children from school or do not encourage school attendance. Frequently children who have been isolated for long periods of time lack the social competence to experience success or enjoyment at school and therefore do not like to attend (Edmundson & Collier, 1993; Ney, Fung, & Wickett, 1993).

TERRORIZING

Terrorizing involves threatening the child with extreme or frightening punishment. Table 5-6 lists parental terrorizing behaviors. The parent intentionally stimulates intense fear, creates an unpredictable and threatening climate, or sets unattainable expectations and punishes the child for not attaining them. The discipline techniques are often arbitrary or beyond the child's ability to understand. The parent may tease or scare a young child in the name of humor, but the results terrorize and confuse the child. The parent may discipline the child by playing on fears that are normal for that age, such as loud noises or the dark. The terrorizing parent uses the feared situation "to scare the child into behaving." Parents may tell preschool children that if they don't behave the "monsters will drag [them] away in the night," or the night-light is "watching and if [they're] not good, the night-light will zap [them]." One of the normal fears of adolescents is that their peers will see them as different or that they will not fit into social settings. The terrorizing parent threatens the adolescent with public humiliation. These children are torn between a sense of loyalty and a sense of fear and apprehension. These children depend on the people that are terrorizing them; they want the abuse to stop but also want to be a part of the family where they long for affection and attention (Wolfe, 1999).

CASE EXAMPLE

Sam's dad has repeatedly threatened Sam and other family members with a gun, a bullwhip, and a switchblade. Sam has never seen them used on a family member, but regularly hides so that he cannot be found in case his dad comes home mad.

RESULTING CHARACTERISTICS

Terrorizing parents play mind games with older children. These games are designed to be no-win situations, where the child becomes very anxious, fearing the consequences. When parents place the child in the middle of arguments, as often happens in divorces, the child also becomes terrorized by this no-win situation. A child may be blamed for everything that goes wrong in the family, regardless of whose behavior is inappropriate. Constant criticism often leaves children so traumatized that they will not act because they fear they will be criticized for any behavior (Higgins & McCabe, 2000; Wolfe, 1999).

Table 5-6. Parental Terrorizing Behaviors

- Threatening and frightening child with guns, knives, whips, etc.

- Using bizarre means of discipline

- Making child feel excessively guilty

- Behaving chaotically to frighten child

- Laughing at or ridiculing child when frightened, or putting child down for expressing normal fears

- Punishing child by playing on normal childhood fears

- Refusing to comfort infant in distress

- Disciplining child inconsistently and capriciously

- Continually threatening suicide or abandonment

- Threatening to harm others in child's presence

- Knowingly permitting child to view or be involved in violent behavior

- Routinely engaging in fights and frightening behavior in front of child/domestic violence

- Failing to recognize the impact of domestic violence on children and failure to remove the child from the violent environment

- Binding and/or gagging child

- Permitting others to terrorize child or exposing the child to on-going domestic violence

- Failing to provide shelter, consistency, and safety for child

---

RITUALISTIC ABUSE

Ritualistic or multiple-victim/multiple-perpetrator abuse is among the most damaging forms of abuse. It is the systematic, bizarre misuse of the child physically, socially, sexually, and emotionally by a group of adults and includes some supernatural or religious activities. Ritualistic abuse is carefully integrated and linked with a symbol of overriding power, authority, and purpose, such as a religion or pseudoreligion. In this type of abuse, children are routinely involved in ceremonial sexual activity with adults, with other children, and, to a lesser extent, with animals. Use of bondage, excessive threats, and force can be present. This activity is usually performed in front of other adults and children. Children are physically tortured, drugged, and forced to ingest drugs, human and/or animal feces, urine, blood, and flesh. They are buried alive in boxes and bound to crosses, and some stories are told of sacrificing children to the devil (Young, Sachs, Braun, & Watkins, 1991).

The children involved in this activity, as well as the adults, are removed from normal social interaction and activity, and are taught a very antisocial value system. The "family" environment is one of absolute control by one individual. The children are told that what is happening to them is punishment for their bad behavior or sin and that they must cleanse themselves during the ceremonies. Children are constantly told that they are of no value except for how they can be used by the "all-powerful one," the group leader (Miller-Perrin & Perrin, 1999; Young et al., 1991).

In ritualistic abuse cases, children are systematically terrorized into participation and silence. Initially, the identified victim appears normal and denies any ritualistic involvement or multiple-perpetrator activity. Over time, when the child feels safe, the child is often able to recall memories and can describe experiences to a therapist or other trusted individual.

The following are commonly used methods of terrorizing children to silence in ritualistic abuse:

Preschool children are given a "mock operation." The child is laid blindfolded and nude on a table. The stomach is brushed with either a local anesthetic or a very cold liquid. Then a sharp pointed object is used to draw an outline on the child's stomach. The child is told that an animal is being placed in his stomach, and if he tells anything that has happened to him, the animal or demon will eat the child up to protect the secret. The child may be drugged to drowsiness before the "operation" and then given additional drugs to induce sleep. On waking, the child is asked what has just happened to check for effectiveness and to begin the terrorizing.

Children of any age can be systematically programmed so that when they hear a specific word or see a specific thing they will forget everything they know, or they will remember specific bizarre threats made against them if they tell anyone what has happened. The word or object is usually something that the child frequently hears or sees, such the word "light" or a postal truck.

Children are taught to believe that others can "read" their minds to know what they are thinking. They are also taught to believe that "good is bad and bad is good; hate is smart and love is dumb."

OVEREXPOSURE TO COMMUNITY AND DOMESTIC VIOLENCE

Exposure to community and domestic violence has serious negative effects on children. The impact on a specific child varies with the length of time the child is exposed, age and developmental stage of the child, other support in the life of the child, other risk factors in the family, and the presence of other stressors such as poverty, homelessness, and substance abuse. Recent brain research has demonstrated changes in the brain functioning of young children exposed to domestic violence. These changes result in different processing of information in the brain. Exposure to chronic or extreme domestic and/or community violence may result in symptoms consistent with posttraumatic stress disorder (PTSD). These PTSD symptoms include emotional numbing, increased arousal, avoidance of any reminders of the violent event, or obsessive and repeated focus on the event, depression, and/or violent behaviors.

It is important to note that the negative impact of violence on children begins in infancy and is cumulative. Infants and toddlers who witness violence in their homes or community show excessive irritability, immature behavior, sleep disturbances, emotional distress, fears of being alone, and regression in toileting control and language. Parents too often deny that young children even know that the domestic violence is occurring. As these children continue to live with this violence, they grow more anxious, experience more sleep disturbances, and have difficulty attending to required tasks and mastering age-appropriate skills. In school these children perform poorly, have emotional problems, experience difficulty with peers, and begin to form aggressive and delinquent behaviors. (Osofsky, 1999).

The impact of the terror of domestic violence changes the lives of exposed children forever, and the impact of violence grows each time the cycle repeats. Estimates are that as many as 3.3 million American children are exposed to domestic violence each year. These children are learning to settle disputes with violence, that might makes right, and that it's okay to beat people you "love." All too often these ideas are further reinforced by the movies, television shows, and videos the child also watches. The American Psychiatric Association statistics estimate that the typical child watches up to 28 hours of television per week. Many children are being terrorized within their own homes where they should be learning trust, security, and love (Osofsky, 1999).

CORRUPTING
Parental corrupting/exploiting behaviors (Table 5-7) teach and reinforce antisocial or deviant patterns that tend to make the child unable to function in a normal social setting. In milder forms, the parents convey approval of or encourage the child's precocious interest and/or behavior in the areas of sexuality, aggression, violence, or substance abuse. In the more serious forms, the parents continue to encourage and reinforce as the child's antisocial behavior grows more intense and destructive to self, others, or property. Reinforcing or ignoring delinquent behavior is parental corrupting behavior.

Corrupting can begin with rewarding the child for sexual contact, creating drug dependence, encouraging violence toward peers, laughing at antisocial behaviors, and continuing to encourage these behaviors as they grow more habitual and serious. Common parental corrupting behaviors include allowing adults to use their children for sexual activity such as prostitution and child pornography, allowing children to sell and deliver drugs, and encouraging drug use. In ritualistic abuse cases, children often reveal, after they feel very safe, that they were encouraged to have sex with younger children.

Parents who knowingly allow children to engage in any illegal activity are corrupting those children. Corruption is also occurring, however, when parents merely fail to teach their children the social skills necessary for successful interaction in the world around them and leave them vulnerable to learn inappropriate behaviors from those who would take advantage of them.

In families where parents are corrupting their children, the parents could be repeating the parenting cycle by passing on the type of parenting they received.

Parents who themselves have antisocial behaviors commonly transmit those values, actions, and attitudes to their children. These parental behaviors result from events or series of events in their own lives. Research suggests that most antisocial and criminal behavior is a consequence of child maltreatment (Miller-Perrin & Perrin, 1999).

CASE EXAMPLE

Sixteen-year-old Katrina's mother has had a series of boyfriends living in the home for many years, most of whom have had substance abuse problems. Both alcohol and drugs are common in the home. Katrina tells her friends that she can supply them with almost any drug they want any time they want them. She has her own car and no curfew. This year her school attendance record has been poor, but she has notes from her mother to "excuse" each absence.

RESULTING CHARACTERISTICS

Children who are mistreated during the first year of life fail to develop a basic sense of trust and therefore see the world around them as negative. They believe that people are not to be trusted or valued. These children frequently are taught that you have to take care of yourself—"take or get taken." This lack of respect for others leads them to have no respect for themselves. The consequence of corrupting children is that they demonstrate antisocial behavior from an early age. These children have a pseudo-mature behavior, unlike the normal behavior of age mates. They are "street-smart kids." From a very young age, they demonstrate few positive emotions and are unable to play in an age-appropriate manner. They often are rewarded for stealing and assaulting peers. As a result, they are unaware that their behavior is inappropriate. Commonly these families

---

Table 5-7. Parental Corrupting Behaviors

- Allowing and/or forcing child to watch pornographic materials
- Teaching child sexually exploitative behaviors
- Teaching child illegal/antisocial behaviors
- Knowingly allowing others to teach illegal activity to child
- Praising child for antisocial/delinquent behavior
- Positively responding to child's antisocial behavior
- Assisting child in delinquent behavior
- Teaching children how to avoid legal consequences of antisocial behavior
- Failing to discipline child for delinquent behavior
- Teaching child that "bad is good and good is bad"
- Giving drugs or other contraband to child
- Exposing child to harmful influences or situations
- Using child as a spy, ally, or confidant in parent's romantic relationships, or marital or divorce problems
- Failing to teach child socially appropriate/legal behaviors

devalue formal public education; they fail to send their children to school on a regular basis or fail to discourage school absences, further isolating the children from learning appropriate social skills, values, and attitudes.

VERBALLY ASSAULTING

Verbally assaulting a child with constant name-calling, harsh threats, and sarcastic put-downs that continually lower the child's sense of worth through humiliation is a type of emotional abuse. Table 5-8 lists parental verbally assaulting behaviors. In the verbally assaultive family, words are used to humiliate and control. The child is repeatedly told of the things that he is doing wrong without regard for what he does well. The child is often unfavorably compared with other family members or with downcast individuals. The child is regularly called derogatory names. The verbal put-downs and attacks can occur in the privacy of the home. Frequently, however, the child is publicly told what he has failed to do and how worthless he is. The verbally assaultive behavior is so pervasive in the family's functioning that child care professionals routinely hear the verbal assaults. These verbal assaults are usually delivered in a loud voice, which further accents their negativity.

Table 5-8. Parental Verbally Assaulting Behaviors

- Continually attacking child verbally, especially in loud voice
- Failing to protect child from verbal attacks of others
- Constantly belittling child
- Excessively criticizing child
- Routinely humiliating child
- Openly telling child that he or she is worthless and no good
- Scapegoating child
- Calling child derogatory or demeaning names
- Cursing at child
- Continually yelling at child
- Falsely attributing negative behavior to the child

CASE EXAMPLE

Phil is 3 years old. He had been developing normal language, but a radical change has occurred. The neighbor is worried; she hears Phil's dad continually telling Phil to shut up all of that chattering and not to talk when the television is on. "No one wants to hear you talk; we want to listen to the television." Phil's mom is telling all her friends, in front of Phil and whomever else is around, that he is "just retarded, can't talk, and the most awkward child [she] has ever seen."

RESULTING CHARACTERISTICS

As a consequence of verbal battering, children have a flat or negative affect, low self-esteem, and, occasionally, self-mutilating behavior. These children are withdrawn and shy, and have no sense of initiative. The children feel they are incapable of any achievements. They are unable to recognize positive social feedback when it is given to them. In some families, one child is scapegoated and routinely verbally assaulted or is the brunt of routine family sarcasm while other children receive no emotional abuse. Scapegoated children are at high risk for failure to thrive, childhood depression, and suicide. Usually, the child exhibits poor posture and a flat affect, or excessive acting-out behavior (Elkind, 1982).

The Second National Family Violence Survey reports that children who experience frequent verbal aggression from parents register elevated rates of physical aggression, delinquency, and interpersonal problems. Other research reports that these children describe less enjoyment in life and more problems with sexual behavior, anger, and aggression. Verbal aggression seems to be transmitted from one generation to the next more commonly than physical abuse (Barnett, Miller-Perrin & Perrin, 1997).

OVERPRESSURING

Primarily a middle class phenomenon, overpressuring parents consistently have inappropriately high expectations for their children. Elkind (1982) described the tendency of many parents today to be more concerned about a child's intellectual achievements than his or her psychological well-being. Children are expected to perform intellectual tasks early to prevent being labeled "normal" or "average" as compared to peers. Instead of facilitating cognitive development as intended by the parent(s), this parental behavior actually impairs both cognitive and emotional development. Table 5-9 lists parental overpressuring behaviors. Overpressuring begins when parents toilet train too early or attempt to teach very young children to read, count, and work on computers. It continues with inappropriate "pressuring and hurrying" throughout the child's life. Graduating tenth rather than first in the high school class or earning a merely above-average ACT score, for example, is seen as failure by the parent. The parent views the child's consistently coming in second in sports or other competitions as not really trying, rather than having done a good job. The overpressured child is praised and valued for what is accomplished but not for just being himself or herself and doing well.

CASE EXAMPLE

Sara's parents expected her to be "Ivy League material." She was expected to do well in everything (playing the piano, sports, and academics), but she was average. Her parents regularly expressed their expectations and disappointment with her level of achievement, her appearance, and her choice of friends. At 15, she was convinced that she was a failure and attempted suicide "to save her parents the embarrassment," the note said.

AGE-INAPPROPRIATE TOILET TRAINING

Beginning to toilet train too early says to the child, "you are not acceptable as you are and need to change." Often parents combine the age-inappropriate toilet training with terrorizing and threats of what will happen to the child if he does not gain control of his bowels and bladder. These children may later be seen in the physician's office with extreme constipation as the child tries to gain control of his or her environment through control of body functions. When children repeatedly hear parents or grandparents say, for example, "Your father or mother was potty trained at 9 months," they feel the pressure to be toilet trained, but may still lack the muscle control. The children feel inferior because they are unable to perform as wanted by these significant

---

Table 5-9. Parental Overpressuring Behaviors

- Expressing excessively advanced expectations of child

- Excessively criticizing appropriate behaviors; calling them inadequate

- Punishing child for acting in age-appropriate manner; calling it "immature"

- Ostracizing child for not achieving far above normal abilities

- Not providing assistance with remedial work; refusing to acknowledge that child would need assistance with such "simple" materials

- Refusing to provide age-appropriate experiences; insisting on providing experiences that are too advanced

- Beginning toilet training very early and insisting that child control body functions

- Comparing child to those who are very advanced, consistently leaving child "poor by comparison"

- Routinely buying toys that are far too advanced for child, with clear expectations that the toy will be used inappropriately, setting the child up for almost certain failure

- "School-shopping" for private/public schools that will allow child to be placed in advanced placement classes that are not appropriate for the child's ability

---

adults. To the child, this is a subtle but consistent put-down for not performing at the same level as the parent. When this put-down is combined with other forms of overpressuring, the results are frequently stress-related illnesses and excessive anxiety.

RESULTING CHARACTERISTICS

Parents can set high standards for their children and still demonstrate acceptance and love. Nurturing parents demonstrate positive feelings to their children, recognize their achievements, and convey pride. Overpressuring parents, however, fail to demonstrate that they feel acceptance, love, and pride toward their children. As a result, the overpressured child feels worthless, discouraged, lazy, unreliable, unacceptable, and inferior. The child feels inadequate or unacceptable as she is because her parents are always trying to change her. The child's identity is in terms of accomplishments rather than based on an appreciation of self. Stress-related illnesses are common in these children. Because they lack parental support and good self-esteem, they are more vulnerable to negative experiences. These children commonly suffer from depression and are at high risk for eating disorders, suicide, and poor peer relationships throughout their lives.

◆ CAUSES OF PSYCHOLOGICAL ABUSE

Many theories exist regarding the causes and correlates of child abuse. The four theories discussed here are (1) the psychiatric approach, (2) the social approach, (3) the developmental approach, and (4) the ecological approach.

PSYCHIATRIC APPROACH

The psychiatric approach to psychological abuse of children assumes that the perpetrating parent suffers from some mental illness. Perhaps 10% of all maltreating parents are psychopathic or sociopathic. Studies of mentally ill patients show they are at high risk for failing to meet a child's psychological needs because of the amount of effort they must expend to meet their own emotional needs. As compared to a control group, psychologically abusive parents have shown significantly more psychosocial problems, more difficulty coping with stress, more difficulty building relationships, and more social isolation. According to one study, psychologically abusive parents described themselves as having poor child management techniques and being victims of child maltreatment themselves. The mother who is overwhelmed with her own depression and psychologically stressed after childbirth lacks the physical or emotional energy to give the child what is needed. The parent preoccupied with the death of a parent, sibling, or spouse may also be unable to meet a child's needs. Although postpartum depression and grief tend to be short term and reversible, they negatively impact the parent-child relationship and can adversely affect the developing child. Mothers who are psychologically unavailable to their children appear to impair both the socioemotional and cognitive development of the children. Psychological abuse stemming from the mental illness of parents is one possible explanation but explains only a small number of psychological abuse cases.

SOCIAL APPROACH

Social approach theory places emphasis on the role of stress as a force impacting the family dynamics and causing psychological abuse. Nearly 60% of all abuse cases are associated with stress. Social stress interacting with other variables leads to aggression in the form of psychological abuse. Family stressors include limited resources, problems at work, death of the significant other, unemployment, health problems, overcrowding, isolation, substance abuse, high levels of mobility, poverty, and marital problems.

Individuals respond differently to stress. Women as a group demonstrate a tendency toward depression rather than violence as a response. Men as a group respond to stress with violence. Stressed women usually are psychologically unavailable to their children, thus ignoring, rejecting, or isolating them. Stressed men, on the other hand, tend to physically or verbally assault their children. The family's socialization to violence determines whether such abuse is physical or verbal.

Since all parents experience stress, the following mediating variables can assist in identifying which parents are more likely to abuse their children:

1. Presence or lack of appropriate coping mechanisms

2. Degree of family integration or isolation

3. Presence or absence of positive social networks

These mediating variables and the underlying causes of the stress determine the length and degree of the psychological abuse and, consequently, the amount of damage to the child's development.

DEVELOPMENTAL APPROACH

The developmental approach to psychological abuse is based on a theory that parenting attitudes and behaviors parallel Piaget's stages of cognitive development and Kolberg's stages of moral development. The stages require increasing cognitive sophistication and moral reasoning. At the lower developmental level, behavior is marked by immediate, direct, and unmodulated responses to external stimuli and internal need states. At higher levels of maturation, behavior is characterized by the appearance of indirect, ideational, conceptual, and symbolic or verbal behavior. Parents at the higher levels are more apt to use words and reasoning as part of parenting. Parents at the higher levels look at each child as an individual and at what is best for that individual. Parents at the lower levels are more impulsive, directive, and physical in their parenting. Parents at the lower levels parent from their own point of view and to make themselves feel good. Abusive parents, therefore, are parenting at their developmental level.

The orientations toward the parent-child relationship are egoistic, conventional, individualistic, and analytic orientations. Following each description is an example of parental reasoning at each of these cognitive-developmental stages.

EGOISTIC

The parent at this developmental level approaches child care tasks in terms of maximizing parental comfort in the long run. The parent responds to external cues from the child which affect the parent's emotional and physical comfort. The child's intentions and motivations are recognized, but not as separate from the child's actions. They are only perceived in relation to parental needs.

Examples:
What do you feel children need most from their parents?

Love and attention.

When you say love, what do you mean?

Holding them, telling them you love them, making them behave so they won't get on that dope and stuff when they get older. I want my kids to feel proud of me. I know eventually when they get older maybe I'll fail, but I'm gonna try my darndest when they're younger and just hope they don't turn out that way.

CONVENTIONAL (NORMS) ORIENTATION

The child's actions and inferred intentions in relation to the parents' preconceived expectations are the basis for parental activity and understanding of the child. The child is understood to have internal states and needs which must be acknowledged, but the parent conceives of the child's subjective reality in a stereotypical way. The child is not seen as unique, but as a member of the class of "children," and the parent draws upon tradition, "authority," or conventional wisdom, rather than solely upon the self, to form expectations and practices. The parent and child are understood to have well-defined roles which are their responsibility to fulfill. The parent-child relationship is conceived as mutual fulfillment of role obligations.

Examples:
What do you feel children need most from their parents?

Love.

Explain.

Just letting them know you love them. Letting them know you care, that you are concerned about what they do, and just trying to be the best parent you can.

Why do you think that is most important, conveying that love?

Because if children know they have love, then they are secure.

INDIVIDUALISTIC (CHILD) ORIENTATION

Each child is recognized to have unique as well as universally shared qualities and is understood in terms of his or her own subjective reality. The parent tries to understand the child's world from the child's particular point of view and conceptualizes the parent-child relationship as an exchange of feelings and sharing of perspectives, rather than only fulfillment of role obligations.

Examples:
What do you feel children need most from their parents?

Love and time. They need to have their needs considered, that they aren't always happy with things that we do and with the things that we want to make them do and with the things we want to make them happy. You have to look at them and if they don't tell, you have to ask them. You have to really try to find out what each child wants and what is going on in his head.

ANALYTIC (SYSTEMS) ORIENTATION

The parent can view the relationship between parent and child as a mutual and reciprocal system and understand that the child has a complex psychological self-system. The parent can understand that the motives underlying a child's actions may reflect simultaneous and conflicting feelings. The parent can also recognize that there may be ambivalence in his or her own feelings and actions as a parent, yet he or she still loves and cares for the child. Individuals and relationships are understood not only in terms of their stable elements, but as a continual process of growth and change. The parent-child relationship is built not only on shared feelings, but on shared acceptance of each other's faults and frailties as well as virtues, and on each other's separateness as well as closeness.

Examples:
What do you feel children need most from their parents?

I will say love and you will say to me, "What do you mean by love?" and I will say, "I think it is an acceptance, unqualified, for what that person is in time." It has nothing to do with grades or cleanliness. I would like her to be clean and tidy, but it has nothing to do with love and feeling that someplace in this world you are loved for what you are by the people who know you best and nevertheless love you. I think that it is something that will help the children begin to love themselves.

What do you mean to begin to love themselves?

Well, I think that people can be so cruel to themselves, "Oh, I'm dumb, I'm stupid." Words which tear down instead of build up. And I think one way to serenity about the way you are and the way you see the world, even if life is difficult, is if you can be gentle with your errors and failures and see them as part of a process. Then I think you will have a kind of stability and mental health that is a legacy from parents who love you unqualified (Newberger & Cook, 1983).

ECOLOGICAL APPROACH

The ecological theory of psychological abuse of children involves all of the various aspects of a family's life and the surrounding community. Parents bring various influences to the parent-child relationship, including their marital experiences, how they understand and implement their roles as parents, and their relationships with their own parents. In the case of re-marriage, new values, beliefs, and history are introduced, and it is necessary for each family member to adapt. How each parent was raised plays a significant role in determining what parenting skills they possess and will use. Knowledge of child development will enhance parenting skills, but some parents may still be more effective at particular developmental stages. The mental health and ability of all individuals in the family will play an important role in the choices and actions of both parents and children. The child may also have a history that did not involve his or her parents. Perhaps the child was reared by a grandmother for the first three years of his life, or one parent was away in the military or working. The child's health, temperament, gender, and ordinal position in the family, and the status of family bonding and relationships are also critical aspects of the ecological theory that can influence parenting choices and actions. In families, each child is parented uniquely, based in part on their own temperament, personality, ability level, and appearance. Verbally assaulting a strong-willed child may seem justified to parents who lack the knowledge and temperament to work with the child. Other parents may ignore a child with challenging behaviors, failing to provide adequate emotional nurturing, guidance, and recognition of his or her needs. Children with special needs are sometimes ignored, rejected, isolated, and verbally assaulted because the parent is inadequately skilled to provide for such needs.

Economic and geographical changes also influence the parent/child relationship. Voluntary or involuntary job changes (e.g., getting a better job, being laid off) introduce stress on the family, which may result in child abuse. Each family varies in its social context and support system. For instance, a higher degree of family isolation and lack of resources dramatically influences parenting values and abilities. If a family moves to another town, the parents may lose the social support system of relatives and friends which helped them care for their children. They may also have to adapt to a lower level of community resources. It is important to recognize that isolation and lack of resources will vary throughout anyone's life. Still, these ecological aspects may heighten a stress level in the family and can result in abuse.

Society also influences parental choices and actions. Does the community offer general acceptance of individual differences or does it demand conformance? Are children or adolescents terrorized into conforming when they question adult authority and beliefs? The answers to these questions will identify critical influences that the community or society may have on parenting choices. In short, the interaction of all the influencing child-parent-family-societal factors helps determine the type of parenting conducted by parents or their surrogates. (Belsky, 1991; Garbarino, Guttmann, & Seeley, 1987; Garbarino & Garbarino, 1994; Kent & Waller, 1998).

♦ IDENTIFYING PSYCHOLOGICAL ABUSE

Psychological abuse, although the core of all types of maltreatment, is very difficult to specifically identify and diagnose. With careful multidisciplinary documentation, each professional can provide a valuable part of the total picture. Many young psychological abuse victims, especially ritualistically abused victims, may initially have few overt indicators. The complete picture becomes evident as the child feels safe with more professionals. The assessment of the child's situation begins with a professional seeing some minor abnormalities and then becoming more concerned as he or she obtains additional information. Psychological abuse generally results in reduced cognitive and emotional function. Identifying reduced cognitive function is more easily accomplished than determining reduced emotional development and function. Although both impairments are usually present, it should not be assumed that cognitive ability is always reduced.

BEHAVIORAL INDICATORS
The psychologically abused child exhibits a wide range of behaviors, including apathy, crying and irritability, refusal to be calmed, and avoidance of eye contact with adults, especially parents.

NEGATIVE OR FLAT AFFECT
Emotionally maltreated infants commonly show a negative affect to anyone in the environment. They also fail to grimace or show pain when appropriate, such as not crying after a fall or an injection. They don't respond as other children would when things such as toys or food are taken away from them. In situations where a normal child would cry or seek comfort, these children have no affect, appearing indifferent.

FAILURE TO THRIVE
In extreme cases of psychological abuse, the infant can undergo the process of nonorganic failure to thrive characterized by insufficient weight gain, impaired health, slow physical growth, retarded language development, distorted social responses, irritability, an anxious attachment, apathetic solitude, and catatonia.

PASSIVITY
Abused children can appear numb to environmental stimuli. If left alone with familiar objects, they do not have normal, age-appropriate play skills and do not demonstrate normal pleasure and satisfaction from either solitary play or play with adults. They are excessively passive and obedient.

NEGATIVE SELF-IMAGE
Young children who have experienced psychological abuse demonstrate a negative view of their world and themselves. They see themselves as unworthy and view the world as a hostile place. They are fearful, angry, anxious, aggressive, and sometimes violent. They may engage in both physically and socially self-destructive behavior. They are often depressed, withdrawn, passive, and shy, exhibiting poor interpersonal communication skills. These children are often suicidal. They may frequently complain of headaches and sleep disturbances.

Children who externalize their feelings tend to be disobedient, impulsive, and overactive. They lack self-control and often are violent toward other people and their environment. Maltreated children who are aggressive exhibit a continuous and generalized aggression. The aggression is a state of being rather than a response to a specific action or individual. They behave according to impulses rather than social norms. Children who internalize their feelings are withdrawn, indifferent, submissive, and hostile.

ABNORMAL RESPONSES

Some psychologically maltreated children have low levels of social responsiveness or hesitant response patterns. They approach unfamiliar adults indiscriminately, seeking attention while avoiding physical contact with them. Other psychologically maltreated children cling to adults other than their parents and remain distant from peers. In both instances, the child's social behavior can be situationally inappropriate. In most instances, the child is unable to respond to environmental rewards, such as children asking them to join in group activities, smiles, and verbal praise. The child is often indifferent to positive feedback about his or her own success and responds negatively with social challenges or peer rejection.

Maltreated children respond negatively to parents or attempt to avoid the parent to avoid more maltreatment. The child may also try to take care of the parent's needs to reduce the instance and degree of maltreatment in the future. In the home, as in other social environments, the child may rebel and aggressively act out, or may withdraw and attempt to escape physically or emotionally.

BEHAVIOR EXTREMES

Child abuse victims characteristically exhibit behavior at the extremes of the normal spectrum. These children have no moderation in their behavior. One child can be at both extremes on the spectrum in different areas of behavior but is more likely to be consistently on one end of the spectrum in all areas of development.

CHILD AND FAMILY ASSESSMENT

The early indicators of psychological maltreatment should alert child care professionals to possible problems, prompting early intervention and treatment. It is estimated that only 5% to 7% of abuse comes to the attention of child protective services, and that more psychological abuse goes unidentified than any other form of abuse (Claussen & Crittenden, 1991; Green, 1988). Assessment tools combined with observational data from all professionals who work with a child and his or her family can give an accurate evaluation of family functioning. Most cases of psychological abuse are mild and will not enter the protective services system; instead, the family in trouble will seek assistance with their own problems. If protective services and the courts become involved, the case should include professional summaries from a variety of professionals and an assessment by a psychologist with at least three of the assessment tools listed in Table 5-10.

Although many different professionals can observe behavioral indicators of psychological abuse, assessment for state involvement either by the protective services agency or the courts commonly requires that the case records include assessment by a licensed psychologist. The multidisciplinary assessment of child maltreatment involves a psychologist who has specialized training in administering developmental tests to evaluate (1) the child's cognitive developmental level, (2) the child's personality characteristics, and (3) the quality of the parent-child interaction. The most commonly used instruments for personality assessment include the Child Abuse and Trauma Scale (CATS), the Minnesota Multiphasic Personality Inventory (MMPI), the Rorschach Test, the Thematic Apperception Test, and the Draw-a-Person Test. A variety of instruments can be used for assessing infant, child, and adolescent psychological maltreatment and parent-child interaction. There are a number of scales and inventories for professionals to use in evaluating several areas relevant to maltreatment, including the child, level of stress, and parenting knowledge. A multi-disciplinary approach is needed in the evaluation and treatment of these cases.

Table 5-10. Instruments Used to Assess Psychological Maltreatment and Child-Parent Interaction

- Guidelines for Psychosocial Evaluation of Suspected Maltreatment in Children and Adolescents (National Psychological Maltreatment Consortium & American Professional Society on the Abuse of Children [APSAC], 1995)
- CARE Index (Crittenden, 1998)
- Psychological Maltreatment Rating Scales (PMS), (Brassard, Hart, & Hardy, 1993)
- Conflict Tactics Scales (Straus, 1979)
- Record of Maltreatment Experiences (ROME) (McGee, Wolfe & Wilson, 1990)
- Bayley Scales of Infant Development (Bayley, 1969)
- Tennessee Self-Concept Scale (Fitts, 1991)
- State-Trait Anxiety Inventory (Rohner, Saavedra, & Granum, 1978; Spielberger, 1971; Spielberger, Gorsuch, & Wishene, 1970).
- Child Abuse and Trauma Checklist (Sanders & Becker-Lausen, 1995)
- Child Behavior Checklist (Achenbach, 1978; Achenbach & Edelbrock, 1979)
- Child Assessment Schedule (Hodges, 1982)

PARENTAL AND ENVIRONMENTAL INDICATORS

Most researchers and practitioners caution against overemphasis on identifying potential child abusers. Professionals, however, should be aware of parental behaviors and family dynamics that may indicate psychological abuse. Emotionally abusive parents as a group share some common characteristics (Table 5-11), although non-abusive parents can also have some of these same characteristics. If parents have some of the identified characteristics, it does not mean that they are or will become abusive parents, but it denotes the potential for abuse.

Summarized national reporting data on psychological maltreatment from the National Center on Child Abuse and Neglect indicated that parents were reported as perpetrators in 90% of reported cases (Department of Health and Human Services [DHHS], 1998). The gender distribution of reported cases indicated that females (57%) were slightly more likely to be reported than males (43%). Parents were most likely to be Caucasians (DHHS, 1998). These parents exhibited more psychosocial problems, more difficulty coping with stress, more difficulty building relationships, and more social isolation than non-abusive parents. The mothers demonstrated a lack of support networks, greater levels of perceived stress, marital discord, and alcohol and drug use (Hickox & Furnell, 1989). Although all types of abuse can occur in homes at all income levels, families with very low incomes (annual income less than $15,000) were significantly more likely to be reported for psychological maltreatment than families with higher incomes (Sedlak & Broadhurst, 1996).

Table 5-11. Characteristics Common to Psychologically Abusive Parents

- Psychologically abused as children
- Stressed
- Lack of appropriate coping skills
- Mental illness, e.g., schizophrenia, character disorder, depression
- Angry
- Hostile
- Ambivalent toward parenthood
- Few resources (financial, social)
- Inappropriate expectations of children
- Lack of knowledge of normal child development
- Marital problems
- Lack of impulse control
- Chemically abusive
- Perpetrates domestic violence and/or knowingly allows child to live in violent home

---

PARENTS MALTREATED AS CHILDREN

Not all maltreated children grow up to abuse their children. Parents who were maltreated as children, however, lacked role models of appropriate parenting and can suffer from lowered self-esteem, higher anxiety levels, and a more negative view of the world—all conditions that may have a negative impact on their child-rearing practices.

Because individuals involved in criminal activity are at higher risk to corrupt and/or terrorize their children, a parent's history of mental illness or violent criminal behavior should be considered a risk factor by protective service workers and other professionals. Repeated instances of domestic violence usually include repeated instances of child maltreatment. The confusion and general dysfunction within the home often distracts law officers from recognizing and reporting the presence of child maltreatment within the environment.

PARENT-CHILD INTERACTION PATTERNS

A recent study identified the following pattern of parent-child interaction that consistently appeared in psychological abuse cases:

1. Verbal communication between mother and child was virtually one-way, with the mother using words as commands rather than initiating or allowing dialogue.

2. The mother repeatedly gave confusing messages to the child about what was wanted; contradictions sometimes occurred within seconds.

3. The mother carried out activities for the child (for example, putting clothes on a doll) at the child's instigation. This was done without involving the child in the task, and consequently did not lead to play or the teaching of skills.

4. The child was not involved in "doing things together with baby." The situation provided numerous missed opportunities for activities likely to provide environmental benefit for the child and also facilitate interaction between the child and her younger brother (Furnell, 1986).

Psychologically abusive parents, like all maltreating parents, have a negative view of their children and their children's behavior. This negative view of their children will be obvious to professionals working with the family. Some of the characteristic responses of abusive parents to their infants are listed in Table 5-12. The negative attitudes toward infants will persist as the children grow and develop if conditions remain the same. Professionals can observe similar parent-child interaction, with children of any age. As compared to control groups of parents, the abusive parent sees the infant as purposefully acting in ways to "get even with" or "annoy" the parent. This may be due to the parent's lack of knowledge about child growth and development, as well as the parent's alexithymia and lack of trust of others. Table 5-13 summarizes parental behaviors that may indicate emotional abuse.

Table 5-12. Characteristic Responses of Abusive Parent to Infant

- Seems excessively irritated by baby's crying

- Exhibits repulsion and irritation at having to change diapers

- Describes the child in negative terms, e.g., ugly, deformed

- Does not show concern for child's needs

- Disciplines (spanks, slaps, yells at) infant under 6 months for bad behaviors

- Does not talk to the child

- Tells others of disappointments with appearance, gender of infant

- States that the infant cries or does things "on purpose to irritate or to get even with" parent(s)

- Plays very little with child

- Is very concerned about how soon infant will have control of bowels and bladder

- Calls the child derogatory names, e.g., little bastard, loser, freak

- Describes domestic violence during pregnancy

Table 5-13. Parental Behaviors That Indicate Potential for Psychological Abuse

- Seldom shows emotions; when present, emotions tend to be negative
- Routinely ignores or denies child's basic needs
- Belittles child or calls child derogatory names in public
- Consistently yells at child rather than talking in normal tone of voice
- Isolates child from normal contact with peers and community
- Routinely ignores inappropriate behavior of child
- Punishes child instead of defining appropriate behavior
- Routinely verbally assaults child in public
- Behaves violently toward family members in child's presence
- Consistently demonstrates inappropriate expectations from child
- Demonstrates a lack of basic knowledge of normal child development
- Demonstrates sadistic behavior toward child
- Threatens child with guns, knives, bondage, abandonment
- Routinely humiliates child in public or in front of peers
- Scapegoats child
- Consistently demonstrates impulsive behavior
- Routinely places own needs before child's to child's detriment
- Consistently uses bizarre or frightening forms of punishment
- Teaches child antisocial or criminal activity
- Knowingly allows child to engage in antisocial or criminal activity
- Sexualizes activities with child
- Consistently criticizes or calls child a "baby" when child behaves in age-appropriate manner
- Begins toilet training very early and harshly disciplines child for "accidents"
- Demonstrates jealous behavior toward child
- Has diminished capacity due to mental retardation, psychopathology, substance abuse
- Feels that his or her life is out of control
- Has history of violent behavior
- Lives in poverty
- Describes self as "no good"
- Lacks parental warmth toward child

♦ CONSEQUENCES OF PSYCHOLOGICAL ABUSE

Consequences of psychological abuse vary with the child's age, relationship to the abuser, and level of development of the self at the time the abuse occurs. Table 5-14 lists some of the common consequences of psychological abuse. The consequences of maltreatment are evident in differing behaviors as the child progresses through different developmental stages. When psychological abuse is combined with sexual maltreatment, the psychopathology appears to be most evident before puberty. Disturbances in body functions as a result of maltreatment are most evident in children under the age of 4 years, whereas psychoneurotic conflicts mostly manifest during adolescence. Behavior disorders and delays in development of motor skills appear at all ages. Longitudinal research has prospectively related psychologically unavailable caregivers and verbally hostile caregivers to the development of child deviance and delay (Young et al., 1991).

Ignoring and rejecting a child's basic needs appears to result in children who are destructive, impulsive, low in ego control, passive, low in impulse control, less flexible, less creative, less persistent, and who avoid their mothers. Young children who have experienced maternal rejection often exhibit symptoms by the age of three years, and have difficulty controlling aggression, respond inappropriately to distress in others, and exhibit self-isolating tendencies. Young children lack the self-esteem and trust necessary to explore the environment or attend to cognitively oriented tasks. Individuals view themselves as they believe "significant others" view them. Because parents are the most significant others of young children, rejected children view themselves as unworthy of love and inadequate as individuals. Negative self-esteem and negative self-adequacy lead children to be less tolerant of stress, less emotionally stable, emotionally insulated, more dependent (clingy, intensely possessive), more defensive, more emotionally detached, and angrier. (Downs & Miller, 1998; Erickson & Egeland, 1987; Hart & Brassard, 1989; Higgins & McCabe, 2000).

INCREASED VULNERABILITY

Threats, trauma, or deprivation in a child's life increases vulnerability to other maltreatment, exploitation, bullying, and poor interpersonal relationships. For instance, the emotionally deprived child is more vulnerable to negative experiences in day care than are children from enriched home environments. Children can overcome the experiences of physical assault or sexual abuse, provided they have been nurtured and valued by psychologically supportive parents.

EATING DISORDERS

Anorexia nervosa, bulimia, obesity, and other eating disorders in individuals at all ages are a common consequence of emotional abuse. The food behaviors of an abuse victim can include refusing to eat or holding food in the mouth but refusing to swallow, gulping food down, scavenging, stealing, and hoarding. These children are enuretic and encopretic; loose stools are common. Victims of psychological abuse commonly attach more emotional than physical significance to food.

LANGUAGE DELAY

Most maltreated children demonstrate some degree of language delay. The infants with better infant-mother attachment, however, consistently demonstrate better linguistic output and general language development.

Table 5-14. Consequences of Psychological Abuse

- Psychiatric disorders—depression, character disorder, borderline personality disorder
- Multiple personality disorder, attention deficit disorder
- Violent behavior, especially toward family members
- Self-destructive behaviors
- Antisocial and delinquent behaviors, often violent
- Increased vulnerability
- Delayed language development
- Delayed cognitive development
- Delayed motor skills development
- Decreased exploratory activity
- Relationship problems
- Low self-esteem
- Negative view of self and others
- Sleep disorders
- Eating disorders
- Nonorganic failure to thrive
- Learned helplessness

DELAYED COGNITIVE FUNCTIONING

Maltreated children are delayed in their cognitive functioning. Children who have been verbally assaulted are less persistent in exploring their environment and have increased difficulty with problem-solving and task completion. These skills are necessary for learning to occur. The abusive environment appears to encourage the development of aggressive behavior as an adaptive coping strategy. Cognitive-affective imbalance in maltreated children can cause them to interpret ambiguous stimuli as being threatening and aggressive. Maltreated children are more likely than other children to interpret behavior as aggressive and respond in a like manner. This results in difficulty when interacting with their peers. Perhaps this can explain why maltreated children have more negative expectations of interpersonal relationships.

ATTACHMENT DISORDERS

Parental threats to abandon the child or commit suicide are rejecting forms of psychological abuse and can have pathogenic effects on the child's attachment mechanism. These pathological conditions can emerge as early as the preschool years and manifest as childhood borderline disorders, attention deficit disorders, dissociative disorders, and childhood depression. Children of psychologically unavailable mothers tend to be more aggressive, less involved with peers, unpopular with peers, nervous, overactive, and lower overall in academic performance. Psychological abuse of children as a result of mothers being psychologically unavailable appears to impair both the socio-emotional and cognitive development of the children. Interaction with their mothers is frequently characterized by negativity, noncompliance, lack of affection, and a high degree of avoidance.

◆ TREATMENT AND SERVICES

Few interventions or treatment services are uniquely designed for psychological maltreatment. Most families with a variety of problems need multi-service interventions, including a combination of the following: individual, group, and family counseling; social support services; behavioral skills training to eliminate problematic behavior; and parenting education including family safety, accident prevention, and nutrition. Children from these environments may also need developmentally appropriate educational services, including speech and language therapy, motor skills development, and environmental enrichment. Children who have lived with psychological maltreatment need a careful medical evaluation to ensure that medical problems do not exist in combination with the many other problems. Because children with disabilities are overly represented among the children identified in child protective services, the treatment team must carefully observe the child.

Research is still needed to determine the effectiveness of specific interventions for all types of child maltreatment. However, treatment of psychological abuse is underrepresented in the outcome literature. As resources for intervention diminish in the public sector, more information is needed on how to most effectively use the limited resources.

◆ SUMMARY

Following psychological abuse, children experience impairment in all areas of development. The impairment can be minimized when the child has secure parental attachment, when the abuse is not combined with other forms of maltreatment, and when the abuse is mild or takes place over a short period of time. However, in all cases, some impairment occurs in all areas of development. The child's self-esteem is lowered. The child enjoys life less and either becomes withdrawn and passive or aggressive and hostile. Cognitive and language ability are also delayed. Physically, the child's growth and motor abilities may be delayed. Ritualistic or multiple-victim/multiple-perpetrator abuse leaves the most profound impairment because it is systematically planned, is continuous, and involves multiple types of maltreatment, including "brain-washing" of the child.

◆ REFERENCES

Achenbach, T. M. (1978). The child behavior profiles. I: Boys aged 6-11, <u>J Consult Clin Psychol, 46,</u> 478-488.

Achenbach, T. M., & Edelbrock, C. S. (1979). The child behavior profiles. II: Boys aged 12-16 and girls aged 6-11 and 12-16, <u>J Consult Clin Psychol, 47,</u> 223-233.

Barnett, O. W., Miller-Perrin, C. L., & Perrin, R. D. (1997). <u>Family violence across the lifespan: An introduction.</u> Thousand Oaks, CA: Sage Publications.

Bayley, N. (1969). <u>Manual for the Bayley Scales of Infant Development.</u> New York: Psychological Corporation.

Belsky, J. (1991). Psychological maltreatment: Definitional limitations and unstated assumptions. <u>Developmental and Psychopathology, 3,</u> 31-36.

Brassard, M. R., Hart, S. N., & Hardy, D. B. (1993). The psychological maltreatment rating scales. <u>Child Abuse and Neglect, 17</u>(6), 715-730.

Claussen, A. H., & Crittenden, P. M. (1991). Physical and psychological maltreatment: Relations among types of maltreatment. <u>Child Abuse and Neglect, 15</u>(1-2), 5-18.

Crittenden, P. M. (1992). Children's strategies for coping with adverse home environments: An interpretation using attachment theory. <u>Child Abuse and Neglect, 16,</u> 329-343.

Crittenden, P. M. (1998). CARE-Index: Revised coding manual. Unpublished manuscript, available from the author.

Department of Human and Health Services. (1998). <u>Study findings: Study of national incidence and prevalence of child abuse and neglect</u> (DHHS Publication No. ADM 20-01099). Washington, DC: Government Printing Office.

Downs, W. R., & Miller, B. A. (1998). Relationships between experiences of parental violence during childhood and women's psychiatric symptomatology. <u>Journal of Interpersonal Violence, 13</u>(4), 438-455.

Edmundson, S. E., & Collier, P. (1993). Child protection and emotional abuse: Definition, identification and usefulness within an educational setting. <u>Educational Psychology in Practice, 8,</u> 4.

Elkind, D. (1982). <u>The hurried child: Growing up too fast too soon.</u> Reading, MA: Addison-Wesley Publishing Co.

Erickson, M. F., & Egeland, B. (1987). A developmental view of the psychological consequences of maltreatment. <u>School Psychology Review, 16,</u> 156-168.

Fitts, W. H. (1991). <u>Tennessee Self Concept Scale, Manual.</u> Los Angeles, CA: Western Psychological Services.

Furnell, J. R. (1986). Emotional abuse of children: A psychologist's contribution to legal establishment, <u>Med Sci Law, 26</u>(3), 179-184.

Garbarino, J., & Garbarino, A. (1994). <u>Emotional maltreatment of children</u> (2nd ed.). Chicago, IL: National Committee to Prevent Child Abuse.

Garbarino, J., Guttmann, E., & Seeley, J. W. (1987). <u>The psychologically battered child: Strategies for identification, assessment, and intervention.</u> San Francisco, CA: Jossey-Bass, Inc.

Green, M. (1988). Vulnerable children, vulnerable mothers. <u>Contemporary Pediatrics,</u> 102-106.

Hart, S. N., & Brassard, M. R. (1989). <u>Developing and validating operationally defined measures of emotional maltreatment: A multimodal study of the relationships between caretaker behaviors and child characteristics across three developmental levels</u> (Grant No. DHHS 90CA1216). Washington, DC: Department of Health and Human Services and National Center on Child Abuse and Neglect.

Hickox, A., & Furnell, J. R. (1989). Psychosocial and background factors in emotional abuse of children. Child Care Health Dev, 15(4), 227-240.

Higgins, D. J., & McCabe, M. P. (2000). Relationships between different types of maltreatment during childhood and adjustment in adulthood. Child Maltreatment, 5(3), 261-272.

Hodges, K. K. (1982). The Child Assessment Schedule (CAS) diagnostic interview: A report on reliability and validity. J Am Acad Child Psychiatry, 21, 468-473.

Kent, A., & Waller, G. (1998). The impact of childhood emotional abuse: An extension of the child abuse trauma scale. Child Abuse and Neglect, 22(5), 393-399.

McGee, R. A., & Wolfe, D. A. (1991). Psychological maltreatment: Toward an operational definition. Development and Psychopathology, 3, 3-18.

McGee, R. A., Wolfe, D. A., & Wilson, S. K. (1990). A record of maltreatment experiences. Unpublished manuscript. London, Ontario: University of Western Ontario.

Miller-Perrin, C. L., & Perrin, R. D. (1999). Child maltreatment: An introduction. Thousand Oaks, CA: Sage Publications.

National Psychological Maltreatment Consortium & APSAC Task Force on Psychological Maltreatment. (1995). Guidelines for psychosocial evaluation of suspected maltreatment in children and adolescents. N. Charleston, SC: APSAC.

Newberger, C. M., & Cook, S. (1983). Parental awareness and child abuse: A cognitive-developmental analysis of urban and rural samples. Am J Orthopsychiatry, 53, 512-524.

Ney, P. G., Fung, T., & Wickett, A. R. (1993). Child neglect: The precursor to child abuse. Pre and Perinatal Psychology J, 8, 95-112.

O'Hagan, K. P. (1995). Emotional and psychological abuse: Problems of definition. Child Abuse and Neglect, 19, 449-461.

Osofsky, J. D. (1999). The impact of violence on children. Future Child, 9(3), 33-49.

Portwood, S. G. (1999). Coming to terms with a consensual definition of child maltreatment. Child Maltreatment, 4(1), 56-58.

Rohner, R. H., Saavedra, J. M., & Granum, E. O. (1978). Development and validation of the personality assessment questionnaire: Test manual. Ann Arbor, MI: ERIC Clearinghouse on Counseling and Personnel Services.

Romeo, F. F. (2000). The educator's role in reporting the emotional abuse of children. Journal of Instructional Psychology, 27(3),183-184.

Sanders, B., & Becker-Lausen, E. (1995). The measurement of psychological maltreatment: Early data on the child abuse and trauma scale. Child Abuse and Neglect, 19(3), 315-323.

Sedlak, A. J., & Broadhurst, D. D. (1996). Third National Incidence Study on Child Abuse and Neglect. Washington, DC: US Department of Health and Human Services.

Spielberger, C. D. (1971). Trait-state anxiety and motor behavior. J Motor Beh, 3, 265-279.

Spielberger, C. D., Gorsuch, R. L., & Wishene, R. E. (1970). The trait anxiety inventory. Palo Alto, CA: Consulting Psychologists Press.

Straus, M. (1979). Measuring intrafamilial conflict and violence: The conflict tactics (CT) scale. Journal of Marriage and the Family, 45, 633-644.

Wolfe, D. A. (1991). Preventing physical and emotional abuse of children. New York: The Guilford Press.

Wolfe, D. A. (1999). Child abuse: Implications for child development and psychopathology. Thousand Oaks, CA: Sage Publications.

Wright, S. A. (1994). Physical and emotional abuse and neglect of preschool children: A literature review. Australian Occupational Ther J, 41, 55-63.

Young, W. C., Sachs, R. G., Braun, B. G., & Watkins, R. T. (1991). Patients reporting ritual abuse in childhood: A clinical syndrome report of 37 cases. Child Abuse and Neglect, 15, 181-189.

Chapter 6

MUNCHAUSEN SYNDROME BY PROXY

MARCELLINA MIAN, M.D.C.M.
JENNIFER COOLBEAR, PH.D.

Munchausen syndrome by proxy (MSBP), or factitious disorder by proxy (FDP), is a very serious and potentially fatal form of child abuse (Hall, Eubanks, Meyyazhagan, Kenney, & Johnson, 2000; Meadow, 1990; Rosenberg, 1987). FDP differs from other forms of child maltreatment in that the caregiver intentionally falsifies or exaggerates a medical history, or induces symptoms in a child in order to assume the sick role indirectly and health professionals participate, albeit unwittingly, in harming the child (American Psychiatric Association, 1994; Donald & Jureidini, 1996; Zitelli, Settman, & Shannon, 1987). Medical knowledge and multidisciplinary cooperation are key to the diagnosis of FDP, which is part of a spectrum of disorders in which a pediatric condition is falsified (Ayoub & Alexander, 1998; Mian, 1995; Libow & Schreier, 1986; Southall, Plunkett, Banks, Falkov, & Samuels, 1997).

In recent years health professionals are more likely to suspect FDP, and find the complex and apparently discordant features of these cases a diagnostic challenge. The factor that alerts them that they may not be dealing with a straightforward medical condition is that the child's persistent or recurring illness does not progress or respond to treatment in the way that the condition usually does, has unusual features, and has few objective findings (Meadow, 1977; Rosenberg, 1987). Overall, the child's case is often characterized as "bizarre" and the differential diagnosis begins to include diseases that are extremely rare and certainly rarer than FDP (Rosenberg, 1987).

Because the vast majority of perpetrators are mothers, the word "mother" or the female pronoun is often used in this chapter when describing the alleged perpetrator. This does not exclude the possibility that other caregivers (e.g., grandparent, father) may engage in FDP behavior. The caregiver who raises most concern is the ever-present mother with medical knowledge who is interested in having more tests and more treatment for her child, rather than appearing concerned that her child's condition remains undiagnosed (Hall et al., 2000; Rosenberg, 1987). The passive or distant father adds to the concern (Ayoub & Alexander, 1998; Guandolo, 1985; Libow & Schreier, 1986).

Yet not all situations that fit the above features are cases of FDP, and, in many instances, making a precise diagnosis is unimportant, because any situation in which a child is presented for medical care with false information poses significant risks to the child's well-being (Ayoub & Alexander, 1998; Libow & Schreier, 1986; Meadow, 1995). Therefore, the critical factor is determining if the child is in need of protection. Central to that determination is establishing whether or not the child is being presented repeatedly for medical testing or treatment the child does not need, for a condition the child does not have or has to a lesser extent than reported, regardless of the underlying reason. Once that finding has been made, assessment of the caregiver may clarify if this is a case of FDP, or one of the other Pediatric Condition Falsification (PCF) syndromes in which other underlying causes are at play (Ayoub & Alexander, 1998).

PCF may be due to the caregiver being inexperienced or overanxious and misinterpreting or misreporting the child's condition; e.g., a mother who is convinced that her newborn's periodic breathing represents life-threatening apnea and brings the infant to medical attention repeatedly, despite reassurance that the baby is normal (Meadow, 1995). Often there is a history of significant psychosocial dysfunction in these mothers' lives (Libow & Schreier, 1986). Alternately, caregivers may disagree with the treatment plan provided by the healthcare system (Ayoub & Alexander, 1998). By presenting their child as having deteriorated under the care prescribed, they hope to change the care plan to the one of their choice, e.g., continued vomiting reported or induced in a child with reflux who is being treated conservatively, in order to force surgical correction. Some caregivers are delusional and believe the child suffers from a non-existent malady (Meadow, 1995). Other parents are so enmeshed with their children that they need them to be dependent and close, and fabricate illness in order to keep the child at home (Meadow, 1999). Abusive parents or those who do not feed their children adequately so that they fail to thrive also have reason to misrepresent the child's history to divert suspicion from the true diagnosis. Parents may also present their children for medical care in order to have access to drugs or be eligible for financial assistance or some other secondary gain (Ayoub & Alexander, 1998).

♦ PRESENTATION

Boys and girls are equally affected with PCF and have been diagnosed from one month of age up to the end of the pediatric age group (Rosenberg, 1987). Older children may actually be colluding with the caregiver/perpetrator or may have developed Munchausen syndrome or factitious disorder in their own right (Libow, 2000). The mortality rate of FDP has been cited as 9% (Rosenberg, 1987). Although this may be inaccurate, the fact that most of these deaths occur in the hospital setting is of grave concern to health professionals.

PCF can mimic a variety of medical conditions or injuries and almost all pediatric sub-specialists can be stymied by a child's clinical picture. The most frequent presenting symptoms are bleeding, seizures, apnea, vomiting, and undiagnosed persistent symptoms (Hall et al., 2000; Rosenberg, 1987). Although these symptoms may be very serious, doctors do not usually observe them in the office and must rely on history alone to formulate a management plan. Very significantly, these symptoms can all be induced, particularly in the hospital setting. In fact, greater reliance on interventionist methods in hospitalized children (e.g., central venous lines, gastrostomy tubes) facilitates the routes of access for producing symptoms of PCF as is illustrated in Figure 6-1 (Hall et al., 2000).

The perpetrator may use a variety of methods alone or in combination to harm a child and deceive medical personnel (Hall et al., 2000; Meadow, 1977; Meadow, 1999; Rosenberg, 1987). A caregiver may exaggerate or fabricate episodes of illness or falsify signs of sickness (e.g., heat a thermometer to simulate fever, or introduce blood into a sample of the child's to simulate rectal or vaginal bleeding). Alternately, a caregiver may actually choke the child, or disconnect the intravenous line to produce bleeding or to introduce foreign substances into the bloodstream. In some cases, the child may be brought to the attention of health care professionals, child protection personnel, or law enforcement for behavioral concerns or allegations of abuse rather than medical conditions, but the principles discussed here remain the same (Schreier, 1996; Schreier, 2000; Stevenson & Alexander, 1990).

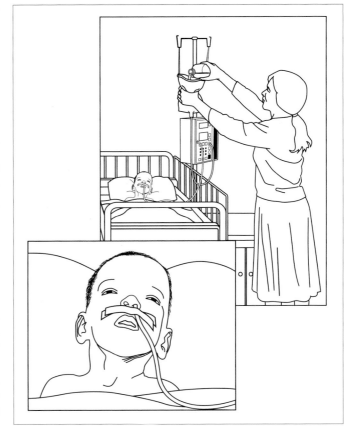

Figure 6-1. *Infant with failure to thrive. The mother is diluting the high-calorie formula being fed by nasogastric tube.*

◆ EVALUATION ISSUES

The medical evaluation and management of cases suspected of being PCF center on establishing the origin of the child's illness (i.e., whether there is an organic cause, falsification, or a combination of the two). Indeed, adding to the difficulty in the diagnosis of PCF is the fact that children may have a component of bona fide medical illness as well as elements of fabrication and deception. The following are key elements of evaluation (Mian, 1995):

1. All diagnostic considerations must take second place to the *child's safety and protection* (Rosenberg, 1987).

2. *Good communication* is key among health care providers and other professionals, including child protection and law enforcement authorities. Parents are normally considered part of the healthcare team, and health professionals often communicate with each other through them. This affords the caregiver/perpetrator involved in FDP an excellent opportunity to conduct the child's care. Therefore, in suspected FDP, only the responsible physician should communicate with the parent, relaying information pertaining to the consultants.

3. *Vigilant observation* of everything that concerns the child's condition and care allows for accurate diagnostic correlations. This observation must be strict, meticulous, and constant. All circumstances surrounding the child and his or her symptoms must be noted, such as the caregiver's arrival and

departure, and whether or not the caregiver is present when the child's symptoms occur or are reported. In cases where administration of a drug or infectious agent is a possibility, the time between administration and onset of symptoms must be calculated in order to establish the critical time during which the parent's presence would be a relevant factor. The child's health record must be carefully protected from possible interference. For example, all recordings should be written in pen and initialed to prevent alteration. A separate covert chart may need to be kept by health personnel during the time that FDP is an active concern. Otherwise, a parent may read the child's record and foil observation or diagnostic plans. All specimens must be collected under direct supervision. Unlike the usual practice of asking the parent to collect certain specimens (e.g., a urine sample), in suspected FDP all specimens must be collected by or in the presence of a health care professional. All equipment used must be identified by serial number and checked should the parent report a malfunction.

The danger in this kind of vigilance is that the health care team may begin to read significance into insignificant events and interpret even innocent comments (e.g., "I like to stay close to my baby") or events as corrupt.

4. *Judicious testing* will minimize unnecessary intervention and harm to the child. Choice of testing should be based on diagnostic necessity, low morbidity and specificity in distinguishing between the organic diagnosis in question and PCF. Testing which relies to any extent on parental observation or requires parental contribution must be avoided or undertaken with cautious consideration. Personnel carrying out these tests must be alerted to provide maximal supervision.

5. *Gathering all relevant information regarding the child's past medical history* begins with sources named by the parent, but the health insurer's files may identify previously unknown healthcare providers. The records require careful review for the limits of objectivity for each diagnosis made on the child. Diagnoses associated with supportive laboratory testing, diagnostic imaging, and pathology specimens yield a very high degree of objectivity, while those based on physical examination alone (e.g., otitis media) are less reliable. Attention must be paid to inconsistencies in the history provided by a parent to different practitioners, aspects of these accounts suggestive of fabrication, and the possible role the caregiver/perpetrator may have played in having a diagnosis made or in directing treatment. Iatrogenic symptoms need to be so identified (e.g., diarrhea due to antibiotics). Interviews of individuals who are said to have witnessed the child's symptoms may corroborate or deny the caregiver's history of symptoms. Interviewing day care personnel about one toddler's alleged seizures revealed that they had witnessed behavior that they would have identified as normal toddler hesitation between activities, had it not been for the mother's identification of these as seizures.

6. *Medical information regarding siblings and parents* may provide evidence of other instances of child maltreatment, unexplained deaths, or fabricated illness (Alexander, Smith, & Stevenson, 1990; Rosenberg, 1987; Southall et al., 1997). The maternal history may reveal elements of factitious disorder in the mother herself (Meadow, 1990; Rosenberg 1987). Members of the family may admit that the mother has always said she was sick, and that they didn't believe her.

7. *The behavior or statements of the mother or other caregiver that is suspected of harming the child* can provide some useful information, particularly in terms of demonstrable lies. However, caution must be taken in interpreting these data, since no characteristic of the abuser's behavior has been found helpful in differentiating between cases of suspected FDP that were confirmed by video surveillance and those that were not (Hall et al., 2000).

8. *Reasoned unbiased correlations* of the data gathered and an understanding of how they best fit together will assist in determining if the diagnosis is one of organic disease, PCF, or a combination of the two.

9. A *multidisciplinary approach* has the advantage of incorporating a breadth of expertise that can carefully consider FDP and other diagnostic possibilities, including rare conditions. A team can develop an initial overall management plan and revise it as needed. The team will provide objectivity, as well as support, to its members. Ideally, the team will be headed by a pediatrician (i.e., a specialist with expertise in children and FDP), and will include the responsible physician, a nurse, a specialist in the field of the organic diseases in the differential diagnosis, a psychiatrist/psychologist, an ethicist, a hospital administrator, and a member of the hospital security service (Mian, 1995).

Healthcare professionals who have been involved with the child for the longest time are likely to have difficulty in entertaining the possibility of FDP, since this implies that they have been duped and have participated in maltreating the child (Rosenberg, 1987). These difficult cases often cause dissension within a healthcare team and strategies need to be developed to cope with that (Blix & Brack, 1988; Sullivan et al., 1991; Zitelli et al., 1987).

COVERT VIDEO MONITORING

One of the important decisions to be made is whether or not video surveillance would contribute to making the correct diagnosis (i.e., differentiating between organic disease and FDP). The benefits of covert video monitoring (CVM) are shorter time from suspicion to diagnosis and protection (i.e., prevention of further episodes) and objective evidence in cases that are otherwise hard to prove (Hall et al., 2000; Southall et al., 1997). Just as importantly, CVM may demonstrate that an organic illness and not FDP is responsible for a child's symptoms (Hall et al., 2000).

Despite its benefits, CVM should not be used as a screening tool, but only as a way of confirming or denying real concerns about FDP. Institutions that admit children with complex diagnostic problems benefit from having a unit with CVM capabilities. There is published experience that can guide the establishment of such a unit (Hall et al., 2000; North Staffordshire Hospital Trust, 1996) and assist in articulating clear criteria for the implementation and use of CVM. Important considerations are the child's safety, visibility of the child and suspected action, parental expectation of privacy, and applicable laws on covert surveillance. It is essential that the video recording be simultaneously monitored so that any activity which is dangerous or harmful to the child can be interrupted. An example of a mother seen inducing a harmful condition is illustrated in Figure 6-2.

♦ REPORT TO THE AUTHORITIES

Like all other forms of child maltreatment, FDP fits into the mandated duty to report where such duty exists. The threshold for reporting is crossed when the

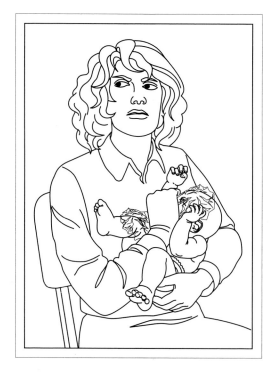

Figure 6-2. *Mother seen holding plastic wrap on her infant's face to produce apnea. She looked furtively about to make sure no one was nearby. The infant struggled forcefully until she lost consciousness.*

medical investigations indicate that the diagnosis of FDP is among the top two or three differential diagnoses. Child protection and law enforcement professionals can add valuable information from interviews with significant others, as well as gather evidence of equipment or drugs available to the suspected abuser. They can also assist in obtaining medical records from other sources.

When the family is notified about the involvement of child protection or law enforcement officials must be carefully planned. Having the authorities involved well before any intervention with the family allows them to become acquainted with the entity of FDP, familiarize themselves with the complex facts of the case, strategize on how and when their resources should be deployed, and prepare for legal intervention as necessary. Once a report is made, the authorities should become part of the multidisciplinary team to optimize case management and ensure communication and coordination of interventions.

◆ CONFRONTATION OF THE CAREGIVER/PERPETRATOR

Confrontation requires careful planning (Mian, 1995). Once there is sufficient diagnostic certainty to warrant intervention for the child's protection, the parents, including the suspected perpetrator, must be confronted with the information. It is best if the least number of professionals who can effectively discuss the facts of the case are present for this meeting. The psychiatrist must be available in case the caregiver decompensates. Child protection and law enforcement may be present from the beginning of this meeting. It is preferable to meet with the caregiver/perpetrator and the non-offending parent(s) separately. Occasionally the non-offending parent(s) can be notified early and take part in the planning strategy.

The meeting should begin by stating that its purpose is to discuss the diagnosis of FDP and the implications for the child's safety. Next, the proposed management plan should be discussed. Further action depends on the parents' response. Some offenders admit their actions, while others deny them. The non-offending parent may choose to believe his or her spouse rather than the evidence presented or may decide to protect the child. Child protection measures depend on these reactions and whether or not the police decide to charge the caregiver/perpetrator.

◆ PSYCHOPATHOLOGY OF THE CAREGIVER/PERPETRATOR

In FDP the relationship with medical practitioners is used to meet a variety of self-serving psychological needs (Ayoub & Alexander, 1998; Parnell, 1997a). It is not specified in the DSM-IV diagnostic criteria what psychological needs are met by this behavior. It has been suggested that some individuals may thrive on being perceived by a medical practitioner as the devoted parent of a sick child.

Others may have a need to manipulate or deceive authority figures or those perceived as being powerful (Ayoub & Alexander, 1998; Meadow, 1995; Schreier, 1996). It does appear, however, that FDP behavior is a complex and multifaceted problem. At any given time there may be several factors motivating a caregiver's behavior, and these motives may change over time (Parnell, 1997a; Schreier & Libow, 1993).

Several authors have observed that caregivers who engage in FDP behavior have had early relationship experiences (i.e., childhood relationships with their own caregivers) that have had a negative impact on their ability to form healthy adult relationships (Polledri, 1996; Schreier & Libow, 1993). Many caregivers who engage in this behavior have childhood histories of maltreatment, and early experiences of emotional abuse, neglect, and deprivation are not uncommon (Eminson & Postlethwaite, 1992; Fisher, 1995; Meadow, 1990; Polledri, 1996; Samuals & Southall, 1992; Schreier & Libow, 1993).

Schreier and Libow (1994) suggest that caregivers' medical help-seeking behavior through their children may originate from a need to be in a relationship with the physician(s). These relationships are potentially warm and nurturing, and it may be the first time these caregivers are valued and acknowledged by an authority figure. These relationships are an opportunity to have unmet childhood needs met as an adult (Schreier & Libow, 1994). Caregivers who engage in FDP behavior pose as the kind of parents that physicians find likable (e.g., devoted, medically knowledgeable), and the physicians become the audience for the behavior. Schreier and Libow (1994) suggest that feelings of longing for this type of relationship co-exist with feelings of anger and rage at not having these needs previously met. The relationships with physicians, therefore, are ambivalent.

Others have suggested that caregivers' early experiences of rejection and deprivation may result in a "latent murderousness" that becomes reactivated into ". . . a perversion of the maternal instinct" when the adult becomes a caregiver (Polledri, 1996, pg. 552). There may be a disturbed psychological boundary between the mother and the child whereby the mother's own somatic concerns "spill over" onto the child, a disorder of empathy, or a disturbance of parent-child attachment (Bools, 1996; Day, 1997; Rosenberg, 1987; Schreier, 1992). These caregivers may also have a history of only being nurtured in the context of disease (Rosenberg, 1987).

Personality or characterological disturbances are commonly noted by those who have worked extensively with this population (Bools, Neale, & Meadow, 1994; Parnell & Day, 1997; Schreier & Libow, 1993). Other disturbances may include coexisting factitious or somatoform illness, self-harm behavior, substance abuse, antisocial attitudes or beliefs, and eating disorders (Bools et al., 1994; Polledri, 1996; Rosenberg, 1987; Schreier & Libow, 1993). Psychosis is less common, but may be present (Ayoub & Alexander, 1998; Bools et al., 1994; Rosenberg, 1987; Schreier & Libow, 1993).

Systematic research that would provide a more complete understanding of why certain individuals engage in this type of behavior while others do not is lacking. Research is undoubtedly hindered by the fact that those who engage in MSBP behavior often deny their involvement and refuse treatment. Until recently data have not been gathered using standardized measures and protocols, and there have been no empirical studies comparing FDP samples to other clinical samples (Parnell & Day, 1997; Schreier & Libow, 1993). Therefore, many of the hypotheses about FDP behavior are based on information gathered from very small samples or individual case studies.

It is important to recognize that many individuals experience early histories of abuse, neglect, and/or emotional deprivation, but never engage in FDP behavior. There is no psychological profile or set of criteria that can definitively confirm or exclude the presence of FDP (Ayoub & Alexander, 1998; Parnell, 1997a; Rosenberg, 1987). There are likely to be many individuals who fit the FDP profile who have never engaged in FDP behavior, and those who have engaged in FDP behavior who do not fit a common profile. Normal assessment profiles for perpetrators are not uncommon (Parnell, 1997b). Thus, it is important to assess each individual case thoroughly, and to interpret information cautiously. Psychopathology or individual dynamics of the parent should not be viewed as the only causal factor to be considered. It is likely that several factors (parent, child, family, social/medical environment) contribute to the final outcome.

◆ ASSESSMENT

The purpose of a psychiatric/psychological assessment is to gather information that will be helpful in establishing the level of risk to the child and in making treatment and management recommendations for the alleged perpetrator, the child, and the family. A single interview is unlikely to be adequate to determine the factors contributing to the perpetrator's behavior and a superficial understanding of the motivations of the perpetrator may place the child at further risk (Neale et al., 1991; Rosenberg, 1987). The assessment should be completed by a mental health professional or team of professionals who have knowledge and experience in areas of adult psychopathology (e.g., personality disorders), parent-child relationships, child development, child psychopathology, and factitious disorders.

COMPONENTS OF THE ASSESSMENT

The list of topics to be covered is not meant to be exhaustive; rather, the purpose is to provide an overview of some of the issues to be addressed during the assessment. Depending on when the assessment is requested, the parent, child, and/or family may be more or less cooperative with the assessment process (e.g., after confrontation the offending parent and/or family members may be very angry or distressed). Also, the nature of the parent-child relationship (e.g., very enmeshed) may result in parental crisis (e.g., becoming suicidal) at the thought of separation from the child.

INTERVIEW WITH THE PARENT
Information about the Child

Interview(s) should be conducted with the caregiver/perpetrator to gather information about the child and to assess the caregiver's reaction and response to the child's illness. Obtaining a thorough developmental history of the child will determine whether the child is meeting developmental milestones and will provide an opportunity for the interviewer to begin assessing the caregiver-child relationship (e.g., does the caregiver empathize with the child, does the caregiver sound overwhelmed and burdened by the child).

The developmental history would include a history of the pregnancy (e.g., was the pregnancy planned, caregiver's physical/emotional health during the pregnancy, medical complications during the pregnancy); the child's early development (e.g., developmental milestones, physical growth, temperament); the child's current social, emotional, behavioral, and cognitive functioning; the child's history of maltreatment (e.g., physical, sexual, emotional abuse; neglect); the child's exposure to domestic violence; significant separations from caregivers; and the quality of the caregiver-child relationship (e.g., caregiver's attitude toward child, parenting style, appropriateness of expectations).

Information about the Caregiver

The purpose of this part of the interview is to develop an understanding of the caregiver's early experiences of being cared for and his or her experiences of significant relationships. This part of the interview involves a shift from the focus on the child to the parent and therefore may be more threatening for the parent.

Information about the caregiver's own developmental history is gathered. This includes the family constellation and quality of relationships in the caregiver's family of origin, style of parenting the caregiver was exposed to, history of maltreatment (e.g., physical, emotional, sexual abuse; neglect) or exposure to domestic violence, and significant separations from caregivers or significant losses (e.g., death of a parent). It is also important to determine how illness was dealt with when the caregiver was a child. Information should also be gathered about the caregiver's academic and employment history, psychiatric illnesses, mental health problems (e.g., substance abuse, self-harm/attention seeking behavior), and relationship history (e.g., length, stability, quality of relationships).

Assessment of the caregiver's current functioning includes gathering information about social, emotional, and cognitive functioning, quality of the relationship with his or her current partner, quality of relationships with extended family, recent stressors in the family (e.g., job loss, death in the family), and community supports. A psychological test battery, including standardized instruments assessing a variety of domains (e.g., personality, cognitive), may be used to augment the information gathered from direct interviews with the parent.

INTERVIEW WITH THE CHILD

In some cases the child will be old enough to be interviewed as part of the assessment process. If the child is too young to be interviewed, information can be gathered by speaking with individuals who interact with the child and by direct observation of the child in a variety of settings (e.g., interacting with the parent, other family members, and medical personnel). Depending on when in the process the child is interviewed, he or she may or may not be living with or seeing the caregiver. These significant disruptions must be considered when gathering and evaluating information from the child.

Interviewing a child can provide useful information about how he or she perceives the current situation and thoughts and beliefs about self, caregiver(s), and family. It also provides an opportunity to assess whether the child has colluded with the parent to any extent and whether the child is ready or willing to discuss the role the parent has played in the illness. On direct questioning, children have revealed the source of their illness (Mian, 1995; Waller, 1983). A woman who suffered from MSBP as a child at the hands of her mother reported she would have disclosed this abuse as an adolescent had she been asked the cause of her illness (Bryk, personal communication, October 16,

2000; Bryk & Siegel, 1997). However, these children do not come forward voluntarily with the information. Children can provide information about family constellation and quality of relationships within the family (e.g., parents, siblings, grandparents, etc.), academic and social functioning, experience of being "ill," perceptions of their parents' response to "illness," and family beliefs about illness.

Depending on the nature of the concerns, formal intellectual, psychological, and developmental assessments of the child using standardized protocols may be helpful.

PARENT-CHILD OBSERVATIONS

These observations should be conducted by mental health professionals who have considerable experience conducting parent-child observations. Caregiver-child interactions in these cases can appear quite appropriate. Experience in observing the subtle nuances of parent-child interactions may result in a very different evaluation of the quality of the parent-child relationship.

Structured observations as well as observations of the parent-child dyad engaging in day-to-day activities (e.g., mealtime, bedtime, bathing, diaper changes) can provide a wealth of information. Things to consider while observing parent-child interactions are the ability of the parent to read the child's cues, the caregiver's sensitivity to the child's needs, whether or not the caregiver's expectations are developmentally appropriate, and caregiver and child response to separations (e.g., when the child must go for a medical procedure or test). Although the assessor should make every effort to observe these interactions directly, nursing notes can be very useful.

COLLATERAL INFORMATION

It is important to gather information about the child, parent, and family from other professionals who have been involved with them. This may include obtaining the child's academic/daycare records, documentation of past and/or current involvement with a child protection agency, documentation from other mental health agencies/professionals involved with the parent, child, and family (e.g., therapist, child counselor), documentation from other community agencies, and the caregiver's education and employment. Family members (e.g., spouse, siblings, grandparents) may provide useful information about the broader context within which the FDP behavior has occurred.

◆ LONG-TERM PLANNING

CHILD PROTECTION

In most cases protection involves removal of the child(ren) from the home to ensure safety (Rosenberg, 1987; Southall et al., 1997). Plans to keep the child in the home must be made with great care and involve exclusion of the possibility that the perpetrator will provide any physical care to the child. Court-ordered foster placement or supervision may be difficult to obtain, however, if the evidence of FDP is not clear or if the legal professionals do not have a good understanding of the entity. This is especially true if the perpetrator presents well and denies any culpability. There are many difficulties associated with the management of FDP cases. There are often delays and differing opinions when making the diagnosis, which in turn delays the onset of intervention. Also, many cases require long-term intervention but many professionals do not have the mandate to stay involved for several years (Kelly & Loader, 1997). The lack of stability of these families makes it difficult to maintain consistency of the professionals involved (Neale, Bools, & Meadow, 1991).

MEDICAL CARE
Arrangements must be made for the child's medical care to be provided by one physician so that real illnesses can be treated as needed.

MENTAL HEALTH TREATMENT
PERPETRATOR
Very little is known about long-term treatment efficacy with individuals who engage in FDP behavior. Few perpetrators willingly participate in counseling, and those who do often do so to fulfill requirements imposed by the courts and/or child protection services. Much of what is known is based on a small number of cases where perpetrators have acknowledged their behavior and willingly engaged in therapy. These cases are described as being very difficult to manage, and they are often associated with poor outcome because these individuals have personality characteristics that are highly resistant to therapeutic change (Parnell & Day, 1997; Schreier & Libow, 1993; Schreier & Libow, 1994). The denial, deception, and manipulation inherent in their pathology make these individuals poor candidates for treatment (Parnell & Day, 1997; Polledri, 1996; Schreier & Libow, 1993). Successful treatment outcome also depends on the skill and experience of the therapist, as these perpetrators can be very manipulative and often evoke intense emotional reactions in those working with them (Fisher, 1995; Kelly & Loader, 1997; Neale et al., 1991; Parnell & Day, 1997; Polledri, 1996; Schreier & Libow, 1993; Schreier & Libow, 1994). Goals of treatment include the following:

- preventing further abusive behavior toward the child victim (or other children)

- the parent acknowledging and accepting responsibility for the MSBP behavior, and demonstrating that they are motivated to make necessary changes in their lives

- the parent demonstrating an ability to genuinely empathize with the child's experience, acknowledge the physical and psychological harm done to the child, and be supportive of the child victim

- the parent displaying an ability to place the child's needs before his or her own needs

- the parent demonstrating insight into the dynamics (e.g., individual, marital, familial) that contributed to the behavior

- helping the parent develop healthier strategies (i.e., other than seeking medical attention) for eliciting support and having needs met, and helping the parent develop a support network (e.g., from friends, family)

- the parent demonstrating an ability to form healthy relationships in place of previously dysfunctional ones

CHILD
Intervention with the child victim varies greatly depending on several factors, including the child's age and developmental level, the length and severity of the

abusive behavior, and the nature and extent of family dysfunction and child psychopathology. Knowledge of normative child development (e.g., cognitive, behavioral, socioemotional), child psychopathology, and experience working with high-risk and maltreated children will be imperative.

Issues that may need to be addressed include the following:

1. Trust. These children, like children who have been subjected to other forms of maltreatment at the hands of their caregivers, may have difficulty establishing a trusting relationship with another adult.

2. Disruptions in the parent-child attachment relationship. Lack of sensitive and responsive care, especially at times when the child is ill, frightened, or hurt, is likely to result in an insecure attachment.

3. Children may have developed distorted perceptions of themselves. For example, they may have developed beliefs about being ill that have impaired their development and have prevented them from engaging in age-appropriate activities.

4. Maladaptive beliefs. Children may develop the maladaptive belief that their needs are only met through illness and may develop their own somatic symptoms and illness behavior (Day & Ojeda-Castro, 1997; Kelly & Loader, 1997).

◆ CASE EXAMPLES
DEFINITE FDP

This baby was admitted at age 4.5 months weighing 4.5 kg. His birth weight was 4.17 kg. The history was that he had had difficulty breast feeding and had been cup and finger fed. Mother reported intermittent vomiting and 2 to 3 loose green stools per day. He was then given nasogastric feedings with an elemental formula; despite being given 170 kcal/kg/day he failed to gain weight. Physical examination revealed no abnormalities other than being thin. In the hospital, his mother was always in attendance and gave him all his feedings. A complete work-up for organic causes of failure-to-thrive proved negative, except for one high calorimetry reading. He was initially given nasogastric (NG) feedings at 200 kcal/kg/day but failed to gain weight. The blanket on his bed was frequently wet. The baby then began to lose weight to 4.22 kg, and the suspicion of FDP arose. He was moved to a 4-bed observation unit and total parenteral nutrition was started. Ten days later his weight was 4.74 kg. At this time Child Protective Services was alerted. He was placed back on NG feedings and moved into a room with CVM capability. Within 24 hours, the mother was seen emptying the formula bag and refilling it with water. Electrolyte analysis confirmed dilution of the formula in the infusion bag. The mother was confronted and admitted to diluting the formula, but said she did not know why she had done it. She was charged and incarcerated. The child was made a ward of the state and placed in the care of his father and maternal grandmother. He was discharged 2 weeks later, after normal oral feedings, weighing 5.28 kg.

PCF OR FDP

This 21-month-old boy was admitted with a history of recurrent seizures and apnea since age 14 days, according to his mother. He had been admitted numerous times for observation and had had several complete medical work-ups. He had never been observed to have any spells of any kind, and his tests were all normal. Concerns arose of possible FDP. More thorough history taking from this single mother revealed that she had had an abusive childhood, had had the baby when she was 16, and had few social supports. She said the baby had started to say words at 6 months but would lose and then reacquire some language after his spells. She described many challenging behaviors in the child, including temper tantrums and feeding and sleeping difficulties, and she lacked insight into what precipitated them. Nurses had noted her inability to comfort the boy when he was upset. She had not established any routines for the child's care. In the hospital she was observed trying to rouse him when the nurse had settled him to sleep, possibly in an effort to precipitate one of the "spells." No other production of illness was observed. There was some evidence of fabrication or exaggeration in that the mother reported she had been told to have the boy's ears checked daily because he had had 17 ear infections. These were not documented. Child Protective Services was involved. It was explained to the mother that the child did not appear to have any underlying medical illness and that repeated investigations and hospitalizations were detrimental to the boy's development and emotional well-being. The plan was to discharge the child to the mother with medical care being provided by a single source, while the mother availed herself of parenting courses. Child Protective Services would remain involved to monitor the situation.

♦ REFERENCES

Alexander, R., Smith, W., & Stevenson, R. (1990). Serial Munchausen by proxy. Pediatrics, 86, 581-585.

American Psychiatric Association (1994). Diagnostic and statistical manual of mental disorders (4th ed.). Washington, DC: Author.

Ayoub, C. C., & Alexander, R. (1998). Definitional issues in Munchausen by proxy. The APSAC Advisor, 5, 7-10.

Blix, S., & Brack, G. (1988). The effects of a suspected Munchausen's syndrome by proxy on a pediatric nursing staff. General Hospital Psychiatry, 10, 402-409.

Bools, C. N. (1996). Factitious illness by proxy. Munchausen syndrome by proxy. Br J Psychiatry, 169(3), 268-275.

Bools, C. N., Neale, B. A., & Meadow, S. R. (1994). Munchausen syndrome by proxy: A study of psychopathology. Child Abuse and Neglect, 18, 773-788.

Bryk, M., & Siegel, P. T. (1997). My mother caused my illness: The story of a survivor of Munchausen syndrome by proxy. Pediatrics, 100, 1-7.

Day, D. O. (1997). The middle therapeutic stage. In T. F. Parnell and D. O. Day (Eds.), Munchausen by proxy syndrome (pp. 183-192). Thousand Oaks, CA: Sage.

Day, D. O., & Ojeda-Castro, M. D. (1997). Therapy with family members. In T. F. Parnell and D. O. Day (Eds.), Munchausen by proxy syndrome (pp. 202-215). Thousand Oaks, CA: Sage.

Donald, T., & Jureidini, J. (1996). Munchausen syndrome by proxy: Child abuse in the medical system. Arch Pediatr Adolesc Med, 150, 753-758.

Eminson, D. M., & Postlethwaite, R. J. (1992). Factitious illness: Recognition and management. Archives of Disease in Childhood, 67, 1510-1516.

Fisher, G. C. (1995). The role of psychiatry. In A. L. Levin and M. S. Sheridan (Eds.), <u>Munchausen syndrome by proxy: Issues in diagnosis and treatment</u> (pp. 369-397). New York: Lexington.

Guandolo, V. L. (1985). Munchausen syndrome by proxy: An outpatient challenge. <u>Pediatrics, 75,</u> 526-530.

Hall, D. E., Eubanks, L., Meyyazhagan, L. S., Kenney, R. D., & Johnson, S. C. (2000). Evaluation of covert video surveillance in the diagnosis of Munchausen syndrome by proxy: Lessons from 41 cases. <u>Pediatrics, 105,</u> 1305-1312.

Kelly, C., & Loader, P. (1997). Factitious disorder by proxy: The role of child mental health professionals. <u>Child Psychology & Psychiatry Review, 2,</u> 116-124.

Libow, J. (2000). Child and adolescent illness falsification. <u>Pediatrics, 105,</u> 336-342.

Libow, J. A., & Schreier, H. A. (1986). Three forms of factitious illness in children: When is it Munchausen syndrome by proxy? <u>American Journal of Orthopsychiatry, 56</u>(4), 602-611.

Meadow, R. (1977). Munchausen syndrome by proxy: The hinterland of child abuse. <u>Lancet, 2,</u> 343-345.

Meadow, R. (1990). Suffocation, recurrent apnea, and sudden infant death. <u>Journal of Pediatrics, 117,</u> 351-357.

Meadow, R. (1995). What is and what is not Munchausen syndrome by proxy? <u>Arch Dis Child, 72,</u> 534-538.

Meadow, R. (1999). Mothering to death. <u>Arch Dis Child, 80,</u> 359-362.

Mian, M. (1995). A multidisciplinary approach. In A. L. Levin and M. S. Sheridan (Eds.), <u>Munchausen syndrome by proxy: Issues in diagnosis and treatment</u> (pp. 271-286). New York: Lexington.

Neale, B., Bools, C., & Meadow, R. (1991). Problems in the assessment and management of Munchausen syndrome by proxy abuse. <u>Children & Society, 5,</u> 324-333.

North Staffordshire Hospital Trust, Staffordshire Social Services, Staffordshire Police (1996). Guidelines for the multi-agency management of patients suspected or at risk of suffering from life-threatening abuse resulting in cyanotic apnoeic episodes. <u>J Med Ethics, 22,</u> 16-21.

Parnell, T. F. (1997a). Defining Munchausen by proxy syndrome. In T. F. Parnell and D. O. Day (Eds.), <u>Munchausen by proxy syndrome</u> (pp. 9-46). Thousand Oaks, CA: Sage.

Parnell, T. F. (1997b). Guidelines for identifying cases. In T. F. Parnell and D. O. Day (Eds.), <u>Munchausen by proxy syndrome</u> (pp. 47-67). Thousand Oaks, CA: Sage.

Parnell, T.F., & Day, D.O. (Eds.). (1998). <u>Munchausen by proxy syndrome.</u> Thousand Oaks, CA: Sage.

Polledri, P. (1996). Munchausen syndrome by proxy and perversion of the maternal instinct. <u>The Journal of Forensic Psychiatry, 7,</u> 551-562.

Rosenberg, D. (1987). Web of deceit. <u>Child Abuse and Neglect, 11,</u> 547-563.

Samuals, M. P., & Southall, D. P. (1992). Munchausen syndrome by proxy. <u>British Journal of Hospital Medicine, 47,</u> 759-762.

Schreier, H. A. (1992). The perversion of mothering: Munchausen syndrome by proxy. <u>Bulletin of the Menninger Clinic, 56,</u> 421-437.

Schreier, H. A. (1996). Repeated false allegations of sexual abuse presenting to sheriffs: When is it Munchausen by proxy? <u>Child Abuse and Neglect, 20,</u> 985-991.

Schreier, H. A. (2000). Factitious disorder by proxy in which the presenting problem is behavioral or psychiatric. <u>Journal of the American Academy of Child and Adolescent Psychiatry, 39,</u> 543-544.

Schreier, H. A., & Libow, J. A. (1993). <u>Hurting for love: Munchausen by proxy syndrome.</u> New York: Guilford.

Schreier, H. A., & Libow, J. A. (1994). Munchausen by proxy syndrome: A modern pediatric challenge. <u>Journal of Pediatrics, 125,</u> 110-115.

Southall, D. P., Plunkett, M. C. B., Banks, M. W., Falkov, A. F., & Samuels, M. P. (1997). Covert video recordings of life-threatening child abuse: Lessons for child protection. <u>Pediatrics, 100,</u> 735-760.

Stevenson, R. D., & Alexander, R. (1990). Munchausen syndrome by proxy presenting as a developmental disability. <u>Developmental and Behavioral Pediatrics, 11,</u> 262-264.

Sullivan, C. A., Francis, G. L., Bain, M. W., et al. (1991). Munchausen syndrome by proxy: 1990. A portent for problems? <u>Clinical Pediatrics, 30</u>(2), 112-116.

Waller, D. A. (1983). Obstacles to the treatment of Munchausen by proxy syndrome. <u>Journal of the American Academy of Child and Adolescent Psychiatry, 22,</u> 80-85.

Zitelli, B. J., Settman, M. F., & Shannon, R. M. (1987). Munchausen syndrome by proxy and its professional participants. <u>Am J Dis Child, 141,</u> 1099-1102.

Chapter 7

VIOLENCE AMONG CHILDREN

JAMES J. WILLIAMS, M.D.

"Guns are common as water around here," a 15-year-old boy said. As a student at a school where a shooting had occurred, he had not shot at anybody nor did he carry a gun to school, but felt that he may have to. "I don't want to shoot anybody," he said, "but I have to protect myself and they had better not bully me or my friends" (Interview by the author).

Deeply disturbing as they are, these stories of school violence unfortunately have little shock value for us today. Violence impacts a child's development in many complex ways, but that tends to be ignored in our society, which treats troubled youth with a demonizing and punitive approach. We find in these stories a common readiness to use violence as a means to achieve an end in an interpersonal conflict. Many young people feel trapped by the violence around them. Violence harms all in its path, including victims, perpetrators, and witnesses. Instead of fearing for our children, we are becoming fearful of them. A relatively self-sustained victimiza-

tion develops in all who are touched by violence. Throughout our lives, the manner in which we are treated influences the manner in which we consider others. The Golden Rule, or like version, transcends all cultural and religious traditions and is enshrined in our hearts: "Do unto others as you would have them do unto you." Stories of violence may produce a perverse reformulation: "Treat others as you fear they would treat you," in which victim is difficult to distinguish from victimizer.

Violence springs from the human quality which makes us most ourselves—our ability to associate with and relate to one another. Poor or damaging relationships are at once the source and outcome of interpersonal violence, resulting in a repetitive cycle of victim and victimizer. Violence emerges when stressors overwhelm the ability to cope. The youthful perpetrator may feel isolated, particularly from adults who might provide support during a crisis, while there is often peer support for violence. In many

situations, violence may seem to be the only available option. We have learned that this circuit may be interrupted, particularly when the child has meaningful relationships with significant, caring adults. Parents who give unconditional love and attention are the most important factors in providing a child with a secure and violence-free life. Conversely, the loss or absence of such a relationship is a significant source of a child's pain and suffering. Physical or emotional pain, repeatedly inflicted and unmoderated, is a very powerful and direct source of human violence. Nearly all other risk factors for generating violence stem from this primary defect.

◆ MODELS OF VIOLENCE

There are a few models to study the emergence and scope of violence. One, the cycle of violence hypothesis, maintains that the experience of violence perpetuates its expression and transmission to succeeding generations (Spatz-Widom, 1989). Such expressions may range from condoning violent discipline or developing hostile thought patterns to delinquency, violent crime perpetration, or premature death. This hypothesis appeals to the intuitive sense that "what goes around, comes around." The cycle of violence hypothesis cannot predict which individuals will become violent. It has been useful in alerting us to the fact that violence, though transmitted through the generations of families as a learned behavior, is by no means inevitable. Violence may be interrupted in its transmission by certain protective or resiliency factors.

In the public health model, the many forms of violence are seen as amenable to a systematic, science-based analysis. Healthcare providers have a major role to play in its detection and treatment. Exposure to violence is common for large segments of our population, especially the young. It has become so pervasive that we cannot view it solely as a criminal justice problem, involving a few maladjusted individuals who need to be incarcerated or placed into a "program." Instead, many different professional disciplines deal with violence in the structured framework of victim, offender, and weapon. Violence and its causes have a natural history that may be at least partially studied with the tools of surveillance, epidemiology, intervention, and reevaluation. Control is sought in terms of interventions that change victim susceptibility, change offender characteristics, eliminate or reduce weapons, and modify the environment, especially drugs. Three levels of prevention or intervention strategy are proposed for each factor: primary, secondary, and tertiary (Table 7-1). Primary prevention aims to make general interventions before violence occurs; secondary prevention aims to reduce the level of violence once it has been detected and decrease its threat to others; tertiary prevention aims to reduce the harm caused by existing violence or ensure rehabilitation after it has already happened.

◆ SCOPE OF THE PROBLEM

Violence in American society has gained the nation's attention and concern. Substantial economic and social burdens are brought on society as a result of violence (Miller, Fisher, & Cohen, 2001). Large numbers of our young people are being exposed to it from abusive parents in the home, neighborhoods with high crime rates and severe poverty, violent or abusive peers at school, and the mass media that glorifies violent behavior. The levels of violence today are far above what one would expect. They have increased rapidly within all youth age groups. Inner-city neighborhoods throughout the nation have been experiencing violence of epidemic proportions for the past two decades, and violence has spread itself toward the suburbs in the past decade. Why are so many young people acting violently today? Is an even greater outbreak in the offing as our children become adults? What can be done about a problem that seems to be so intractable and complex? There are no simple answers.

CHILDREN WHO DIE BY HOMICIDE/SUICIDE

The toll of child and youth deaths is seen in the daily media. The combined U.S. homicide and suicide rate for youth (under age 20 years) is about 15 people per day. This exceeds the rates of the next 25 industrialized nations by a factor of 16 and is nearly double the U.S. rate of a decade ago (Centers for

Table 7-1. Examples of Violence Prevention Strategies in a Public Health Model

	Primary (directed to general population before violence occurs)	Secondary (directed to populations at risk or with early signs of violence)	Tertiary (directed to populations already affected by violence)
Perpetrator (change characteristics)	• Parent training • Reduce or eliminate corporal punishment • Improve educational & health care opportunities • Violence prevention & awareness education, conflict resolution • Violence anticipatory guidance • Enhance child resilience factors • Promote academic achievement	• Home visitation programs for at-risk families • Intervention to improve educational, health, social services for at-risk children • Reduce or eliminate corporal punishment • Violence prevention & awareness education, conflict resolution • Mentors/early intervention relationships for at-risk children • Job training for at-risk youth • Mentor parents/family skills training • Promote academic achievement • Gang resistance • School/community interventions	• Intervention with bullies • Imprisonment, diversion program, probation • Educational/emotional rehabilitation • Alternative school
Firearms, Other Weapons (reduce)	• Selective ban on firearms	• Firearm reduction • Develop gun safety awareness • Metal detectors at certain schools	• Trace firearms used in crimes through a national registration center
Victim (change susceptibility)	• Parent training • Reduce or eliminate corporal punishment • Improve educational & health care opportunities • Violence prevention & awareness education, conflict resolution • Violence anticipatory guidance	• Home visitation programs for at-risk families • Intervention to improve educational, health, social services for at-risk children • Reduce or eliminate corporal punishment • Home visitation services • Medical services	• Mental health services • Foster care

(Dwyer, Osher, & Wagner, 1998; Hawkins et al., 1998; National Center for Injury Prevention and Control [NCIPC], 2000)

Table 7-1. Examples of Violence Prevention Strategies in a Public Health Model—*Continued*

	Primary	Secondary	Tertiary
	(directed to general population before violence occurs)	(directed to populations at risk or with early signs of violence)	(directed to populations already affected by violence)
Victim (change susceptibility) *continued*	• Enhance child resilience factors • Promote academic achievement	• Violence prevention & awareness education conflict resolution • Mentors/early intervention relationship for at-risk children • Job training for at-risk youth • Mentor parents/family skills training • Promote academic achievement • Gang resistance training • School/community interventions • Intervention with bullies	
Physical & Social Environment (home, neighborhood, school)	• Reduce neighborhood crime, poverty, unemployment • Reduce media violence	• Safe homes/shelters • Increased police presence • Metal detectors at certain schools	• Alter high-crime neighborhoods

Note: primary, secondary, and tertiary interventions vary according to the developmental level of the victim or offender.

Disease Control and Prevention [CDC], 1997a). Gun-related deaths at the hands of male strangers or acquaintances account for nearly all of the increase. Nearly 3,600 children and youth were murdered and 2,100 committed suicide in 1997. Firearms were responsible 67% of the time (NCIPC, 2000; Ward, 1999). Homicide and suicide are respectively the second and third leading causes of death in adolescents. Over twenty percent of high school students seriously contemplated suicide in 1997: 16% made a specific plan, 8% attempted suicide, and 2.6% required medical attention (CDC, 1997b). Homicide is the leading cause of death for African-American youth. It is the fourth leading cause of death for children less than five years old, who are more often killed by a family member in the context of physical abuse (Table 7-2). Adolescent homicides, on the other hand, are usually committed by males of approximately the same age through the impulsive use of guns.

CRIMES COMMITTED AGAINST CHILDREN

Large numbers of our young are involved in violent altercations, in which they

Table 7-2. Juvenile Homicide Victims by Age Group

Weapon	Age of Victim (in years)			Total
	0 - 5	6 - 11	12 - 17	0 - 17
Firearm	10%	42%	75%	51%
Knife/blunt trauma	11%	19%	15%	14%
Personal (hands, feet, etc.)	48%	11%	3%	19%
Other	30%	28%	7%	16%

Between 1980 and 1997, 3 of 4 murdered juveniles age 12 or older were killed by a firearm. Nearly half of the children below age 6 were killed by perpetrators using hands, fists, or feet (Office of Juvenile Justice and Delinquency Prevention [OJJDP], 1999).

are substantially more likely than adults to be injured. Though constituting only 10% of the U.S. population, children under 18 years of age are victims in 25% of the total serious and violent crimes (aggravated assault, robbery, sexual assault). This is two to three times greater than the adult rate (Finkelhor, 2000). Moreover, only the most violent victimizations are likely to be reported to the police; there was about a 50% report rate in 1996. Overall, adolescents are more likely to die of gunshot wounds than of any of all the natural diseases combined (CDC, 1994). Assault-related physical injuries, especially permanent injuries to the brain and spinal cord, have kept pace with the rising youth homicide rate. Ten percent of high school students reported they had been injured by a weapon while on school property in the preceding year (CDC, 1997b). In 1995, children under 17 years of age had 517,000 hospital emergency department visits for assault-related injuries and accounted for nearly half of the 64,000 nonfatal firearm-related injuries (CDC, 1999; Stussman, 1997).

About 20% of adult females and 5-10% of adult males recall being sexually abused as children (Finkelhor, 1994). A majority of reported sexual assaults are of children under 18 years of age, who are victims in 70% of forcible and 95% of non-forcible cases (Crimes Against Children Research Center [CCRC], 1998). Self-report data indicate that one in two sexual assault victims is under 18 years of age, while one in three is under 12 years of age (Kilpatrick, Edmunds, & Seymour, 1992).

CHILDREN WHO ARE ABUSED OR NEGLECTED

In 1998 more than three million children were reported to child protective services agencies for suspected child abuse or neglect; one-third of the cases were substantiated. This is a 160% increase since 1980. About 1,100 children died due to maltreatment in 1998, of which 42% died due to neglect and 54% died due to physical abuse. In 24% to 45% of the deaths, the families were already known to child protective services because of a current or past problem (Weise

& Daro, 1994). Parents were perpetrators 87% of the time (US Department of Health and Human Services [USDHHS], 2000).

CHILDREN WHO WITNESS FAMILY OR COMMUNITY VIOLENCE

Approximately 3 to 10 million children per year witness the abuse of their mothers; such children suffer from both short- and long-term adjustment problems, including post-traumatic stress, increased anxiety, poor school performance, increased aggression, impaired self-esteem, and withdrawn behavior (Jaffe, Wolfe, & Wilson, 1990). Boys who witness family violence are at increased risk of abusing their own partners as adults (Straus & Gelles,1990). Nearly half the men who abuse their female partners also abuse their children (Walker, 1989). In reports of abused children to protective service agencies, 11% to 45% of the mothers are themselves victims of violence (Children's Defense Fund [CDF], 2000).

CHILDREN AND YOUTH WHO COMMIT CRIMES

Juveniles aged 14 to 17 years have been involved as perpetrators in 25% of the serious violent crimes annually over the past 25 years; the rates rose steeply from 1983 to 1993 as the numbers of offenders in each age group increased substantially and proportionately. The numbers have since dropped by 40%, but the arrest and incarceration rates remain at unprecedented levels. Homicides by juveniles doubled in this period: murdered strangers or acquaintances accounted for nearly all of the increases. By 1997, more than 1,700 juveniles were implicated in 1,400 homicides: 56% of the victims were acquaintances, 34% were strangers, and 9% were family members. Serious and violent juvenile offenders are also disproportionately victims of violence themselves, having multiple problems at home, at school, and with drug and alcohol abuse (Loeber & Farrington, 1999).

CHILDREN WHO ARE AFFECTED BY DRUGS/ALCOHOL

More than 500,000 infants are born each year drug-exposed and many more are alcohol-exposed. They are compromised by their mothers' behaviors and are at risk for poor development and maltreatment. The largest proportion of child abuse reports occur among mothers who abuse drugs or alcohol (Famularo, Kinscherff, & Fenton, 1995). Children's protective services estimate that 40% to 80% of their family caseloads are in this category (CDF, 2000).

CHILDREN IN A CULTURE OF VIOLENCE

Corporal punishment is the most common form of violent behavior inflicted on U.S. children today and is a deeply embedded element in our culture. A large majority of American parents, as much as 90%, physically punish their children or agree that it is sometimes justifiable, though not necessarily at a high frequency or intensity. In studies using the Conflict Tactics Scales (CTS), Straus argues that there is a correlation between the common behavior of corporal punishment and the behavior involved in criminal assaults and homicides, though it is seldom perceived as such by the public (Straus, 1994; Straus, 1996). Corporal punishment has harmful consequences for the individual and society, and is also a risk factor for the more severe attacks of physical abuse (Straus, 2000). It is a form of violent socialization that gives contradictory messages to children. Corporal punishment teaches the child to suppress empathy, and may paradoxically enhance the value of what is being punished, thus, introducing the undesirable behavior as an option to the desired action (McCord, 1996).

Bullying, or peer abuse, is another type of violence and intimidation perpetrated against children. In one survey, 8% to 10% of students in middle and high school experience bullying (National Center for Educational Statistics, [NCES], 1998). When asked about the causes of youth violence, they invariably list violence in the home and bullying at school (Horn, 2000). Adults must understand that the shame inflicted by bullying is, in itself, a cause of violence among youth.

Media violence is another source of violent ideas for children. The media and some video games and toys reflect and create societal norms that contribute to the promotion of violence. Men and women tend to be stereotyped in media programming: women are often depicted as young, passive, and physically desirable, while men are relatively more powerful and violent. Children's television programming rarely shows the realistic and logical consequences of violence. Children begin to show a definite modeling of televised behavior as early as age 15 months. They may show temporary increases in violent attitudes and aggressiveness immediately after viewing violent media content. Young viewers are more likely to adopt the attitude that violence is a justifiable means to settle disputes, especially when portrayed by heroes and authority figures (Strassburger, 1995). The amount of violence viewed in grade school is directly related to aggressive behavior by age 18 years.

Children face serious short- and long-term physical and emotional consequences as victims, witnesses, and perpetrators of violence in contemporary culture (Prothrow-Stith, 1991). While the immediate consequences on victims may involve physical or psychological trauma, the residual effects—emotional and developmental scars—often emerge as problem behaviors in adolescence and adulthood. Violence is an issue that crosses all geographic and socioeconomic boundaries.

◆ Risk and Resiliency Factors in Violence

Although past behavior is the best predictor of future conduct, there are no reliable profiles of risk factors to predict which children are likely to become tomorrow's violent youth. It is a dangerous oversimplification to make a list of attributes shared by a few troubled youths and try to apply it to all in a predictive manner.

The public health model uses certain risk factors for preventive intervention, in a primary (i.e., universal), secondary, or tertiary manner. The various factors operate differently at various developmental periods throughout life and may be divided into individual/behavioral, family, peer, and environmental (school and community) categories (Table 7-3). Not all juveniles exposed to multiple risk factors become delinquents or school dropouts. Important aspects of their lives may protect them against increased risk. Some prevention programs aim to enhance these characteristics, such as having a "resilient" temperament, a positive social orientation, and positive relationships with caring adults, families, schools, and churches.

A recent statement on youth violence by the American Academy of Pediatrics (1999) suggests many ways in which healthcare providers and communities can respond to violence. These include a call for greater advocacy, collaboration with the CDC and other agencies in research on the effectiveness of prevention strategies, supervised educational programs, interventions in current clinical practice, screening, treatment, and referrals.

Table 7-3. Factors in the Development of Abnormally Aggressive Behaviors

Individual Factors That Increase Behavioral Risk

- Male gender

- Attention-deficit hyperactivity disorder

- Below-average IQ

Interpersonal Relationship Factors That Increase Behavioral Risk

- Child abuse and/or neglect

- Inconsistent parenting/discipline

- Severe corporal punishment

- Antisocial behavior in friends

Environmental Factors That Increase Behavioral Risk

- Family violence and discord

- Parental psychopathology

- Parental drug and/or alcohol addiction

- Stressful home life

- Violence in the school or neighborhood

- Poverty

- Large family size

Protective Factors That Reduce Behavioral Risk

- Secure attachment relationship with parent(s)

- Presence of caring and supportive adults outside the family during stressful periods

- Commitment to schooling

- Bonded to prosocial peers

- Sense of community ownership

(Dwyer, Osher, & Wagner, 1998; Hawkins et al., 1998; NCIPC, 2000)

INDIVIDUAL/BEHAVIORAL FACTORS

Violence is a learned disorder. Individual attitudes result from a child's early experiences and development, which are rooted in interactions with parents, family members, teachers, and peers. The origins of violence can primarily be attributed to exposure to conflict-filled relationships and to deficiencies in social problem-solving and other interpersonal skills.

Individual attitude and temperament can influence a child's risk for being injured. When the world is seen as a dangerous place, the normal vulnerability, immaturity, and impulsivity of children may lead to conflict, injury, and death, especially where access to guns, drugs, and alcohol is relatively easy. Children are becoming afraid of each other. Thus, students who have been victimized by violence and who fear attending school are at greater risk of using alcohol and carrying a gun at school (DuRant, Kahn, Beckford, & Woods, 1997). Weapon-carrying is common among high schoolers and is a strong indicator of the youth's tendency and willingness to condone and engage in physical violence. This may further enhance his or her perceptions of vulnerability (Lowry et al., 1998). In one study 20% of 12,000 high school students said that they had carried a weapon on school property in the previous month; 7.6% had carried a gun (CDC, 1997b). Surveys indicate that as many as 50% of juveniles can acquire a handgun if so desired, often within 24 hours (LH Research, 1993). When students who carried a weapon to school were asked why, they gave two main reasons: self-protection and enhancement of social identity, e.g., to impress other students. Even when protection was not a real issue in a particular school, students said they "heard" from other students that they needed to take care of themselves. Individual attitudes toward violence are also strongly influenced by a past history of antisocial behavior. Subsequent delinquent behaviors, such as vandalism, theft, and selling illegal drugs are highly correlated with violent injury (Resnick et al., 1997).

Other problem behaviors, such as alcohol and drug abuse (ADA), increase the risk for interpersonal violent injury. The catalysts for ADA among teens are complex and many. ADA is found at all demographic levels and is more likely in persons who have been developmentally scarred by abuse or exposure to violence (Ireland & Widom, 1994). In one study, one-third of 12,000 high school students reported current (i.e., within the past 30 days) episodic heavy use of alcohol; one-third reported they were offered, sold, or given an illegal drug on school property in the past year; one-quarter reported current marijuana use; 3.3% reported current cocaine use (CDC, 1997b). ADA correlates not only with increased accidental injuries (e.g., motor vehicle crashes), but is also linked to a youth's intentions to use or condone violence (DuRant et al., 1996).

Psychobiological theory postulates that antisocial behavior is a result of post-traumatic stress. Violent behavior results in traumatic neurophysiological changes (Bremner & Narayan, 1998). Abused children show activation of impaired central nervous system stress responses, which may be reactivated when they later experience stress. It is proposed that abuse, neglect, and exposure to family violence set up conditioning effects on nervous system pathways in young children that later influence aggressive and violent behavior (Perry, 1997). This theory suggests that bioneurochemical and emotional linkages may exist between exposure to violence and current substance abuse.

FAMILY FACTORS

The family is the first influential "environmental" factor in a young person's life. Family violence is perhaps the most extreme form of destructive conflict witnessed and experienced by children. The family has been referred to as "the main training ground for violence." Parent factors, such as poor affective bonding, are believed to be at the core of child maltreatment and antisocial behavior. Attachment theory says that social and psychological development is strongly influenced by the quality of parental care. The securely attached child is able to recall empathetic figures to help label and regulate emotional states, especially in times of stress. The maltreated child, on the other hand, is at risk for an insecurely attached relationship, in which the parent is remembered as unresponsive and rejecting. As an adult, such a child may have great difficulty in trying to form secure relationships with his or her children (Buchanan, 1996).

Social learning theory says that modeling and reinforcement play important roles in the development of aggressive behaviors. We learn behaviors by observing others directly in real life (Bandura, 1994). Family violence and poor discipline strongly promote and reinforce child antisocial behavior. Erratic and inconsistent discipline are generally found in homes of children with aggressive behavior problems. Such children have learned to use aversive behavior to manipulate the family environment. Many behave so because of neglecting or rejecting parents, who provoke the child to be demanding and aggressive. They tolerate the child's aggression and fail to set limits. They neglect to notice or reward the child's cooperative behavior. When the child's negative behavior becomes too great for them, they may withdraw from the child or resort to excessive force to beat him or her into submission. Typically by the time they punish, the child's negative behaviors have been under way for some time. In response to punishment, the child may then escalate his aggressiveness to maximum intensity; in reaction, the parents may stop their opposition. In effect, the child learns that his or her behavior will compel attention and possibly capitulation. This further compounds the child's deficits in communication and social skills. If such a home environment is also marked by family violence, even greater conflict may occur when the child attempts to be aggressive in the outside world of school and peers.

Relationships between violent parents emphasize the use of power, threat, coercion, and humiliation. Because accepting the violence is perceived as temporary compliance with the abuser's wishes, it is likely that most children have observed abusive behavior being reinforced. Children who are not directly abused themselves but who witness violence, internalize norms in which violence is acceptable and may be stimulated to aggression against others (Patterson, DeBaryshe, & Ramsey, 1989; Patterson, Reid, & Dishion, 1992). The level of corporal punishment in these homes is also high. In one study, eight times as many women reported using corporal punishment on their children while living with their batterer than those who lived alone or with a nonbattering partner (Harrell, 1993).

PEER AND SCHOOL FACTORS

By mid-adolescence, most children who will manifest serious antisocial behavior have already begun to do so and may be more resistant to change. The problems may come from a background of family violence and/or child abuse, but serious antisocial behaviors at this stage are more influenced by factors outside the family. Relations with peers, school, and neighborhood enhance deficiencies that are already present in the child's social problem-solving and cognitive skills. Many of these children feel that violence leaves them with limited choices and consider it normal to use physical force to obtain what they desire. Their style may be viewed negatively by peers, which eventually leads to their isolation and rejection (Dodge & Coie, 1987; Olweus, 1993). Rejected children are more likely to escalate aggression when they perceive negative feedback from peers, and they are less likely to learn from "prosocial" peers (those who behave constructively with each other).

Antisocial behavior that begins in adolescence is often preceded by earlier academic failure and association with delinquent peers. School bonding is an important prosocial factor at this stage. School is one of the most significant sources of norms and behavior models to which children are exposed. Its learning climate and teaching practices are related to the child's academic success and behavior in the community. Practices that promote social development create many opportunities for success, provide recognition for children, and aid in protecting against associating with antisocial peers.

NEIGHBORHOOD AND COMMUNITY FACTORS

Poverty is *a level of resources that is so inadequate as to prevent participation in expected community activities.* Poverty increases the stressors that impede effective parenting and interfere with normal child development. It results in disempowered families that live with reduced economic and educational opportunities, absent fathers, inadequate or absent health care, poor nutrition, violent neighborhoods, and a limited life potential. From birth, children living in low-income families are at much greater risk of premature death, child abuse and neglect, non-intentional trauma, homicide, and untreated illness. Poverty is a creation of our culture, in which many people still believe that no one needs to be poor as long as one "plays by the rules." Strong traditions in our culture equate the presence of poverty with personal failure and moral inferiority. These attitudes further impede parents struggling with limited resources.

ENVIRONMENTAL FACTORS

Ecological theory emphasizes that child development is influenced by the quality of parental care, which is influenced by the family's social and economic contexts within the neighborhood or community (Bronfenbrenner, 1979). Environmental factors that increase the risk for violence are past or current exposure to violence and community norms that condone violent behavior (Song, Singer, & Anglin, 1998). Child and environment constantly influence each other in ways that lead over time to developmental and behavioral outcomes that are difficult to predict.

Prior victimization due to family or community violence is strongly associated with future perpetration. Witnessing violence has similar effects (Song et al., 1998). Psychopathology theory maintains that child abuse and family violence originate in individual dysfunctional personality structures that are learned and shaped by early childhood experiences. Witnessing family or community violence or being abused undermines a child's ability to trust and regulate emotional states. This results in hostile and insecure persons who have little or no ability to develop healthy relationships.

◆ WHAT WE CAN DO ABOUT VIOLENCE

SCREENING AND EDUCATION BY HEALTHCARE PROVIDERS

Healthcare providers have an important role to play in screening for and educating about violence (AAP, 1999). Providers face many barriers in identifying, treating, and referring victims of violence, not the least of which are their own attitudes. Providers who are aware of the risk factors involved and community resources available will be in a much better position to be useful to their patients.

Screening to predict who might become violent is highly sensitive but nonspecific. Screening during the well-child exam is most meaningful when applied to the following points:

- Exposure to family violence and child abuse

- Exposure to violence in neighborhood, school, and media

- Drug abuse or alcoholism

- Family stressors, e.g., poverty, unemployment

- Child care and the family's social network

- Disciplinary attitudes of the parents

- School bonding, academic performance

- Access to firearms in the home or community

- Association with antisocial peers, youth gangs, fighting

Many relevant healthcare issues coincide with areas where children are at risk. An outline of anticipatory guidance would cover these points:

- Infancy: Inquire about family care and social supports; educate the parent(s) on appropriate skills and disciplinary strategies (after careful inquiry about their views); teach that corporal punishment is less effective than other strategies.

- Preschool years: Encourage parents to spend time with the child, read to the child, teach positive social skills, monitor the child's television viewing, learn what behaviors are age-appropriate, and model nonviolent behavior and conflict resolution; encourage parents to use strategies, such as natural consequences for specific behaviors, and consistency in reacting to a child who knowingly misbehaves; encourage parents to reward the child when he or she behaves appropriately; give advice, when needed, on how to manage assertive and aggressive behaviors in the child.

- School age: Encourage parents to model nonviolent anger management and conflict resolution, encourage development of empathy skills in the child, give the child more responsibilities, continue nonviolent discipline, clearly articulate family rules.

- Adolescence: Encourage the parents to lead the teen toward greater independence, educate the teen on his or her responsibilities, and maintain involvement with their child; address potential areas of conflict, such as driving, curfews, school performance, and substance abuse; encourage the teen to discuss appropriate dating and relationships, and how to avoid and resolve peer and school conflicts.

GUN CONTROL

Firearm-related injuries and fatalities are the most visible and tragic outcomes of the violence experienced by young people. Approximately 200 million guns are privately owned in the U.S. (Kleck & Patterson, 1993). The proliferation and ease of obtaining firearms has contributed greatly to the increased morbidity and mortality associated with this epidemic. The increased numbers of homicides of and by juveniles are nearly completely accounted for by the increases in firearm-related homicides. Youths carry firearms much more commonly than in the past, and the ill effects of violent acts are greatly enhanced when a firearm is involved. Gun control is a controversial topic in American culture. Opponents of gun control argue that guns are needed to provide protection against home intruders, but this has not found support in clinical studies (Kellerman et al., 1993). At a minimum, healthcare providers should focus on gun safety and the risks of gun ownership. Children should not have access to guns; gun ownership should require licensure, similar to a driver's license; persons with past records of violence should not be allowed to own or use a gun; the most lethal types of guns should be banned; and the availability of all guns should be reduced (Adler et al., 1994). If guns were not so available, the extent of killings could be reduced, but reducing the supply of available weapons is by no means an easy task to accomplish and requires a great deal of community mobilization.

ANTI-BULLYING PROGRAMS

Children are exposed in school to numerous instances of assaultive or intimidating behaviors, especially low level harassment and physical abuse from peers. Bullying often has an impact beyond its immediate target, in which even peers who merely witness the abuse also become anxious and distressed. School-based programs for violent and aggressive children teach self-awareness of the level of physiological arousal, teach self-control strategies to cope with anger, and provide teacher training for effective recognition and response to bullying (Johnson Institute, 1996).

FAMILY VIOLENCE PREVENTION

Increased recognition of and willingness to ask about possible family violence by healthcare providers is a necessary first step toward helping families and victims. Increased access to services for victims and perpetrators of family violence and their children should be given high priority. School-based prevention programs for family violence have focused both on teen dating violence and family violence among parents. Topics addressed include exploration of gender roles, personal safety, the law, and social norms that tolerate violence (Institute of Medicine, 1998). Home visitation services and interventions with children have shown some promise but more research is needed. Practice guidelines for healthcare providers include recommendations to screen all women for the possibility of family violence (American Medical Association [AMA], 1992a; AAP, 1998).

COMPONENTS OF VIOLENCE PREVENTION PROGRAMS

Although no single strategy can be relied on in each and every community, interventions should meet certain minimum criteria that are founded on the public health model:

- Comprehensive, community-based, and early in the developmental course of at-risk individuals.

- Science-based public health approaches that target known risk factors and use epidemiological data analyses to identify patterns or risk and protective factors.

- Continuing surveillance to establish and monitor intervention effectiveness and trends in risk factors.

- Integrated delivery of services. They should include, where appropriate, health care, the schools, protective services agencies, and the juvenile justice system.

What sorts of interventions might make sense? There are well-designed programs that show promise. Violence is a learned behavior. So is nonviolence. Studies suggest that many of the social conditions and developmental processes that produce violence can be changed. Careful research has documented a number of components, listed below, that may be added to comprehensive approaches.

Parent Management Training (PMT) is family-focused and teaches parents to identify their child's positive and negative behaviors, communicate clear and consistent expectations, provide appropriate consequences, and reduce reliance on corporal punishment (Smith & Thornberry, 1995). Evaluations of PMT demonstrate substantial and sustained changes, especially when it is a component of a multi-factor program, e.g., Project Head Start or the Seattle Social Development Project (Hawkins et al., 1992; Miller, 1994; Webster-Stratton & Hammond, 1997). Multisystemic Therapy (MST) techniques have also been combined with PMT and successfully applied to reduce abusive parenting (Brunk, Henggeler, & Whelan, 1987).

Functional Family Therapy (FFT) is family-focused and aims to improve communications through a variety of behavioral and cognitive techniques to alter the emotional and blaming elements in family interactions. With 29 years of data and clinical experience, FFT is a well-documented, empirically-grounded program; it has been widely adopted and is commonly used in dealing with antisocial teens and their families. Interventions may be for as much as 30 hours of direct service, provided over a three-month period. Studies have indicated that FFT can reduce arrest recidivism and is cost-effective (Barton et al., 1998).

Social Competence Training (SCT) is a child-focused classroom intervention in which teachers aim to increase children's conversational skills, academic performance, problem solving, and ability to take perspective. SCT has been incorporated into Promoting Alternative THinking Strategies (PATHS) curriculum and the Positive Adolescents Choices Training (PACT) Program with positive results.

Classroom Contingency Training (CCT) is child-focused and aims to adapt successful PMT techniques to elementary and middle school teachers' needs for behavioral management skills in dealing with low-achieving students (Hawkins, Doueck, & Lishner, 1988). CCT has been a component of multi-factor programs, e.g., the Seattle Social Development Project.

Academic skills support is child-focused and aims to improve poor school achievement, which places children at risk for school failure and subsequent antisocial behavior (American Psychological Association [APA], 1993). Academic support has long been part of well-designed programs, such as Fast Track, Success for All, and the Seattle Social Development Project (Conduct Problems Prevention Research Group, 1992; Slavin et al., 1990).

Peer mediation is a child-focused curriculum for elementary through high school students that aims to train young people in "active listening" to defuse potential confrontational situations. It may operate in tandem with conflict resolution education to increase the child's knowledge about the causes and consequences of violence and to improve self-control. Peer mediation and conflict resolution are often components of comprehensive school or community programs.

Family preservation is an intervention offered by child protective service agencies. It consists of an array of time-limited services to families whose children are at risk for abuse, neglect, or out-of-home placement. Such families often have a number of related social problems, such as unemployment, drug and alcohol abuse, poverty, and family violence, that limit their ability to deal with crises. Workers usually have small caseloads and may visit the families several times a week. Depending on the need, services may include counseling, respite care, intensive in-home assistance by parent aides, PMT, budget management, assertiveness training, and help accessing other social and healthcare programs. Family preservation requires careful monitoring. Maintaining a child at home, though cost-effective, is not always of value in light of the potential for further abuse or violence (US Government Accounting Office, [USGAO], 1995).

EXAMPLES OF WELL-DESIGNED PROGRAMS
PRENATAL AND INFANCY
The most pervasive and intractable problems faced by children in our society interfere with parent-child attachment and result from dysfunctional parenting, poverty, and stressful environmental conditions. Any early intervention that attempts to change child function, such as health, nutrition, and cognitive development, or attempts to change family function, such as parent-child interactions, family employment, or access to supports, should be viewed as a violence prevention program.

Home Visiting Programs for families with infants and toddlers. Family functioning is often linked to community circumstances. Successful home visiting programs look at the ways the family's economic and social circumstances affect parenting and development, and attempt to link the family to community services. Home visiting programs are a key element for health and social service agencies' efforts at child abuse prevention for infants. The programs have a special quality that is not found in other programs, particularly the relationship building between home visitor and family. Visitors aim to deliver health education to the mother, reduce her health risk behaviors (e.g., smoking, drinking, drug abuse), and thereby reduce the rate of low birth weight deliveries. Additionally, they may cover how to structure the home environment and relate to the child. Home visiting has been found to be a necessary, though not sufficient, means to improve family functioning. Examples of effective home visiting are the Prenatal/Early Infancy Project in Elmira, NY; Parents as Teachers program; Maternal and Infant Health Outreach Worker Project; and the Yale Child Welfare Project (Clinton, 1992; Olds, Henderson, Chamberlin, & Tatelbaum, 1986; Pfannenstiel & Seltzer, 1985; Seitz, Rosenbaum, & Apfel, 1985). Home visiting has been successfully combined with other services, e.g., the Perry Preschool Project and Project CARE (Berreuta-Clement et al., 1984; Wasik et al., 1990). Home visitation infancy program sites number in the thousands.

In a review, the beneficial effects of the programs were found to be greater for families that had greater risks (Olds & Kitzman,1993). In comparison with control groups, the visited families at follow-up had a lower incidence of serious child abuse, less physician visits for injuries and ingestions, and fewer subsequent pregnancies, with longer intervals between them. Among children of low-income women, there was a lower level of antisocial behaviors at the 15-

year follow-up. These programs focus on individual change and are not broad policy solutions. The programs need to be part of more comprehensive efforts on entrenched problems, such as poverty, neighborhood crime, and violence.

THE PRESCHOOL YEARS

At this developmental stage, programs address risk and protective factors in the family and preschool. They aim to provide support for parenting skills and children's verbal ability, as well as to alleviate both family and community poverty. In practice, several components are combined to address multiple risk factors.

Early childhood education programs are usually center-based and provide a range of emotional and educational supports. They emphasize children's language and social development and promise long-term benefits. *Family support programs,* on the other hand, are parent-focused, home-centered efforts in which home visits are used to aid the family in obtaining needed social services, provide various supports, and encourage the parents to pursue their own educational or occupational goals. At some sites, family support is combined with early childhood education to address multiple risk factors. A variety of approaches may be incorporated by the home visitor, including child care, literacy development (e.g., Reach Out and Read), PMT, parent-child interaction training, and Project Head Start (High et al., 2000). Positive effects have been demonstrated in juvenile delinquency prevention in selected programs more than 5 years after the services (Yoshikawa, 1994). The effects on cognitive ability and parenting preceded the long-term reductions of antisocial behavior. Examples of effective combined programs include the Perry Preschool Project, the Syracuse University Family Research Development Program, the Yale Child Welfare Project, and the Parent-Child Development Centers.

Parent-child interaction training was an intervention for low-income parents who had noted that their preschool child exhibited a behavioral or emotional problem. The parents were taught parenting skills, behavioral management, and constructive play (Strayhorn & Wiedman, 1991). At one-year follow-up, the program children improved significantly more than controls.

ELEMENTARY THROUGH MIDDLE SCHOOL

Violence prevention shifts from the home to the classroom at this stage. Elementary school programs are usually at the level of primary or universal application. The early elementary school years are a developmentally favorable period to curb aggressive behaviors and ensure that children experience early academic success. Successful prevention programs included components such as PMT, promotion of school bonding and academic achievement, CCT and behavioral management, SCT, mentoring, anti-violence curricula, and community service assignments.

Anti-violence curricula and community service. In one study, eighth graders participated in classroom exercises coupled with community service in a local health agency. The program had a positive impact on antisocial behavior of children at high risk for being perpetrators and victims of peer violence (O'Donnell, Struve, & Sandoval, 1999).

Mentoring programs are child-focused interventions which pair paid employees or volunteers with at-risk children over prolonged periods of time; examples are

Big Brothers/Big Sisters of America, Friends of the Children, and Foster Grandparents. These programs take adults who desire to be involved and inject them into children's lives. They also have the potential to enhance empathy for children living in low-income families and achieve greater levels of child advocacy among the general public.

ADOLESCENCE

Family influences still play a role in adolescence, though unfortunately most programs concentrate more on factors that are outside the home. These approaches attempt to alter the course of trends that are already apparent by addressing multiple risk and protection factors simultaneously. Peers are of increasing developmental importance at this stage, and most programs either target peers for change (e.g., prevent the teen from joining with antisocial peers) or target peers as vehicles of change (e.g., peers as mediators).

Positive Adolescents Choices Training (PACT) is an example of a violence prevention curriculum that promotes anti-violence values, conflict resolution, and peer mediation (Yung & Hammond, 1998). It and similar programs have demonstrated decreases in aggressive behavior (Brewer, et al., 1995). PACT's curriculum is specifically aimed at African-American youth and is based largely on SCT. In comparison to control students, PACT students had better impulse control at one-year follow-up.

Positive Action Through Holistic Education (PATHE) was a comprehensive, school-based, 3-year intervention for middle and high school students from low-income families who had behavioral and academic problems. The program aimed to improve student attachment to school, self-esteem, and the learning environment. The intervention included vocational and behavioral counseling, tutoring, peer counseling, a student leadership system, and teacher training in classroom behavioral techniques. Involved families were given support in communication skills about academic and discipline problems. Evaluation revealed declines in self-reported delinquency and drug involvement in the program schools; increases were noted in the control schools (Gottfredson, 1986; Gottfredson, 1990).

Prevent association with antisocial peers. Past efforts in this area have not produced encouraging results (Brewer et al., 1995). *Skills and Mastery Resistance Training (SMART)* is a child-focused, center-based series of multi-factorial programs sponsored by the Boys and Girls Clubs of America and located in housing projects across the country. The programs appear to have positive effects on reducing local drug abuse and trafficking.

Multisystemic Therapy (MST) is an intensive intervention that deals with chronic, violent, or drug-abusing adolescent offenders who are at risk for out-of-home placement (Henggeler, 1997). MST bases its approach on the principle that individuals are simultaneously involved in and affected by mutual systems, including family, peers, neighborhood, and schools. MST therapists are full-time, carry small caseloads (four to six families), and are available all day every day (typically about 60 hours of face-to-face contact over a 4-month period). After an evaluation, interventions are provided across a range of factors known to be related to delinquency within the settings of the adolescent's home, school, and neighborhood. Clients are typically males between 12 and

17 years of age who live in single parent homes that are characterized by multiple needs and problems. They generally have a history of multiple arrests, associate with delinquent peers, have school behavior and academic problems, and abuse drugs or alcohol. Interventions aim to improve parent disciplinary practices, enhance effective relations in the family, improve school performance, engage the youth in prosocial recreational activities, and develop a supportive network of extended family, neighbors, and friends. Family members are treated as collaborators in the treatment planning and delivery with goals primarily driven by the parents. MST is also useful in treating abusive parents (Kazdin, Siegel, & Bass, 1992). MST has its own internal quality control and holds its therapists accountable for the effectiveness of their work. MST has been evaluated in several randomized trials and has shown sustained ability to reduce out-of-home placement, repeat arrests, and psychiatric hospitalization (Bordin et al., 1995). It is also found to be cost-effective.

Prevent gang violence. Juvenile gang members contribute disproportionately to the total volume of criminal violence. A program's efficacy in this area is enhanced by having multiple components, including prevention, social intervention, treatment, police suppression of gun usage and drug dealing, and community mobilization. These are integrated into a cooperative and coordinated approach. Examples of successful programs are ***Chicago's Gang Violence Prevention Program*** and the anti-gang program in Boston (Spergel & Grossman, 1997; US Department of Justice [USDOJ], 1996).

EXAMPLES OF COMMUNITY-WIDE VIOLENCE PREVENTION PROGRAMS

Violence prevention should be linked to components of early intervention and graduated sanctions in a comprehensive community strategy. The OJJDP Comprehensive Strategy for Serious, Violent, and Chronic Offenders; the Weed and Seed Program of the Bureau of Justice Assistance; and the Fighting Back Initiatives of the Robert Wood Johnson Foundation all emphasize community involvement in planning comprehensive strategies to prevent antisocial behavior. ***Communities That Care (CTC)*** is a comprehensive system for planning and implementing risk prevention at the community level. CTC has shown positive results in reducing risk factors in long-term follow-up (Abner et al., 1996; Gottfredson, Gottfredson, & Hybl, 1993; Harachi et al., 1995). Later comprehensive programs, such as SafeFutures, link research findings with state-of-the-art approaches toward preventing juvenile violence (Morley, Rossman, Kopczynski, Buck, & Gouvis, 2000).

Earlier studies identified the need for comprehensive, long-term community-level research to describe the development of antisocial behavior and violence. ***The Project on Human Development in Chicago Neighborhoods,*** sponsored and funded by the MacArthur Foundation and the National Institute of Justice, is attempting to achieve this end (Earls, 1997). Unprecedented in its scope, the Project is a randomized, longitudinal, prospective study that traces Chicago residents from 1994 to 2003 by age cohort from birth through 26 years of age. The whole social and political ecology of 80 Chicago neighborhoods and the personal characteristics of 7,000 randomly selected children, adolescents, and young adults are followed to identify factors that may lead them toward or away from a variety of antisocial behaviors. The impact of exposure to violence and child care on early child development is part of the study.

A preliminary finding of the Project is that "collective efficacy" is a significant ecological predictor of violent crime. Collective efficacy is defined as the level of community trust and common values in which adults are willing to intervene in the lives of others' children to maintain order (Sampson, Raudenbusch, & Earls, 1997). The Project recorded drops in crime in as little as 2 to 3 years when neighbors work together to police their community and supervise and discipline their children. Neighborhoods (in all socioeconomic levels) with a strong sense of collective efficacy had lower rates of violence. Collective efficacy does not downplay the need for external mechanisms of support (e.g., public transportation, housing, nutrition, police suppression of drug dealing, etc.). It emphasizes informal mechanisms by which residents themselves are willing to achieve public order as a dimension of the public life of neighborhoods. Collective efficacy has an impact over and above the traditional risk factors of violence, such as racial injustice, poverty, and residential instability (Hawkins et al., 1998). Collective efficacy is supported elsewhere, for instance, in the finding that the numbers of professional people who live in the community is critical. When their levels declined below a threshold of 5%, indicators of community health, such as the rates for school drop-outs and teen pregnancy, worsened. Community structure was no longer able to exert influence over individual behavior (Bennett, 1994).

◆ CONCLUSIONS

There are no simple answers to the problem of youth violence. Violent behavior arises in a complex context of multiple problems that are chronic and pervasive. Work on multiple fronts is the only hope of changing deeply embedded individual and community behavioral patterns. Evaluations of existing violence prevention programs have shown that comprehensive approaches can have a powerful overall effect. In the infant home visitation program, for example, comprehensiveness might be defined as services for parent and child plus access to or provision of other basic services (e.g., health and child care). Existing visitation programs should not be characterized as one-time inoculations to protect for all time against poor developmental outcome and violence. These programs have shown us how the family is affected in its child-rearing role by context and circumstances, which are complex and interrelated. Major conceptual shifts will be necessary if we are to effectively reduce the national levels of violence. Comprehensive solutions are required that force rethinking of the ways that services are organized and delivered. A public health framework will help guide us in formulating and evaluating programs, but reliance on public health alone will not be sufficient to deal with our problems. Beneath the current violence in America is a long tradition of unacknowledged violence that must be addressed: the genocide of the native American population; the institution of slavery and widespread racism; the serious maldistribution of income; and the increasing militarization of U.S. economy and policy, which sustains the nation's disproportionate consumption of the world's resources (Terris, 1998). "Treatment" of the nation's structural violence will require major political and social shifts (Gil, 1996).

At the beginning of the 20th century, reformers debated whether poverty was the result of an individual's failure. Our culture still proclaims a universal individualism and self-sufficiency that says that if one gets into trouble, it is due to his or her own moral failing. How do we institute comprehensive prevention systems in this culture when reform strategies still center on efforts to change and rescue individuals? We live in environments where toxicity may be societal or structural. At the start of a new century, we are fundamentally challenged to move beyond changing individuals to changing communities and systems. The effective prevention of violence does not depend on the development of any one program. Rather, promising interventions need a more generalized process of community involvement and mobilization within which we move beyond the piecemeal addition of services to systems of community support to reach and help families. To do this across a whole community requires more than just another program. No matter how comprehensive, no one program will have all the resources to strengthen and support families.

ENDNOTES

This chapter uses the following definitions:

Interpersonal violence is intentionally threatened or inflicted force by one person that leads to, or has a high likelihood of leading to, physical or psychological injury or death of another person.

Victimization is the harm done by interpersonal violence, specifically with regard to issues of malevolence, betrayal, injustice, and morality (Finkelhor, 1997).

The *cost of a death* due to a single 22-cent, 9-millimeter bullet has been documented as follows: juvenile hall and jail costs for 1 year for 4 suspects: $85,710; a 2-week trial: $61,000; crime scene investigation: $13,438; medical treatment: $4,950; autopsy: $2,804; state incarceration costs if the four suspects are convicted and serve 20 years: $1,796,625 — total: $1,964,527. Extrapolated costs in terms of lives cut short and loved ones' grief, lost potential and productivity, and resulting damage to the nation's psyche and society are inestimable, but nonetheless real (Arnette & Walsleben, 1998).

Bullying or *peer abuse* is defined as intentional harm inflicted by other children repeatedly and over time within an interpersonal relationship which is characterized by an imbalance of power.

Child abuse is inflicted or threatened interpersonal violence by nonaccidental means. *Child neglect* is harm by an omission of care.

The CTS measures the extent of specific physical assaults and other tactics used in dealing with the conflict separately from presumed causes or effects of maltreatment, regardless of whether the child was injured. The Scale has been useful, for example, in uncovering many more cases of severe physical assault than were previously officially known by child protective workers (Straus & Gelles, 1990).

♦ REFERENCES

Abner, J. L., Brown, J. L., Chaudry, N., et al. (1996). The evaluation of the Resolving Conflict Creatively Program: An overview. Am J Prev Med, 12, 82-90.

Adler, K. P., Barondess, J. A., Cohen, J. J., et al. (1994). Firearm violence and public health: Limiting the availability of guns. JAMA, 271, 1281-1283.

AAP, Committee on Child Abuse and Neglect. (1998). The role of the pediatrician in recognizing and intervening on behalf of abused women. Pediatrics, 101(6), 1091-1092.

AAP, Task Force on Violence. (1999). The role of the pediatrician in youth violence prevention in clinical practice and at the community level. Pediatrics, 103(1), 173-181.

AMA. (1992a). Diagnostic and treatment guidelines on domestic violence. Chicago: AMA.

AMA, Council on Scientific Affairs. (1992b). Violence against women: Relevance for medical practitioners. JAMA, 267, 3184-3189.

APA, Commission on Violence and Youth. (1993). Violence and youth: Psychology's response. Washington, DC: APA.

Arnette, J. L., & Walsleben, M. C. (1998). Combating fear and restoring safety in schools. OJJDP Bulletin, NCJ 267888. Washington, DC: US Department of Justice.

Bandura, A. (1994). Social cognitive theory of mass communication. In J. Bryant and D. Zillman (Eds.), Medical effects: Advances in theory and research (pp. 61-90). Hillsdale, NJ: Lawrence Erlbaum.

Barton, A. J., Gordon, D., Grotpeter, J., et al. (1998). Blueprints for violence prevention, book three: Functional family therapy. Boulder, CO: Center for the Study and Prevention of Violence.

Bennett, A. (1994, December 7). Economists demonstrate that neighbors, not wardens, hold keys to cutting crime. The Wall Street Journal, p. B1.

Berreuta-Clement, J. R., Schweinhart, L. J., Barnett, W. S., et al. (1984). Changed lives: The effects of the Perry Preschool Program on youths through age 19. Monographs of the High/Scope Educational Research Foundation, no. 8. Ypsilanti, MI: High/Scope Press.

Bordin, C. M., Mann, B. J., Cone, L. T., et al. (1995). Multisystemic treatment of serious juvenile offenders: Long-term prevention of criminality and violence. J Consult Clin Psychol, 63, 569-578.

Bremner, J. D., & Narayan, M. (1998). The effects of stress on memory and the hippocampus throughout the life cycle: Implications for childhood development and aging. Dev Psychopathol, 10, 871-885.

Brewer, D. D., Hawkins, J. D., Catalano, R. F., et al. (1995). Preventing serious, violent, and chronic offending: A review of evaluations of selected strategies in childhood, adolescence, and the community. In J. C. Howell, B. Krisberg, J. D. Hawkins, et al. (Eds.), Sourcebook on serious, violent, and chronic juvenile offenders. Thousand Oaks, CA: Sage Publications.

Bronfenbrenner, U. (1979). The ecology of human development: Experiments by nature and design. Cambridge, MA: Harvard University Press.

Brunk, M. S., Henggeler, S. W., & Whelan, J. P. (1987). A comparison of multisystemic therapy and parent training in brief treatment of child abuse and neglect. J Consult Clin Psychol, 63, 569-578.

Buchanan, A. (1996). Cycles of child maltreatment. Cichester, UK: John Wiley & Sons.

CDC. (1994). Homicides among 15-19 year-old males: United States, 1963-1991. Morb Mortal Wkly Rep, 43, 725-727.

CDC. (1997a). Rates of homicide, suicide, and firearm-related death among children in 26 industrialized countries. Morb Mortal Wkly Rep, 46, 101-105.

CDC. (1997b). Youth Risk Behavior Surveillance System (YRBSS) – United States. Washington, DC: US Department of Health and Human Services.

CDC. (1999). Morb Mortal Wkly Rep, 48(45), 1029-1034.

CDF. (2000). The state of America's child yearbook 2000. Washington, DC: Children's Defense Fund.

Clinton, B. (1992). The Maternal Infant Health Outreach Worker Project: Appalachian communities help their own. In Larner, M., Halpern R., and Harkavy, O. (Eds.), Fair Start for Children: Lessons Learned from Seven Demonstration Projects. New Haven: Yale University Press.

Conduct Problems Prevention Research Group (1992). A developmental and clinical model for the prevention of conduct disorders: The FAST track program. Dev Psychopathol, 4, 509-527.

Crimes Against Children Research Center. (1998). National Incident Based Reporting System (NIBRS) 1995 data analysis. Sexual Assault Fact Sheet. Retrieved June 5, 2001 from the Word Wide Web: http://www.unh.edu/ccrc/factsheet.html#3

Dodge, K. A., & Coie, J. D. (1987). Social information processing factors in reactive and proactive aggression in children's peer groups. Journal of Personality and Social Psychology, 53, 1146-1158.

DuRant, R. H., Kahn, J., Beckford, P. H., & Woods, E. R. (1997). The association of weapon carrying and fighting on school property and other health risk and problem behaviors among high school students. Arch Pediatr Adolesc Med, 151, 360-366.

DuRant, R. H., Treiber, F., Goodman, E., et al. (1996). Intentions to use violence among adolescents. Pediatrics, 98, 103-112.

Dwyer, K., Osher, D., & Wagner, C. (1998). Early warning, timely response: A guide to safe schools. Washington, DC: US Department of Education.

Earls, F. J. (1997). Project on human development in Chicago neighborhoods: A research update. OJJDP Research Brief, NCJ 163603. Washington, DC: US Department of Justice.

Famularo, R., Kinscherff, R., & Fenton, T. (1995). Parental substance abuse and the nature of child maltreatment. Child Abuse Negl, 16, 475-483.

Finklehor, D. (1994). Current information on the scope and nature of child sexual abuse. Future Child, 4(2), 31-53.

Finkelhor, D. (1997). The homicides of children and youth: A developmental perspective. In G. K. Kantor and J. Jasinski (Eds.), Out of the darkness: Contemporary perspectives on family violence (pp. 17-34). Thousand Oaks, CA: Sage Publications.

Finkelhor, D. (2000). <u>Online Victimization/Youth Internet Safety Survey.</u> Retrieved June 5, 2001 from the World Wide Web: http://www.unh.edu/ccrc/Youth_Internet_info_page.html

Gil, D. G. (1996). Preventing violence in a structurally violent society: Mission impossible. <u>Am J Orthopsychiatry, 66,</u> 77-84.

Gottfredson, D. C. (1986). An empirical test of school-based environmental and individual interventions to reduce the risk of delinquent behavior. <u>Criminology, 24,</u> 705-711.

Gottfredson, D. C. (1990). Changing school structures to benefit high-risk youths. <u>Understanding troubled and troubling youth: Multidisciplinary perspectives.</u> Newbury Park, CA: Sage Publications.

Gottfredson, D. C., Gottfredson, G. D., & Hybl, L. G. (1993). Managing adolescent behavior: A multiyear, multischool study. <u>American Educational Research Journal, 30,</u> 179-215.

Harachi, T. W., Ayers, C. D., Hawkins, J. D., et al. (1995). Empowering communities to prevent adolescent substance abuse: Results from a risk- and protection-focused community mobilization effort. <u>Journal of Primary Prevention, 16,</u> 233-254.

Harrell, A. (1993). <u>A guide to research on family violence</u> (pp. 27-29). San Francisco, CA: National Council of Juvenile and Family Court Judges for the State Justice Institute (March 25-28, 1993).

Hawkins, J. D., Catalano, R. F., Morrison, D. M., et al. (1992). Seattle Social Development Project: Effects of the first four years on protective factors and problem behaviors. In J. McCord and R. E. Tremblay (Eds.), <u>Preventing antisocial behavior: Interventions from birth through adolescence</u> (pp.139-161). New York, NY: Guilford.

Hawkins, J. D., Doueck, H. J., & Lishner, D. M. (1988). Changing teaching practices in mainstream classrooms to improve bonding and behavior of low achievers. <u>American Educational Research Journal, 25,</u> 31-50.

Hawkins, J. D., Herrenkohl, T. I., Farrington, D. P., et al. (1998). Predictors of youth violence. In R. Loeber and D. P. Farrington (Eds.), <u>Serious and violent juvenile offenders: Risk factors and successful intervention</u> (pp.104-146). Thousand Oaks, CA: Sage Publications.

Henggeler, S. W. (1997). Treating serious anti-social behavior in youth: The MST approach. OJJDP Bulletin, <u>NCJ 155151.</u> Washington, DC: US Department of Justice.

High, P., La Grasse, L., Becker, S., et al. (2000). Literacy promotion in primary care pediatrics: Can we make a difference? <u>Pediatrics, 105</u>(9), 927-933.

Horn, D. (2000, April). <u>Bruised inside: What our children say about youth violence, what causes it, and what we need to do about it.</u> Washington, DC: National Association of Attorneys General.

Institute of Medicine/National Research Council. (1998). <u>Violence in families: Assessing prevention and treatment programs.</u> Washington, DC: National Academy Press.

Ireland, T., & Widom, C. S. (1994). Childhood victimization and risk for alcohol and drug arrests. The International Journal of Addictions, 2(2), 235-274.

Jaffe, P. G., Wolfe, D. A., & Wilson, S. K. (1990). Children of battered women. Thousand Oaks, CA: Sage Publications.

Johnson Institute. (1996). The no-bullying program: Preventing bully/victim violence at school. Minneapolis, MN: Johnson Institute.

Kazdin, A. E., Siegel, T. C., & Bass, D. (1992). Cognitive problem-solving skills training and parent management training in the treatment of antisocial behavior in children. J Consult Clin Psychol, 60, 733-747.

Kellerman, A. L., Rivara, F. P., Rushforth, N. B., et al. (1993). Gun ownership as a risk factor for homicide in the home. N Engl J Med, 329, 1084-1091.

Kilpatrick, D. C., Edmunds, C., & Seymour, A. (1992). Rape in America: A report to the nation. The National Women's Study. Washington, DC: National Institute of Drug Abuse, National Victim's Center, & National Crime Victims Research and Treatment Center at the Medical University of South Carolina.

Kleck, G., & Patterson, E. B. (1993). The impact of gun control and gun ownership levels on violence rates. Journal of Quantitative Criminology, 9, 249-287.

LH Research. (1993). A survey of experiences, perceptions, and apprehensions about guns among young people in America. Boston, MA: Harvard University, School of Public Health.

Loeber, R., & Farrington, D. P. (Eds.). (1999). Serious and violent juvenile offenders: Risk factors and successful interventions. Thousand Oaks, CA: Sage Publications.

Lowry, R., Powell, K. E., Collins, J. L., et al. (1998). Weapon-carrying, physical fighting, and fight-related injury among US adolescents. Am J Prev Med, 14, 122-129.

McCord, J. (1996). Unintended consequences of punishment. Pediatrics, 98(4), 832-834.

Miller, L. S. (1994). Preventive intervention for conduct disorders: A review. Child Adolesc Psychiatr Clin N Am, 3, 405-419.

Miller, T. R., Fisher, D. A., & Cohen, M. A. (2001). Costs of juvenile violence: Policy implications. Pediatrics, 107(1):e3.

Morley, E., Rossman, S. B., Kopczynski, M., Buck, J., & Gouvis, C. (2000, November). Comprehensive responses to youth at risk: Interim findings from the SafeFutures initiative. OJJDP Bulletin, NCJ 183841. Washington, DC: US Department of Justice.

NCES. (1998). Indicators of School Crime and Safety, 1998. Retrieved June 5, 2000 from the World Wide Web: http://nces.ed.gov/pubsearch/pubsinfo.asp?pubid=98251

NCIPC. (2000). Youth Violence in the United States. CDC web site. Retrieved October 1, 2001 from the World Wide Web: http://www.cdc.gov/ncipc/dvp/yvpt/newfacts.htm

O'Donnell, L., Struve, A., & Sandoval, A. (1999). Violence prevention and young adolescents' participation in community youth service. J Adolesc Health, 24(1), 28-37.

OJJDP. (1999). Juvenile offenders and victims: 1999 national report (Chapter 2: Juvenile victims). Retrieved September 14, 2001 from the World Wide Web: http://www.ncjrs.org/html/ojjdp/nationalreport99/chapter2.pdf

Olds, D. L., Henderson, C. R., Chamberlin, R., & Tatelbaum, R. (1986). Preventing child abuse and neglect: A randomized trial of nurse home visitation. Pediatrics, 78, 65-78.

Olds, D. L., & Ktizman, H. (1993). Review of research on home visiting for pregnant women and parents of young children. Future Child, 3, 53-92.

Olweus, D. (1993). Bully/victim problems among school children: Long-term consequences and an effective intervention program. In S. Hodgins (Ed.), Mental disorder and crime (pp.317-419). Thousand Oaks, CA: Sage Publications.

Patterson, G. R., DeBaryshe, B. D., & Ramsey, E. (1989). A developmental perspective on antisocial behavior. Am Psychol, 44, 329-335.

Patterson, G. R., Reid, J. B., & Dishion, T. J. (1992). Antisocial boys: A social interactional approach (Vol 4). Eugene, OR: Castalia.

Perry, B. D. (1997). Incubated in terror: Neurodevelopmental factors in the "cycle of violence." In J. D. Osofsky (Ed.), Children in a violent society, (pp. 123-149). New York, NY: Guilford Press.

Pfannensteil, J. C., & Seltzer, D. A. (1985). New parents as teachers project evaluation report 1985. Jefferson City, MO: Missouri Department of Elementary and Secondary Education.

Prothrow-Stith, D. (1991). Deadly consequences. New York: Harper Collins.

Resnick, M. D., Bearman, P. S., Blum, R. W., et al. (1997). Protecting adolescents from harm: Findings from the national longitudinal study on adolescent health. JAMA, 278, 823-832.

Sampson, R. J., Raudenbusch, S., & Earls, F. (1997). Neighborhoods and violent crime: A multilevel study of collective efficacy. Science, 277, 918-924.

Seitz, V., Rosenbaum, L. K., & Apfel, N. H. (1985). Effects of family support intervention: A ten-year follow-up. Child Development, 56, 376-391.

Slavin, R. E., Madden, N. A., Karweit, N. L., et al. (1990). Success for all: First year outcomes of a comprehensive plan for reforming urban education. American Educational Research Journal, 27, 255-278.

Smith, C., & Thornberry, T. P. (1995). The relationship between childhood maltreatment and adolescent involvement in delinquency. Criminology, 33, 451-477.

Song, L., Singer, M. I., & Anglin, T. M. (1998). Violence exposure and emotional trauma as contributors to adolescents' violent behaviors. Arch Pediatr Adolesc Med, 152, 531-536.

Spatz-Widom, C. S. (1989). The cycle of violence. Science, 244, 160-166.

Spergel, I. A., & Grossman, S. F. (1997). The little village project: A community approach to the gang problem. Social Work, 42, 456-470.

Strassburger, V. C. (Ed.). (1995). Adolescents and the media—Medical and psychological impact. Thousand Oaks, CA: Sage Publications.

Straus, M. A. (1994). Hitting adolescents. In M. A. Straus (Ed.), Beating the devil out of them: Corporal punishment in American families (pp. 35-48). San Francisco, CA: Lexington/Jossey-Bass.

Straus, M. A. (1996). Spanking and the making of a violent society. In S. B. Friedman and S. K. Schonberg (Eds.), The short- and long-term consequences of corporal punishment. Pediatrics, 98(4) Supplement, 837-842

Straus, M. A. (2000). Beating the devil out of them: Corporal punishment in American families and its effects on children (2nd ed.). New Brunswick, NJ: Transaction Publishers.

Straus, M. A., & Gelles, R. J. (1990). How violent are American families: Estimates from the national family violence survey and other studies. In M. A. Straus and R. J. Gelles (Eds.), Physical violence in American families: Risk factors and adaptations to violence in 8,145 families (pp. 95-112). New Brunswick, NJ: Transaction Publishers.

Strayhorn, J. S., & Wiedman, C. S. (1991). Follow-up after one year parent child interaction training: Effects on behavior of preschool children. Journal of American Academy of Child and Adolescent Psychiatry, 30, 138-143.

Stussman, B. J. (1997). National ambulatory medical care survey: 1995 emergency department summary. Advance data from Vital and Health Statistics, No. 285. Hyattsville, MD: National Center for Health Statistics.

Terris, M. (1998). Violence in a violent society. J Public Health Policy, 19(3), 289-302.

USDHHS. (2000). Child maltreatment 1998: Reports from the states to the national child abuse and neglect data system. Washington, DC: US Government Printing Office.

USDOJ. (1996). Youth violence: A community-based response—One city's success story. NCJ 162601. Washington, DC: US Department of Justice.

USGAO. (1995, June). Child welfare: Opportunities to further enhance family preservation and support activities, GAO/HEHS (pp. 94-112). Washington, DC: US Government Printing Office.

Walker, L. (1989). Terrifying love: Why battered women kill and how society responds. New York, NY: Harper & Row.

Ward, J. M. (1999, October). Children and guns: A Children's Defense Fund report on children dying from gunfire in America. Washington, DC: Children's Defense Fund.

Wasik, B. H., Ramey, C. T., Bryant, D. M., Sparling, J. J., et al. (1990). A longitudinal study of two early intervention strategies: Project CARE. Child Dev, 61, 1682-1696.

Webster-Stratton, C., & Hammond, M. A. (1997). Treating children with early onset conduct problems: A comparison of child and parent training intervention. J Consult Clin Psychol, 65, 93-109.

Weise, D., & Daro, D. (1994). Current trends in child abuse reporting and fatalities: The results of the 1994 annual fifty state survey. Working Paper No. 808. Chicago, IL: National Committee to Prevent Child Abuse.

Yoshikawa, H. (1994). Prevention of cumulative protection: Effects of family support and education on chronic delinquency and its risks. Psychol Bull, 115, 28-34.

Yung, B. & Hammond, R. (1998). Breaking the cycle: A culturally sensitive prevention program for African American children and adolescents. In J. Lutzker (Ed.), Handbook of child abuse research and treatment (pp. 319-340). New York: Plenum Publishing.

Chapter 8

PSYCHOLOGICAL AND PSYCHIATRIC ISSUES

BARBARA WHITMAN, PH.D.

The 1962 publication of *The Battered-Child Syndrome* forced both a societal recognition and a societal response to the issue of child maltreatment, a tragedy that had been present—but ignored—for centuries (Kempe, Silverman, Steele, Droegemueller, & Silver, 1962). Since then, child abuse has emerged as a major public health concern. Extensive research has been conducted regarding the prevalence, causes, correlates, consequences, and prevention of child abuse. Yet, despite nearly four decades of intensive efforts, child abuse continues to increase both in prevalence and in severity (Chiocca, 1998; Kaplan, 1999; McCarroll et al., 1999). In 1997, 3,195,000 allegations of abuse were reported to American child protective agencies (National Committee to Prevent Child Abuse [NCPCA], 1997), an increase of 41% since 1988. Of those reported cases, approximately one third were substantiated through agency investigations. Fifty-four percent of these children suffered neglect, 22% were physically abused, 8% were sexually abused, 4% were emotionally abused, and 12% suffered either multiple types or other types of abuse (NCPCA, 1997).

The Federal Child Abuse Prevention and Treatment Act of 1974 (Public Law 93-247) defines child abuse as "the physical and mental injury, sexual abuse, negligent treatment, or maltreatment of a child under the age of 18 by a person who is responsible for the child's welfare, under circumstances which indicate that the child's health and welfare is harmed or threatened thereby." Whether active (abuse) or passive (neglect), when adults harm dependent children, the resulting trauma is pervasive, chronic, and costly. In addition to the immediate medical concerns and costs associated with trauma or neglect, research indicates that children suffering abuse and neglect often concurrently develop behavior and emotional problems, decreased cognitive functioning, impaired academic performance, interpersonal difficulties, and physical problems (including psychologically-induced growth failure, eating disorders, and substance abuse problems) (Briere, 1992). Recent evidence suggests these problems may result, in part, because severe and prolonged child abuse irreversibly alters the developing human nervous system (Joseph, 1999; Stratakis, Gold, & Chrousos, 1995). Even in the absence of medical consequences from the abuse, the concurrently developing conditions (termed *comorbidities*) may negatively impact the affected child's functioning long after the physical effects have healed. Further, treating these comorbidities may require extensive and long-term mental health services for both the affected child and his or her family (Landsverk & Hough, 1996). These services—when available—require a substantial time investment and are financially costly.

These effects are not limited to the childhood years. Studies of adults with a known history of child maltreatment document that the adult years may exhibit a range of negative outcomes, including personality and mood disorders, substance abuse disorders, poor social adjustment, vulnerability to further victimization, and chronic physical health problems (Beitchman et al., 1992; Briere & Runtz, 1990; Fergusson, Lynskey, & Horwood, 1996a; Fergusson, Lynskey, & Horwood, 1996b; Johnson, Cohen, Brown, Smailes, & Bernstein, 1999; Silverman, Reinherz, & Giaconia, 1996). While such disorders are not the *inevitable* outcome of early abuse or neglect, research documents that these outcomes occur significantly more often in adults who were abused as children than in adults with no history of abuse. At the same time, other research documents a significant number of adults who have a history of child maltreatment that was not discovered during childhood and for which they received no treatment (Anderson, Martin, Mullen, Romans, & Herbison, 1993). While many may appear to function adequately as adults, many of these adults pay a significant psychological cost that is reflected in chronic medical, mental health, and relationship difficulties, as well as occupational underachievement.

As research regarding the long-term impact of child abuse accumulates, it is clear that many victims have both their childhood years and their adult lives compromised as a result of child abuse. Further, the evidence suggests that the more severe the abuse, the greater the probability of psychological disorders in adulthood (Fergusson et al., 1996a; Mullen, Martin, Anderson, Romans, & Herbison, 1993; Read, 1998). Even if the physical impact is minimal and transient, the human cost, both to the affected individual and to society, is prohibitive. It is imperative, then, that we identify these children and seek help for them and their families.

It is problematic, however, that identifying those youngsters suffering abuse is rarely straightforward and can be quite complex. There are many reasons for this. Affected children frequently lack recognition that their situation is "not normal." If the affected child does recognize the problem, he or she may have learned to feel guilty and deserving of the abuse, or may feel such shame at the situation that concealment seems only logical. Still others fail to come forward because of a misguided need to protect the abuser, a fear of not being believed, or a fear of reprisal by the abuser. Some victims are simply unable to verbalize what is happening. Living in an abusive environment is stressful, and children, like adults, often evidence stress behaviorally. Aside from the physical effects, coping with the stressful emotions generated by an abuse incident may be noticed in behavioral signals. Since those who serve children frequently observe stress-induced behavior changes among their charges, and since most stress-related behavior change is not the result of abuse, it is imperative that these professionals become familiar with the behavioral and psychological "red flags" that may indicate an abusive situation for a child. They must also act to prevent further harm and the further development of severe psychological consequences for that child.

This chapter provides an overview of the behavioral, emotional, and cognitive disturbances associated with physical, sexual, and emotional abuse in children and the red flags that should alert professionals to the possibility of abuse. Some children exhibit warning signs that are primarily externalizing responses (hostility, aggression, acting out through truancy or shoplifting), and some exhibit signs that are primarily internalizing responses (cognitive difficulties, emotional disturbances). Using this framework, victims of physical abuse more often exhibit externalizing behaviors, while children being sexually and/or emotionally abused more often exhibit internalizing behaviors. While not pure (i.e., children whose primary response is depression may irritably strike out), such a framework can be useful in guiding the observation of stress-related changes and in identifying children for whom more intense observation and intervention may be vital. Further, some behaviors may be generically associated with stress, while others are more clearly associated with abuse. However, let us first consider some characteristics of a child and his or her family that seem to place a child more at risk for abuse.

◆ RISK FACTORS FOR ABUSE

THE CHILD

While no single cause for child abuse has been identified, research over time has yielded a pattern of characteristics that seems to place one child at more risk than another child. For example, younger children, children with a chronically irritable temperament, excessively demanding children, and children with developmental disabilities are more often victims of physical abuse than older children and children without these characteristics (Tharinger, Horton, & Millea, 1990). Physical abuse tends to peak in the 4- to 8-year-old range. Emotional abuse appears to peak in the 6- to 8-year-old range and remain at a similar level through adolescence. While any child is a potential victim of sexual abuse, in general girls are at greater risk than boys by a factor of 2:1. Children seem to be the most vulnerable to sexual victimization during pre-adolescence, particularly between the ages of 8 and 12 years (McNeese & Monteleone, 1996). Some studies estimate that 20% to 25% of women and 10% to 15% of men are sexually abused before they reach adulthood (Berkowitz, 2000). While younger children are not exempt from sexual abuse, older children and adolescents are more likely than younger children to have been subjected to invasive sexual abuse (Beitchman et al., 1992). Younger children, however, are more likely to be abused by a father or stepfather than are older children; the traumatic impact of sexual abuse by a father or stepfather is thought to be greater than abuse by other perpetrators.

THE PARENTS

Although parents across the socioeconomic spectrum abuse their children, there are some characteristics that occur with more frequency among parents who abuse and are therefore considered risk factors. Younger parents are at greater risk than older parents to abuse their children (Freitag, Lazoritz, & Kini, 1998). Single-parent families and families with low incomes are at greater risk for abuse than are two-parent families with greater financial means. Of the single parent families which include a non-marital live-in partner, the partner, rather than the biological parent, is frequently the abuser. Additionally, under-education is a correlate of low income and under-educated parents are at greater risk to abuse than are more highly educated parents. Finally, parental substance abuse significantly increases the risk of abusing for all parents, as does a history of the parent(s) having been abused as children.

◆ COMMON BEHAVIORAL INDICATORS OF STRESS

Behavioral indicators of stress may be acute or chronic. When present, they suggest that a child is having difficulty coping with stress and may need help. Thus, when behavioral indicators of stress are noticed, the source of the stress must be investigated. A clear signal is given when a sudden, unexplained, negative change in behavior is observed. While most of these behavioral indicators are not specific for abuse, an abusive situation may be discovered in investigating the stress that is prompting the child to exhibit these behaviors. Younger children often respond to stress with physical symptoms, including changes in eating and sleeping habits, nightmares, a regression of toileting control (either day or night), an excess of unexplained physical/somatic complaints, the appearance of unexplained or excessive fears, and an increase in clinging behaviors. A sudden increase in activity level and aggressive behaviors in play and in their interactions with others may also occur.

The most commonly observed stress-related behaviors for school-aged children include irritability or a "short fuse," extreme and rapid changes in mood, sleep disturbances, change in school performance, change in peer relationships, aggression, destructiveness, excessive withdrawal, running away, or suddenly acting like a much younger child (Table 8-1). As with younger children, the appearance of vague and unexplained physical/somatic symptoms should raise suspicion of elevated stress. Additionally, more serious behaviors requiring an immediate response include cruelty to animals and/or setting fires.

Older children and adolescents, in addition to mood disturbance, may attempt to run away from home or may try to self-medicate by abusing drugs, while others may seek to escape the stress by trying to kill themselves. Additionally, adolescents may respond to stress by withdrawing from family and friends or may suddenly begin to relate to a "less desirable" peer group than previously was the case. They may evidence deteriorating academic performance or may demonstrate a deterioration in hygiene and appearance.

Table 8-1. General Behavioral Indicators of Stress

• Irritability and "short fuse"	• Marked change in appetite and eating habits
• Unexplained or excessive fears	• A regression of toileting control
• Extreme and rapid changes in mood	• Physical/somatic complaints
• Sleep disturbances	• Cruelty to animals
• Marked change in school performance	• Fire setting
• Negative change in peer relationships	• Drug abuse
• Aggression	• Suicide attempts
• Destructiveness	• Running away
• Excessive withdrawal	• Apathy, unresponsiveness
• Suddenly acting like a much younger child	

In addition to these more "generic" indicators of possible abuse, some behaviors, when present, raise immediate suspicion of abuse, particularly sexual abuse. These include:

- Child is "acting out" sexually: pretending to be performing a sexual act or pretending that his or her dolls are engaged in sexual activity

- Child engages in age-inappropriate intimate exploration or touch or is excessively (and usually inappropriately for his or her age) seductive or promiscuous

- Child masturbates excessively or is overly resistant to appropriate exposure or physical examination of the genital area

When these behaviors are present, the child should immediately be considered a possible victim of sexual abuse. Similarly, although not as dramatic in presentation, many children with bruises resulting from physical abuse wear season-inappropriate clothing to cover their injuries; resist changing clothes for physical or sports-related activities; flinch excessively when an adult moves close, or when touched or bumped suddenly or inadvertantly; or walk and sit as though "stiff and sore." These more specific behavioral indicators of abuse are outlined in Table 8-2.

In addition to these behavioral indicators of stress/abuse, a child who is being abused often exhibits difficulties and deficits in other areas of functioning. These will be explored next, using the type of abuse as a framework.

Table 8-2. More Specific Behavioral Indicators of Abuse

Physical Abuse

- Has unexplained bruises

- Resists changing clothes for physical or sports-related activities

- Walks and sits as though "stiff and sore" and gives vague reasons why

- Wears season-inappropriate clothing to cover bruises

- Flinches excessively when an adult moves close or at a sudden touch or inadvertent bumping

Sexual Abuse

- "Acts out" sexually (i.e., pretends to be performing a sexual act or pretends that his or her dolls are engaged in sexual activity)

- Is excessively (and usually inappropriately for his or her age) seductive or promiscuous

- Resists appropriate exposure or physical examination of the genital area

- Engages in age-inappropriate intimate exploration or touch

- Masturbates excessively

PHYSICAL ABUSE

Physical abuse is child abuse that results in physical injury, including fractures, burns, bruises, welts, cuts, and/or internal injury. Physical abuse often occurs in the name of discipline or punishment and ranges from a slap of the hand to use of an object to inflict pain (National Center on Child Abuse and Neglect [NCCAN], 1988). Physical abuse, with rare exception, occurs reactively. The perpetrator's motivation is to provide a consequence for a real or imagined infraction, but he or she overreacts by using punishment methods that (1) are of a level of severity far exceeding the infraction (e.g., shaking an infant to stop the baby from crying); (2) would never be condoned as appropriate retribution under any circumstance (e.g., placing a child in a tub of boiling water for excessive crying, or burning with cigarettes for some infraction); (3) indicate a complete misunderstanding of a child's developmental abilities; and (4) result from a parent's inability to control his or her own behavior once angered by a child's infraction. The results of physical abuse are usually externally visible if sought.

As previously noted, children who are physically abused tend more often to exhibit "externalizing" behaviors and coping strategies. In the academic arena, research indicates that physically abused children tend to have lower receptive language skills, lower expressive language skills, poorer reading ability, impaired comprehension and abstraction skills, and poorer task management (Swenson & Kolko, 2000). Whether these delays and deficits result from the abuse or were pre-existing risk factors is unclear. Either way, school can then become another arena of under-performance or failure for the victimized child, leading to more abuse.

In addition to having academic difficulties, younger children who are physically abused are more often disruptive and not compliant in class; are sent to the principal's office more often; are truant more often; have difficulty relating to others (including often being openly disliked by others); are more often in trouble for fighting; have an increased number of fights even with those they call friends; demonstrate more negative language both about and toward others; may exhibit "bullying" behaviors; and will show fewer positive emotions than their non-abused peers.

The adolescent who has been or continues to be abused often demonstrates academic difficulties; is more likely to evidence aggression toward others or engage in delinquent behaviors (e.g., shoplifting); more frequently engages in risk-taking behaviors (e.g., physical/daredevil risks, legal risks such as car theft, and drug use); and attempts suicide more often than an adolescent without a history of abuse.

Affectively, physically abused children tend to feel chronically mistrustful, anxious, and angry. In addition, their ability to build relationships with others, who might be able to offer support, is tainted by the mistrust and constant anxiety, often leading to misperceptions that quickly precipitate an expression of the ever-present anger. This expression can be as "mild" as simply being obnoxious and oppositional, or more severe, as in the form of reactive aggression toward others. If the abuse continues over time, these initial feelings of mistrust, anxiety, and anger can solidify into more permanent parts of the child's personality, so that by pre-teen to early adolescent age, evidence of serious personality disorders and psychiatric difficulties in the form of oppositional defiant disorder, conduct disorder, and antisocial personality can be seen (Kaplan & Weeston, 1998). It is then a short step to more adult forms of aggression toward others, ranging from becoming abusive in intimate relationships to serious antisocial aggression, including the use of weapons, substance abuse, and legal problems.

Johnson et al. (1999) described the typical evolution from abused child to deviant adult in a community-based study. This team studied 639 families with children between the ages of 1 and 11 years from two counties in New York. Initial interviews were conducted in 1975; subjects were re-interviewed in 1991 and again in 1993. A history of abuse was obtained from each affected child in both 1991 and 1993, and validated by obtaining substantiated reports of abuse for the study population from the New York State Central Registry for Child Abuse and Neglect. Both the parent and the affected child were interviewed regarding the presence or absence of personality disorders as defined by stringent psychiatric criteria found in the *Diagnostic and Statistical Manual-IV.* In the 639 families, 31 cases of childhood maltreatment were documented; 15 of the 31 cases were physical abuse. An additional 58 people self-reported childhood maltreatment, including 34 cases of physical abuse. On analysis, documented physical abuse was associated with elevated symptom levels of antisocial, borderline, dependent, depressive, passive-aggressive, and schizoid personality disorders. After statistically controlling for a number of possible intervening variables such as parental education, parental psychiatric history, and childhood temperament, a significant association between documented abuse and both antisocial and depressive personality disorders remained. When compared to the rest of the sample with no history of abuse, adults for whom case records document an early history of physical abuse were four times more likely than those who had not been abused to have personality disorders during early adulthood.

SEXUAL ABUSE

The American Academy of Pediatrics (1991) defines sexual abuse as "the engaging of a child in sexual activities that the child cannot comprehend, for which the child is developmentally unprepared and cannot give informed consent, and/or that violate the social and legal taboos of society. Sexual abuse describes a range of behaviors from sexual touching or fondling to forced masturbation to digital or object penetration to sexual intercourse. Exposing a child to exhibitionism or other forms of sexual behavior, or using a child in the production of pornography are also considered forms of sexual abuse, as is inappropriate talk about sex."

Sexual abuse differs from physical abuse in a number of ways, each of which contributes to an overall conclusion that the traumatic impact and long-term sequelae from sexual abuse may be, in many respects, more chronically debilitating than those associated with physical abuse. Unlike physical abuse, which is generally reactive, sexual abuse is almost always purposeful. It requires opportunistic planning, and involves the systematic violation of the trust relationship with the child through a conditioning process while violating a trusting relationship with the child's parent. It is often both invisible in its physical effect and secretive in its occurrence. Further, unlike physical abuse, which always involves the infliction of pain, sexual abuse seldom involves extensive physical pain; indeed, the sexual contact involved can be physically exciting to the victim. It is this latter aspect that often amplifies the impact of the emotional damage.

Behavioral indicators of sexual abuse differ according to the age of the child (Beitchman et al., 1992). Preschoolers most often display some age-inappropriate and/or abnormal form of sexual behavior. This may include sexual play with dolls, insertion of objects into the vagina or anus, masturbation, seductive behavior or requests for sexual stimulation, age-inappropriate or precocious sexual knowledge, or inappropriate touching of others. Less obvious, but nonetheless significant, are the sudden development of inappropriate fears of certain places, particularly the bathroom; a re-initiation of wetting after successful toilet training; nightmares; development of excessive clinging to parents; and the development of passivity and withdrawn behavior.

While age-inappropriate sexualized behavior is almost always an indication of some form of sexual abuse, children quickly learn the unacceptability of this behavior in public places. The cessation of the behavior, however, is not an indication of a cessation of either the abuse or its impact. In fact, unlike the external sexualized behavior that may still be evidenced in the younger grade school child, middle-school age victims of sexual abuse more often tend to exhibit internalizing kinds of trauma-related symptoms that may only be obvious through their impact on the child's academic performance. Studies show that children who are sexually abused have more physical symptoms, attention deficit-hyperactivity disorder, sleep disturbances, suicidal thoughts or attempts, self-mutilation, substance abuse, and dissociative symptoms when compared to non-abused peers. For many, when closely examined, these symptoms occur in a typical constellation now termed "post-traumatic stress disorder." Research indicates that sexually abused children show more post-traumatic stress symptoms even when compared to other children in mental health treatment (Kendall-Tackett, Myers, & Finkelhor, 1993).

The formal description of this constellation of symptoms includes "persistent symptoms of increased arousal," such as sleep disturbance, heightened startle response, poor concentration, and hypervigilance. At the same time, there is evidence of "numbing of general responsiveness to, or avoidance of, current events." This translates to children who appear to be depressed, withdrawn, lethargic, and unable to concentrate on routine tasks while at the same time seeming to be extremely fearful, watchful, and over-reactive to even the slightest noise or change in the environment. If the child also has repetitious nightmares of the abuse or has sudden, unexpected, intrusive memories of the abuse during waking hours (often appearing to the observer as daydreaming), leading to increased anxiety and fearfulness, then a complete "post-traumatic syndrome" is present. When the latter symptom is present, it is as though the sexual abuse is ever-present and victimizing, requiring all the child's attention and energy to ward off or deal with the ongoing fear and anxiety. Thus, during the day, the child must concentrate on not being victimized by his or her own internal representations of the abuse, while at night the child must try to avoid sleep for the same reasons. If, in addition, the abuser is a family member who continues to reside in the home, much energy is expended in avoiding or dealing with the complexities of that relationship and the ever-present possibility of repeat abuse.

Studies of sexually abused adolescents document depression, low self-esteem, suicidal thoughts and/or attempts, and more severe symptoms such as psychotic behavior, including hallucinations. Equally prominent are "acting out" types of behaviors, such as running away, alcohol and drug abuse, and promiscuity.

Additionally, a number of adult psychopathological disorders have been associated with a childhood history of sexual abuse, including chronic post-traumatic stress disorder, multiple personality disorder, eating disorders, (psycho)somatic disorders, depression, anxiety, substance abuse disorders, and dysfunctional or maladpative sexual behavior (Berkowitz, 2000; Briere & Runtz, 1990; Kluft, 1984; McLeer, Callaghan, Henry, & Wallen, 1994; Wonderlich, Brewerton, Jocic, Dansky, & Abbot, 1997). As was noted in the case of physical abuse, there appears to be a direct relationship between the severity of childhood sexual abuse and the severity of adult psychopathology. In a retrospective record study, Read (1998) compared hospitalized psychiatric patients who had been abused as children to other psychiatric inpatients on a number of severity of disturbance measures. Records were examined for a reported history of abuse, involuntary vs. voluntary admission, level of suicidal thoughts on admission, length of admission, and need for protective seclusion. Nine of the 57 men and eight of the 43 women reported a history of sexual abuse. All nine sexually abused men were highly suicidal compared to 15 of the 48 men who had not been sexually abused ($p<0.0001$). The relationship between suicidality and sexual abuse did not reach statistical significance for females. Nonetheless, the length of stay was significantly longer for women with a history of sexual abuse than for their non-abused counterparts (33.7 days vs. 24.8 days). Additionally, there was a strong trend for women who had a history of sexual abuse to have been admitted involuntarily (seven of the eight sexually abused females) and to have been in protective seclusion (five of the eight sexually abused females) when compared to those patients without such history. Sixty percent of those with a history of sexual abuse had had a previous hospitalization during the past 12 months compared to 43% of those with no abuse history. Further, women with a history of childhood sexual abuse were significantly more likely to have been hospitalized for psychiatric reasons before the age of 18 years.

Fergusson et al. (1996b) conducted a prospective study with a cross-sectional assessment of both sexual abuse and mental health outcomes. A total of 1265 children born in Christchurch, New Zealand, in 1977 were studied at birth, at age 4 months, annually to age 16 years, and again at age 18 years. At 18 years, 1019 (80.5%) of the young adults were interviewed in private by trained interviewers who administered a 1.5- to 2-hour interview on a range of mental health issues. As part of this interview, young people were asked whether, before age 16 years, anyone had attempted to involve them in any of a series of 15 unwanted sexual activities. The activities ranged from non-contact episodes including indecent exposure and public masturbation, to incidents involving attempted or completed oral, anal, or vaginal intercourse. From those who answered positively, information was sought regarding the perpetrator and the nature and extent of abuse, including age of occurrence, number of incidents, duration of occurrence, use of force or restraint, when the interviewee became aware that the behavior was abusive, and if the abuse had been previously reported to authorities. One hundred six (10.4%) reported abuse before age 16 years by 132 perpetrators. The rate among females (17.3%) was more than five times greater than that reported by males (3.4%). Those reporting childhood sexual abuse had higher rates of major depression, anxiety disorder, conduct disorder, substance abuse disorder, and suicidal behaviors than the non-abused subjects, a finding that held up even after adjusting for possibly confounding family factors. Those reporting childhood sexual abuse that included attempted or completed intercourse had the highest rates and severity of the disorders. One of the more serious disorders that is found almost exclusively among victims of childhood sexual abuse is multiple personality disorder. The psychological environment necessary for this disorder is a coping mechanism termed "dissociation."

DISSOCIATION AND MULTIPLE PERSONALITY DISORDER

For many children, physically leaving or avoiding the abusive situation may not be possible, particularly if the abuser is a close family member. Thus, for many, the only escape route is a psychological escape known as "dissociation." Dissociation can be defined as "a defensive psychophysiologic process that disrupts the normal connections among feelings, thoughts, behavior, and memories so that for a period of time, certain information is not integrated normally or logically with other information." In essence, to deal with the overwhelming nature of the abuse, the child attempts to psychologically numb himself or herself or to "psychologically be somewhere else." Adults describing their experience of these dissociative episodes often report accompanying "depersonalization" and "out-of-body" phenomena such as "there was a spot on the wall where I routinely went and watched as he raped me."

Repeated entry into a dissociative state to cope with sexual abuse appears to lead to a more general use of a dissociative process as a means of coping with lesser stressors, including those associated with poor school performance or social distress (Putnam, 1993). For the observer, the best indicator of a possible dissociative process is frequent trance-like behavior (Dell & Eisenhower, 1990; Kluft, 1984; Peterson, 1990; Putnam, Guroff, Gilberman, Barban, & Post, 1986). Although some "normal" children occasionally demonstrate trance-like behavior, dissociating children frequently and spontaneously lapse into vacant, trance-like states. A child exhibiting episodes of dissociation may evidence confusingly erratic behavior. He or she may be cooperative and compliant one minute and make a sudden (often seemingly unprovoked) "Jekyll and Hyde" transformation into excessive oppositional and aggressive behavior. When confronted about an aggressive act, the child may have no memory of the act, becoming hurt by the accusation—often vigorously denying having done what others witnessed. In school these episodes may lead to missed information and confusion on the part of the child. The child may appear to have significant learning disabilities and attention disorders, with memory of information and tasks intact at one point and absent at another. Often, when queried regarding their "lack of attention," the child may evidence surprise or deny that such has occurred.

Dissociation becomes pathological when the frequency and/or duration of the dissociative episodes becomes so complete that the link between the feelings, memories, and behavior in the dissociated or protective state becomes completely inaccessible and "unremembered" when in a non-dissociative state. For many children suffering long-term sexual abuse, this "state separation" is a solution to overwhelming trauma. The solution is creative in that the child can maintain his or her love for the perpetrator in one state, the memory of the painful experience and feelings in another, and frequently the angry and aggressive emotions and behaviors in yet another. Once the separation between states is established, each separate state may continue to develop a personality totally independent of the others, thus solidifying the development of a more serious dissociative disorder termed multiple personality disorder (Table 8-3).

Table 8-3. Symptoms of Multiple Personality Disorder

Forgetfulness and amnesia

- Amnesia for recent events such as abuse, schoolwork, tantrums, rage attacks

- Perplexing forgetfulness such as time lost, tardiness with an inability to remember where they just were

- The appearance of items of clothing, toys, school supplies that they have not been given by parents and cannot recall buying (or the unexplained disappearance of such items)

Forgetfulness reflected in interpersonal relationships

- Confusion regarding the names of teachers or peers

- Denial of behavior witnessed by others—often accompanied by a fierce sense of injustice if punished or confronted for lying

- Apparent inability to learn from experience such as discipline or punishment

Affective symptoms

- Severe periodic depression, sometimes including suicidal gestures but with no clear precipitating factor

Somatic symptoms

- Physical complaints and injuries of vague origin, sometimes clearly self-inflicted

Behavioral symptoms

- Subtle alternating personality changes such as a basically shy child exhibiting depressed, angry, seductive, or regressive episodes

- Extreme regressive episodes followed by amnesia, such as frightened thumb-sucking in a pre-teen or sudden and dramatic yet transient loss of language or motor skills

- Frequent angry outbursts without apparent provocation and frequently accompanied by extreme physical strength

- Dramatic fluctuations in conduct and performance (especially in abilities relating to school work, games, and music)

- Continually changing preferences in food, clothing, and social relationships

Daydreaming, sleepwalking, depersonalization (unrelated to seizure disorder)

- Excessive daydreaming, sleepwalking, trance-like behavior, including concentration and attention difficulties

Table 8-3. Symptoms of Multiple Personality Disorder—*continued*
Auditory "hallucinations" and imaginary companions   • Hallucinated voices (either friendly or unfriendly) often attributed to imaginary companions   • Imaginary companion still real to a child over age 6 years

Not all victims of child sexual abuse dissociate, and many authors note that some forms of dissociation are developmentally normal (Putnam, 1993). Even among a severely abused population, not all dissociation leads to multiple personality disorder; many children and adults dissociate emotionally as a coping strategy. This dissociation, however, is limited to the emotional sphere with no loss of continuity and with no apparent demonstration of affect. However, the use of dissociation can become a primary coping mechanism, and the boundaries between dissociative states can become fixed and impenetrable, leading to the development of a multiple personality disorder. If this occurs, then, without rapid and intense therapy, the development of a chronic, unremitting, and totally devastating psychiatric disorder that is refractory to treatment is inevitable. Dramatic representations of this disorder in the popular media demonstrate well the complexity of the disorder, but fall short of demonstrating the psychological and functional devastation to victims and the impact on those to whom they relate.

EMOTIONAL/PSYCHOLOGICAL ABUSE
While emotional trauma occurs as part of all physical and sexual abuse, emotional abuse can also occur independently. Young children who were emotionally or psychologically abused as infants or toddlers can experience difficulty developing appropriate attachments. Similarly, emotional/psychological abuse may also impair the affected child's capacity to develop appropriate emotional responses and can lead to lifelong emotional difficulties (Brothers, 1989; Kent & Waller, 1998). In the extreme, emotional/psychological abuse can shut down physical growth and cognitive development.

While probably the most common form of abuse, emotional/psychological abuse is the most under-reported form of abuse and, except in the most extreme forms, the most difficult form of abuse to substantiate. This is, in part, because we cannot clearly define what constitutes emotional/psychological abuse, except in the most severe forms. The Federal Child Abuse Prevention and Treatment Act 42 (1974) defined emotional abuse as a repeated pattern of caregiver behavior or an extreme incident or incidents of behavior conveying to children that they are worthless, flawed, unloved, unwanted, endangered, or only of value in meeting another's needs. This definition was extended by the American Professional Society on the Abuse of Children (APSAC) (1995), which defined six forms of psychological abuse. These are: spurning; exploiting/corrupting; terrorizing; denying emotional responsiveness; isolating; and unwarranted denial of mental health care, medical care, or education. Common to all definitions is the notion of a repeated pattern or extreme incident(s) of those conditions that convey the message that a child is worthless, flawed, endangered, or only valuable for meeting someone else's needs.

Further complicating the identification of emotional abuse is that, unlike physical and sexual abuse, external physical markers that are specific for emotional/psychological abuse are rare. Most child-evidenced behavioral symptoms of emotional abuse are not significantly different from those indicating physical or sexual abuse. Finally, the evidence that such abuse may be occurring is frequently found not in the behavior of the child, but instead in the behavior of the parent. However, the index of suspicion should be raised when any of the symptoms of abuse previously described are present without an obvious or forthcoming explanation.

When the observer suspects emotional/psychological abuse, the search for red flags must shift focus from the child to the parent. Parental behaviors constituting emotional/psychological abuse can be either active (commission behaviors) or passive (omission behaviors). Pearl (1998) details a number of parental red flag behaviors for the categories of spurning, exploiting/corrupting, terrorizing, denying emotional responsiveness, and isolating (Table 8-4).

While emotional/psychological abuse at any age can significantly damage a child's sense of self and worth, early and severe emotional/psychological abuse can lead to complete growth failure accompanied by developmental and psychological retardation. This phenomenon is termed "psychosocial dwarfism."

Recent studies of young children raised in state-operated residential institutions in Romania demonstrate serious, long-term neurological and developmental difficulties resulting from severe emotional/social deprivation. The social and economic policies of Nicolae Ceausescu were such that families were forced to bear more children than they wanted or could afford. As a result, 2% of the population was committed to state care until the age of 18 years. These figures have not diminished since Ceausescu's death in 1989, due to continuing economic and social instability. Children committed to care in state Leagane (meaning cradles) experience child-caregiver ratios of 20:1, allowing for no more than minimal custodial care. With this level of care, their medical and nutritional needs are basically met, but their psychological and social needs are not met at all. Comparison studies of Romanian children reared in Leagane and those raised in families indicate that the children in Leagane had significant delays in physical and developmental growth, while family-reared children were similar to American children in their psychological performance and physical growth (Carlson & Earls, 1997).

As these children have been adopted, our knowledge of the extent of damage resulting from these environments is rapidly expanding. The severe emotional neglect experienced by many infants in these orphanages results in growth failure of the right prefrontal cortex of the brain, leading to an inability to appropriately attach to the adoptive parents; generalized sensory impairments, such as tactile defensiveness and increased arousal with an excessive startle response; and attention and learning problems. The physiologic stress associated with the environmental deprivation significantly alters brain chemistry, leading to profound failure of linear growth (height) and weight, and further impacts brain development. Although the average age of adoption for many of these children is 18.5 months, their early and severe emotional deprivation has already resulted in attachment disorders, symptoms of post-traumatic stress disorder, and for many, development in the autistic spectrum, including mental retardation (Faber, 2000).

Table 8-4. Parental Behaviors Constituting Emotional/Psychological Abuse

Ignoring behaviors

- Fails to respond to or provide for child's needs

- Does not show affection to or for child

- Does not initiate looking at child or look responsively

- Fails to recognize child's presence

- Does not call child by name

- Fails to stimulate child appropriately

- Is psychologically unavailable to child

- Fails to allow child normal and appropriate privacy

Terrorizing behaviors

- Uses excessive guilt-producing activity

- Engages in chaotic behavior to frighten child

- Uses inconsistent and capricious discipline

- Makes excessive threats and uses psychological punishment

- Threatens with weapons

- Employs bizarre means of punishment

- Ridicules child for being appropriately frightened

- Uses normal fears for punishment (e.g., maliciously encourages fear of dark, dogs)

- Refuses to comfort frightened child

- Threatens suicide or abandonment

- Permits others to terrorize child

- Refuses to provide shelter and safety

Rejecting and verbally assaultive behaviors

- Belittles or ridicules child, uses verbal attacks

- Purposefully and continually embarrasses child

- Publicly and privately humiliates child

- Singles child out for criticism and punishment

- Offers excessive or continuous criticism

- Routinely rejects child's ideas

**Table 8-4. Parental Behaviors Constituting
Emotional/Psychological Abuse—***continued*

- Routinely calls child "dumb," "stupid," and other demeaning names
- Treats child as though he or she is much younger than actual age
- Prevents the development of or sabotages the child's development of peer or other adult relationships
- Makes child perform household tasks beyond his or her level of ability
- Makes child meet parental needs
- Refuses to obtain appropriate medical or other health care for child
- Tells child he or she is worthless or no good

Corrupting behaviors

- Allows or forces viewing of pornography
- Teaches child sexually exploitative behavior
- Teaches child illegal behavior
- Knowingly allows others to teach child illegal behavior
- Teaches, encourages, or praises antisocial behavior
- Assists in delinquent and antisocial behavior
- Fails to discipline for delinquent or antisocial behavior
- Gives drugs or stolen goods to child or uses child in obtaining or using these items
- Uses child as spy, ally, or confidant in parent's romantic relationships or marital or divorce problems

Isolating behaviors

- Separates child from family unit
- Does not allow child to participate in normal family routine and activities
- Does not allow child normal contact with peers
- Does not allow child to participate in social aspects of school
- Avoids appropriate physical contact with child (e.g., hugging)
- Locks child in room, basement, attic
- Punishes child for requests for interaction with family or others
- Refuses child appropriate contact with extended family

Table 8-4. Parental Behaviors Constituting Emotional/Psychological Abuse—*continued*

- Binds or gags child to prevent interaction

- Hides child from outside world

Overpressuring behaviors

- Has excessively advanced expectations and makes unreasonable demands

- Is excessively critical of age-appropriate behaviors

- Punishes child for acting in age-appropriate manner

- Fails to provide needed or appropriate supportive help

- Demands that child exhibit behavior and accomplishments of older child

- Negatively compares child with those older and more advanced

- Provides toys and activities beyond the child's abilities

- Continually sets child up for failure

While not all adoptees are so seriously affected, few are totally unaffected. Fisher, Ames, Chisholm, and Savoie (1997) compared Romanian adoptees who had spent at least 8 months in an orphanage with Canadian-born children with no history of institutional care. The average age of adoption was 18.5 months. After the children had been in their adoptive homes approximately 11 months, parental interviews indicated that the adoptees had a significantly greater number of eating disorders, stereotypic rocking behavior, stereotypic hand flapping, and greater difficulty with withdrawal and anxiety behaviors. Long-term follow-up studies suggest that children spending six months or more in these environments and adopted after age 1 year more frequently have chronic attachment difficulties that continue to have a negative impact on their functioning in adolescence and adulthood.

CASE EXAMPLE

Such abuse is not limited to institutional settings. Consider the case of Leah, which follows:

Leah was brought to a developmental clinic for an assessment of her learning ability by her foster/adoptive parents. The foster/adoptive parents were a professional couple, the husband a minister and the wife a nurse, with one older biological son. Leah was 4 at the time of her initial visit to the clinic. Her foster/adoptive parents reported that Leah had been a part of their family for a year after removal from her biological home due to sexual abuse. They stated that Leah was an extremely difficult and demanding child who seemed unappreciative of all they were doing for her. They were becoming concerned about her physically, however, because she had not grown in height or weight since arriving in their home. In addition, they viewed her as quite oppositional and exhibiting a refusal to learn. Their typical form of punishing Leah for any infraction was to have her march around the dining room table, usually for an hour at a time. Leah's work-up included an extensive physical examination, including endocrine, genetic, and developmental studies. All physical parameters were normal. Developmentally, Leah tested as having an IQ of 65, in the mildly cognitively impaired range. During all work-ups at the clinic, no evidence of any behavioral difficulties were noted. In fact, Leah was appropriately charming and compliant with all staff. Following the evaluation, her foster/adoptive parents returned her to the child-welfare authorities who found another adoptive placement for Leah. She initially grew an inch in the first six weeks, but then seemed to again stop growing. She was returned to the clinic for additional studies, and the young couple with whom she had been placed again reported extremely oppositional behavior. She had also begun to exhibit excessive water drinking, raising concerns for diabetes or other medical conditions. Again all physical parameters were normal. Testing at that point yielded an IQ score of 85, greater than one standard deviation above the previous testing. Again Leah evidenced no oppositional or difficult behavior with any staff. Soon after this visit, this couple gave Leah up as too difficult for them to handle and she was placed with another couple in their late 30s with no children of their own. After six months in this family, Leah returned to the clinic for additional testing to determine her need for special education services as she entered first grade. This couple indicated that upon entering their family, Leah had indeed evidenced some difficult behaviors, but that with consistency and constant assurance that she would remain in their home no matter how poorly she behaved, Leah began to settle down and become more compliant. She had grown six inches in six months and had added weight appropriate to her increase in height. Leah's testing at that point indicated an IQ score of 100, with some unevenness in her language skills, but nothing serious enough to require special education intervention. Leah returned to the clinic yearly for the next 3 years. At her final visit, Leah's weight and height were at the 75th percentile for age and her IQ score was 140, more than twice her initial assessment and in the area of superior intelligence. Leah's family had adopted her and had obtained a long-term therapist for her so they would be appropriately prepared if Leah needed therapeutic support when she entered adolescence.

Although such severe abuse is rare, careful studies of these children is instructive in demonstrating the impact of emotional abuse not only on psychological development but also on physical development, brain and mental development, and psychological functioning. At a minimum, continued emotional/psychological abuse can lead to an impaired capacity to enjoy life; excessive passivity that can impact the ability to effectively get needs met; extreme shyness; poor social interactions; a poor sense of self; and a fear-driven tendency toward being a loner—further exacerbating feelings of loneliness, unhappiness, and powerlessness, and suspiciousness regarding any human interaction. In essence, early abuse and deprivation lead to adult behavior that continues the deprivation and often the sense of continuing abuse.

◆ Factors Influencing Outcome

Thus far we have focused on common comorbidities accompanying physical, sexual, and emotional abuse. While most victimized children evidence some degree of emotional trauma, there are a number of factors that influence the long-term impact resulting from the abuse. Among these are the age of first abuse, length of time abused, severity of any given episode of abuse, relationship to abuser, type of abuse (e.g., physical, sexual), whether the abuse was ever reported by the child to a responsive adult, intervening treatment, and removal to alternative living environments. In addition, with appropriate treatment, many children can show remarkable resilience. Above-average cognitive abilities, high self-esteem, an internal sense of the ability to positively affect their environment (internal locus of control), an external attribution of blame (the perpetrator was at fault, I am not defective), the presence of spirituality and/or involvement with a religious community, high ego controls (ability to understand and not feel vulnerable to environment), involvement in extracurricular activities or hobbies so that isolation is not debilitating, and the presence of a caring, supportive adult combined with positive family changes have all been related to a child's ability to recover from abuse trauma (Heller, Larrieu, D'Imperio, & Boris, 1999). A closer examination of the factors that help a child recover from abuse shows that they are, in many ways, the opposite of the factors that raise a child's risk for abuse. Thus it appears that ultimately our approach to this issue must not only address the child, but must also focus on the larger context in which the child lives.

◆ REFERENCES

American Academy of Pediatrics Committee on Child Abuse and Neglect Policy Statement. (1991). Guidelines for the evaluation of sexual abuse of children. Pediatrics, 87, 254-260.

APSAC Task Force on Psychological Maltreatment. (1995). Guidelines for psychosocial evaluation of suspected maltreatment in children and adolescents. N. Charleston, SC: APSAC.

Anderson, J., Martin, J., Mullen, P., Romans, S., & Herbison, P. (1993). Prevalence of childhood sexual abuse experiences in a community sample of women. J Am Acad Child Adolesc Psychiatry 32(5), 911-919.

Beitchman, J., Zucker, K., Hood, J., DaCosta, G., Akman, D., & Cassavia, E. (1992). A review of the long-term effects of child sexual abuse. Child Abuse & Neglect, 16, 101-118.

Berkowitz, C. (2000). The long-term medical consequences of sexual abuse. In R. Reece (Ed.), The Treatment of Child Abuse (pp.54-94).Baltimore, MD: Hopkins University Press.

Briere, J. (1992). Child Abuse Trauma: Theory and Treatment of the Lasting Effects. Newberry Park, CA: Sage Publications.

Briere, J., & Runtz, M. (1990). Differential adults symptomatology associated with three types of child abuse histories. Child Abuse & Neglect, 14(3), 357-364.

Brothers, L. (1989). A biological perspective on empathy. Am J Psychiatry 146(1), 10-19.

Carlson, M., & Earls, F. (1997). Psychological and neuroendocrinological sequelae of early social deprivation in institutionalized children in Romania. Annals of the New York Academy of Sciences, 807, 419-428.

Chiocca, E. (1998). Child abuse and neglect: Part 1. A status report. Journal of Pediatric Nursing, 13(2), 128-130.

Dell, P.J., & Eisenhower, J.W. (1990). Adolescent multiple personality disorder: a preliminary study of eleven cases. J Am Acad Child Adolesc Psychiatry, 29, 359-366.

Faber, S. (2000). Behavioral sequelae of orphanage life. <u>Pediatric Annals,</u> <u>29</u>(4), 242-248.

Federal Child Abuse Prevention and Treatment Act of 1974, Public Law 93-247. <u>U.S. Statutes at Large,</u> 88, 4-8.

Fergusson, D., Lynskey, M., & Horwood, J. (1996a). Childhood sexual abuse and psychiatric disorder in young adulthood: I. Prevalence of sexual abuse and factors associated with sexual abuse. <u>J Am Acad Child Adolesc Psychiatry,</u> <u>34</u>(10), 1355-1364.

Fergusson, D., Lynskey, M., & Horwood, J. (1996b). Childhood sexual abuse and psychiatric disorder in young adulthood: II. Psychiatric outcomes of childhood sexual abuse. <u>J Am Acad Child Adolesc Psychiatry, 34</u>(10), 1365-1374.

Fisher, L., Ames, E. W., Chisholm, K., & Savoie, L. (1997). Problems reported by parents of Romanian orphans adopted to British Columbia. <u>International Journal of Behavioral Development, 20,</u> 67-82.

Freitag, R., Lazoritz, S., & Kini, N. (1998). Psychosocial aspects of child abuse for primary care pediatricians. <u>Pediatric Clinics of North America,</u> <u>445</u>(2), 391-402.

Heller, S., Larrieu, J., D'Imperio, R., & Boris, N. (1999). Research on resilience to child maltreatment: Empirical considerations. <u>Child Abuse and</u> <u>Neglect, 23</u>(4), 321-338.

Johnson, J., Cohen, P., Brown, J., Smailes, E., & Bernstein, D. (1999). Childhood maltreatment increases risk for personality disorders during early adulthood. <u>Arch Gen Psychiatry, 56</u>(7), 600-606.

Joseph, R. (1999). The neurology of traumatic "dissociative" amnesia: Commentary and literature review. <u>Child Abuse & Neglect, 23</u>(8), 715-727.

Kaplan, J. (1999). Child and adolescent abuse and neglect research: A review of the past 10 years. Part 1: Physical and emotional abuse and neglect. <u>J Am</u> <u>Acad Child Adolesc Psychiatry, 38</u>(10), 1214-1222.

Kaplan, S., & Weeston, T. (1998). Psychopathology and the role of the child psychiatrist. In J. Monteleone and A. E. Brodeur (Eds.), <u>Child maltreatment:</u> <u>A cinical guide and reference</u> (2nd ed.) (pp. 281-299). St. Louis, MO: GW Medical Publishing, Inc.

Kempe, C.H., Silverman, F.N., Steele, B.F., Droegemueller, W., & Silver, H. K. (1962). The battered-child syndrome. <u>JAMA, 181,</u> 17-24.

Kendall-Tackett, W., Myers, L., & Finkelhor, D. (1993). Impact of sexual abuse on children: A review and synthesis of recent empirical studies. <u>Psychol</u> <u>Bull, 113,</u> 164-180.

Kent, A., & Waller, G. (1998). The impact of childhood emotional abuse: An extension of the child abuse and trauma scale. <u>Child Abuse & Neglect, 22</u>(5), 393-399.

Kluft, R. (1984). Multiple personality in childhood. <u>Psychiatric Clinics of</u> <u>North America, 7</u>(1),121-134.

Landsverk, J., & Hough, R. (1996). Type of maltreatment as a predictor of mental health service use for children in foster care. <u>Child Abuse & Neglect,</u> <u>20</u>(8), 675-688.

McCarroll, J., Newby, J., Thayer, L., Ursano, R., Norwood, A., & Fullerton, C. (1999). Trends in child maltreatment in the US army, 1975-1997. Child Abuse & Neglect, 32(9), 855-861.

McLeer, S., Callaghan, M., Henry, D., & Wallen, J. (1994). Psychiatric disorders in sexually abused children. J Am Acad Child Adolesc Psychiatry, 33(3), 313-319.

McNeese, V., & Monteleone, J. (1996). Sexual abuse in children. In J. Monteleone (Ed.), Recognition of child abuse for the mandated reporter (2nd ed.) (pp. 31-53). St. Louis, MO: GW Medical Publishing, Inc.

Mullen, P. E., Martin, J. L., Anderson, J.C., Romans, S. E., & Herbison, G. P. (1993). Childhood sexual abuse and mental health in adult life. British Journal of Psychiatry, 163, 721-732.

National Center on Child Abuse and Neglect. (1988). Study findings: National study of the incidence and prevalence of child abuse and neglect. Washington, DC: US Department of Health and Human Services.

National Committee to Prevent Child Abuse. (1997). Current trends in child abuse reporting and fatalities: The results of the 1997 annual fifty state survey, paper number 808. Chicago: Author. Retrieved October 11, 2001 from the World Wide Web: www.join-hands.com/welfare/1997castats.html

Pearl, P. (1998). Psychological abuse. In J. Monteleone and A. E. Brodeur (Eds.), Child maltreatment: A clinical guide and reference (2nd ed.) (pp. 371-396). St. Louis, MO: GW Medical Publishing, Inc.

Peterson, G. (1990). Diagnosis of childhood multiple personality disorder. Dissociation, 3, 3-9.

Putnam, F. (1993). Dissociative disorders in children: Behavioral profiles and problems. Child Abuse & Neglect, 17, 39-45.

Putnam, F., Guroff, J.J., Gilberman, E.K., Barban, L., & Post, R.M. (1986). The clinical phenomenology of multiple personality disorder: A review of 100 recent cases. Journal of Clinical Psychiatry, 47, 285-293.

Read, J. (1998). Child abuse and severity of disturbance among adult psychiatric inpatients. Child Abuse & Neglect, 22(5), 359-368.

Silverman, A., Reinherz, H., & Giaconia, R. (1996). The long-term sequelae of child and adolescent abuse: A longitudinal community study. Child Abuse and Neglect, 20(8), 709-723.

Stratakis, C.A., Gold, P.W., & Chrousos, G.P. (1995). Neuroendocrinology of stress: Implications for growth and development. Horm Res, 43,162-167.

Swenson, C. C., & Kolko D. (2000). Long-term management of the developmental consequences of child physical abuse. In R. Reece (Ed.), The treatment of child abuse (pp. 135-154). Baltimore, MD: Hopkins University Press.

Tharinger, C., Horton, B., & Millea, S. (1990). Sexual abuse and exploitation of children and adults with mental retardation and other handicaps. Child Abuse and Neglect, 14, 301-312.

Wonderlich, S., Brewerton, T., Jocic, Z., Dansky, B., & Abbot, D. (1997). Relationship of childhood sexual abuse and eating disorders, J Am Acad Child Adolesc Psychiatry, 36(3), 1107-1115.

Chapter 9

TO REPORT OR NOT TO REPORT...

IS THAT THE ONLY QUESTION?
CHILD MALTREATMENT AND SOCIAL WORK
RESPONSIBILITIES IN ACUTE HEALTHCARE SETTINGS

WILLIAM TIETJEN, M.S.W., L.S.W.

Mandatory reporting of suspected child maltreatment to public welfare agencies has been required of health professionals since the mid-1960s. The initial legal intervention flowed from the pioneering work done earlier in that decade and the resulting societal awareness of a duty to protect children from serious forms of victimization (Helfer & Kempe, 1987). As recognition of this national tragedy increased, so did the development of knowledge about how to identify and intervene with children and their families so that subsequent acts of maltreatment might be avoided. Many models of reporting, intervention, and treatment have emerged over the decades. It has become clear that this work cannot be successful without a firm understanding of both the laws that guide child protection and child welfare services and the clinical phenomenon itself. A critical ingredient for society's competence with this challenge is the capacity of multiple individuals and organizations to coalesce in order to prevent child maltreatment by building strong families and communities.

◆ TO REPORT OR NOT TO REPORT

The healthcare social worker's interactions with a family in which maltreatment is suspected demonstrates a significant and equal obligation to the objectives of child welfare and child protection. This is not a statement that separates child welfare from child protection services, but rather one that joins them as components of the same legal and clinical equation. Such a framework engages multiple professionals and organizations in a transcending partnership that relates to both child and caregiver over the course of time. From this perspective, a social worker's first duty is to explore what is needed for the safety and well-being of these vulnerable clients. Second, the social worker responds to these needs with the information and resources needed to ensure families can be competent as caregivers who will provide for this safety.

When a suspected maltreatment assessment rises from a "concern threshold" to a "reporting threshold," initiating involvment of a Child Protective Services (CPS) agency, the objectives of this assessment are not altered (Giardino, Christian, & Giardino, 1997). In fact, the task then becomes how private and public organizations that are community servants in child welfare and child protection will join to serve the needs of the child and caregiver. Viewing this as a trans-organizational process challenges both the mandated reporter's organization and the CPS agency to actively shape their interactions with mutual clients so that both child welfare and child protection can occur. "To report or not to report?" should never be the first or only question asked by healthcare organizations in situations of suspected child maltreatment.

◆ PURPOSE

In the acute healthcare setting, the purposes of identifying suspected child maltreatment are as follows:

1. To provide the required medical care and treatment

2. To understand the immediate causality of the suspected maltreatment and introduce a plan for safety

3. To establish whether or not the situation rises to the level of a mandatory report to a CPS agency and file accordingly

In this order of responsibilities, the reporting of suspected child maltreatment is a secondary duty that is fulfilled only after the primary medical care and treatment obligations have been met.

Embedded in this series of activities is the requirement that all team members maintain a therapeutic relationship with both the child and the caregiver. The necessity for a constructive relationship is based on the premise that no matter what the cause or ultimate disposition of the case may be, the mutual positive experience in such a relationship will provide the best opportunity for an accurate assessment of the situation and the introduction of effective treatment. Respectful interactions build the requisite partnerships to ensure the best outcomes (Ternell & Edwards, 1999).

The social worker contributes to the interdisciplinary practice of child maltreatment through the use of core knowledge and the standards of the profession. Social workers routinely have both opportunity and obligation in the course of their work to intervene to prevent child maltreatment and to treat children and families at risk. They also have the same legal duty to report child maltreatment as other health professionals. The mechanism for fulfilling this mandate is generally outlined in institutional policy and protocol. The professional practice is further described through discipline values and ethics that are captured in the National Association of Social Work (NASW) Code of Ethics (1996) and the National Association of Social Work (NASW) Standards for Child Protection (1981).

Table 9-1 contains the requisite professional behavior, skills, and attributes for social work practice (Bosak & Tietjen, 1996).

Social work's clinical opportunity to intervene in child maltreatment is derived from practice-based principles that emphasize the "individual well-being in a social context and the well-being of society" (NASW Code of Ethics, 1996). With the emphasis on population management in today's healthcare environment, many social workers find that their routine work with children and families who have either acute or chronic illnesses extends over a long term. The social work clients may include families with a current index of maltreatment risk or ones in which maltreatment was previously identified and successfully treated. This framework of practice provides the social worker with the opportunity to be alert for "prevention interventions" that seek to ensure child safety by coaching caregivers to improve their capacities to be competent

> **Table 9-1. Essential Behavior, Skills, and Attributes for Social Work Practice**
>
> **Professional presence**: The ability to be aware of personal influence and its effects on individual and group interactions.
>
> **Critical thinking**: The professional ability to analyze a situation without laboring in irrelevant data. Such analysis accounts for clinical and systems issues concurrently.
>
> **Assertiveness**: A demonstrated ability to effectively communicate professional information both in written and verbal forms.
>
> **Conviction**: The demonstration of passion, desire, and enthusiasm to practice social work and the continuing development of skills for excellent performance.
>
> **Accountability**: The ability to make thoughtful and thorough professional recommendations and to be confident in one's decision-making.
>
> **Change agent/ risk taker**: The social work profession is about change, and successful practitioners are ones who have an ability to influence the change process and not be overrun by it.
>
> **Hopefulness**: A "can do" attitude. The ability to see the opportunities and potential in any situation. The capacity to persevere even in the face of ambiguous or conflictual information.

in their roles with the child. When done well, the logical conclusion of this routine preventative work is that child maltreatment is avoided in the first place.

◆ HEALTHCARE SOCIAL WORKER DUTIES

How does the social worker complete his or her duties when participating in an interdisciplinary assessment of suspected child maltreatment? It is done through the careful and sensitive use of a professional relationship with caregivers. This effective working rapport provides for continuous mutual learning between the professional and the caregivers so that the interdisciplinary assessment and care planning can occur most effectively. This professional relationship maintains a focus on the present and a view toward the future that prepares the caregiver for a transition to an improved level of caregiving. The social worker also provides pertinent information and resources in an understandable manner throughout the course of care.

What does the social worker contribute to interdisciplinary assessment and care planning? The social worker contributes a psychosocial assessment that is derived from caregiver data. The assessment is a professional conclusion, with recommendations, that is determined through the application of knowledge about child maltreatment to the specific case.

The social work assessment addresses several key questions for team decision-making:

1. What transpired that caused the child to be presented for medical care? Is the explanation logical and plausible?

2. What other stressors and supports have been in the life of this family? What are the influences of these factors on the situation now? Can they be used positively to ensure safety?

3. Does the caregiver demonstrate an appropriate awareness of the present concerns or danger for the child? Is there both the capacity and the willingness to change the situation?

4. Does this situation rise beyond a "concern threshold" to a "reporting threshold," bringing the local CPS agency into the decision-making team (Giardino, Christian & Giardino, 1997)? What are the recommended approaches in meeting both the medical care requirements and the legal obligations for involving a CPS agency?

♦ THE CLINICAL PROCESS

Kerson has described a framework for the examination of social work practice in health care that applies to child maltreatment (1997). Her "practice in context" approach is built on theoretical constructs that use general systems theory as their base. At the center of the model is an examination of the relationship between the social worker and the client. In that work, she notes that it is the power of the relationship to be "catalytic and enabling" that can make a difference in clients' lives. This energy comes not only from the ability to examine the client and the circumstance, but, more importantly, from the transaction between the client and the provider. A study of the child maltreatment scenario presents a context that is defined by law and by both public agency and organizational mission. A closer examination of this scenario shows that it is what happens between provider and client that can create the vehicle through which the parties can accomplish their goals. This applies to the most contentious and most benign of transactions, and it requires purposeful activity, judgment, and responsibility on the part of the provider (Kerson, 1997).

PREPARATION

The involvement of a social worker in an interdisciplinary assessment requires that the worker become familiar with the presenting information. Such information can be obtained from the physician, nurse, or medical record. The purpose of this pre-interview work is to become familiar with as much as is known or speculated by members of the team in order to establish a preliminary line of psychosocial inquiry. The social worker should be alert to his or her personal response to what has been reported so that it does not interfere with the professional approach to the caregiver. Since an interdisciplinary assessment requires a set of relevant facts, the social worker should predetermine a general line of exploration and be prepared to ask follow-up questions while listening carefully for new areas of inquiry. The social worker should enter into conversation with a caregiver fully prepared to convey a firm command of what exact assessment and care-planning activities will take place and why they are necessary.

INTRODUCTION/ENGAGEMENT

After completing preparation for the initial interview, the social worker begins the function of mutual learning. The social worker should start by establishing his or her identity and role in the process, in addition to determining who the clients are and what they need in order to be constructive participants in the assessment. A simple introduction by name and title is a first step. The caregiver must understand the distinction between the healthcare social worker role that is part of the interdisciplinary medical team and the healthcare social worker role in a CPS agency. The initial moments of the interview are a good time to ask about any previous work with the CPS agency and to explain how the medical organization works in collaboration with the CPS staff. Directness, without ambiguity, is essential. The discussion should be conducted in a nonjudgmental manner that actively invites the caregiver's participation. Attention to verbal and non-verbal cues should also contribute to a relatively positive flow in communication. The social worker should be aware of any developmental, cultural, and linguistic differences and should take them into consideration during the interview.

Having established his or her identity with the caregiver, the social worker should explain the purpose of the interview and what part he or she will be playing with the interdisciplinary team. In this exchange, it is essential to describe the overarching concern for the care and safety of the child and to explain that the caregiver's participation in the assessment is crucial.

Although the caregivers are a part of the assessment process, they do not have absolute decision-making authority with respect to reporting. This apparent paradox can pose a dilemma for the social worker who obtains the unqualified participation by the caregivers through any tacit or unspoken agreement not to involve public agencies. While any information obtained will be used to provide care and treatment, these same disclosures may require that a mandatory report be filed with a CPS agency. A caregiver misunderstanding that if he or she cooperates, no report will be made, should be explored and countered sensitively so as to avoid such problems. Despite the professional's view that the CPS report represents an opportunity for child welfare services, the caregiver may see this as intrusive or coercive.

DATA GATHERING

The social work data collected for the interdisciplinary assessment should include the caregiver explanation about what happened to the child, its meaning to the family, and their understanding of what must happen to make the situation safe for the child.

There are many data compilations that can be used to standardize the psychosocial assessment process (Krugman, 1987; Monteleone, 1996). Inglis (1997), for example, provides a listing as depicted in Table 9-2.

Professionals should anticipate receiving cooperation from the caregiver by acting as if cooperation is simply expected. To do this, it is important to determine what the caregiver wants to say or know about what is happening, to pace conversations comfortably, and to use open-ended questions designed to determine what has happened and what the caregivers need to ensure their

---

Table 9-2. Psychosocial Assessment: Caregiver Questions

Identifying information

    Names, ages, and addresses and phone number(s) of caregiver(s) and child

    Local or referring physician or healthcare professional

Presentation

    Caregiver behavior and appearance

    Caregiver mental status/developmental level

    Evidence of drug or alcohol use

    Ethnic/cultural background

Nature of problem

    How and when did child become injured/ill? (caregiver's description of problem)

    Has this happened before?

    Has your child been injured in the past? If so, when and how? Determine each injury.

    What made caregiver decide to seek medical care?

Family history

    A. Household composition

        Who lives at home?

        With whom does child spend most of his or her time?

        Where do other family members/caregiver(s) reside? (if child is cared for by others)

        Were there other living arrangements in the past (i.e., another caregiver)? If so, why?

    B. Caregiver information

        Who is the primary caregiver?

        With whom does the child spend time?

        Does the caregiver have other responsibilities? If so, what?

        Do caregiver(s) have a history of substance abuse?

    C. Family structure

        Are biological parents, siblings, extended family involved in child's care? How?

Table 9-2. Psychosocial Assessment: Caregiver Questions—*continued*

Who is legal guardian, if not natural parent or caregiver?

Who cares for child when caregiver goes out?

What is a regular day like for the child?

What time does everyone in the family get up?

What do you do in the morning? in the afternoon? in the evening?

Child's history

When does child eat? sleep?

What does child like to do?

Does he or she seem normal for age?

Who does child play with?

How would you describe your child? Describe behavior.

What do you do when your child misbehaves?

What developmental milestones has child achieved? (be specific)

Does your child have any special needs concerning his or her care?

School

Where does child go to school?

Is child in the usual grade for age?

What grades does the child get?

Are there any problems at school with child, other children, or teachers? If so, how are they handled?

Does the child get along with peers?

Environment

Describe the housing situation.

Is there a history of conflict or violence in the home?

Describe employment/financial support.

Is transportation available to family?

Social support

Who helps the caregiver when needed: family, friends, community?

Other social agencies: Has CPS been involved in the past or present? If so, why?

Adapted from Inglis, 1997.

child's well-being. The social worker is responsible for setting the atmosphere through the appropriate use of space, timing, and tone of voice. Clients should be allowed appropriate expressions of anger with redirection as needed. They should be informed continuously about all that is going on in the assessment and the professional interpretation of their situation. All these steps are designed to allow the maximum caregiver participation within his or her capabilities.

TEAM DECISION-MAKING

The social worker condenses the findings from the interview for the interdisciplinary team. While it may be possible to present the full interview, the healthcare social worker should be able to present the relevant facts and professional conclusions about the following points:

- The cause of the child's need for medical attention

- The caregiver capacity to understand the risks and dangers

- The probability that the caregiver will take appropriate actions to ensure the child's safety

- A recommendation about the requirement to report to CPS along with a plan to communicate that to the caregiver

- A recommendation for a transition plan to the next level of care

COMMUNICATION

Recommendations from the assessment, including the social worker's findings and conclusions, should be shared with the caregivers. This should include information about the medical care plans and plans for psychosocial services, including the involvement of the CPS agency. There should be clear direction provided to the caregiver about the steps that will be taken, what will be done for the child and the caregiver, and what the caregiver must do in order to continue to be an active participant in the process.

TRANSITION

As a child and caregiver leave the care of the initial team of professionals, they should be prepared for the next levels of care, whether these occur inside the healthcare organization or in the community. This includes a description of what will happen for the child and family and the identification of other professional parties who may become involved. If a decision has been made to report to the CPS agency, the healthcare social worker should consider making the verbal report in the presence of the caregiver and showing the written report to him or her. If a CPS agency staff member is to be involved at the healthcare organization, the healthcare social worker can introduce that individual to the family. Presenting a review of the team's findings, the course of care with the family, and a summary of expected goals and outcomes would be an important clinical bridge that allows an effective transition of care. Table 9-3 provides a review of the clinical process steps.

♦ SOCIAL WORK FUNCTIONS

The role of the healthcare social worker in a case of suspected child maltreatment is to obtain sufficient psychosocial data so the interdisciplinary team can establish an appropriate plan of care for a child and his or her caregiver. This clinical process has therapeutic opportunities throughout its

Table 9-3. Outline of the Clinical Process
• Preparation
• Introduction/engagement
• Data gathering/synthesizing
• Team decision-making
• Communication
• Transition

course. One of the first lessons in social work practice is that assessment and treatment occur simultaneously. Nowhere is this adage as important as in the work of evaluating a case of suspected child maltreatment. Gathering data to formulate a conclusion about reporting to the CPS agency without simultaneously attending to the immediate and long-term psychosocial needs of a family is not likely to lead to success for either objective.

The healthcare social worker intervenes using a framework of client-focused functions. The social worker establishes an effective working rapport with clients by focusing on the overall tasks in a maltreatment assessment: mutual learning, the provision of information and resources, and transition planning.

MUTUAL LEARNING
The work of assessment and care planning results from a partnership between the social work professional and the client. Listening to questions and concerns allows both the caregiver and the social worker to actively participate in the care planning. In this process of mutual learning (or assessment), the social worker assists the client in identifying his or her own needs and creating plans for meeting them. Safe and adequate care plans are developed with an understanding of the client's problems and strengths.

INFORMATION AND RESOURCES
Wise decisions and good choices are made when clients have adequate information available to them. This relates not only to community resource planning but also to situations in which a client may feel uncertain or frightened about what is immediately ahead. In cases of suspected child maltreatment, caregivers need continuous information during the initial health care assessment and treatment phases. They need to know what the assessment will entail and why, who will be involved in the assessment, and how they can be effective participants.

TRANSITION PLANNING
The work of reconstructing positive relationships can be interrupted by critical medical, psychosocial, or developmental events. If clients learn how to anticipate transitional events, they can be prepared to master them. For suspected child maltreatment, the transitions can include hospitalization for immediate medical care, the establishment of a safety plan, a referral for voluntary child welfare services, the filing of a mandatory child abuse report for investigation (as needed), and the introduction of the CPS personnel.

◆ SOCIAL WORK SERVICES

The healthcare social worker who has organized his or her work using the functions just outlined will employ a combination of services in all interactions with the caregiver. The services include assessment of psychosocial functioning, counseling for care planning and decision-making, social work treatment, and providing information and resources.

ASSESSMENT OF PSYCHOSOCIAL FUNCTIONING

Through an effective working relationship with the caregiver (and the child, if that is developmentally and clinically appropriate), the social worker obtains information on what has happened to the child. The social work professional analyzes this information using current knowledge about the dynamics of child maltreatment and makes a recommendation to the interdisciplinary team. The social worker's psychosocial assessment is used along with the medical findings to make decisions for care and treatment as well as to decide whether to report the incident to the CPS agency. This assessment is not done in the same manner as the investigation that is completed by a CPS agency. The healthcare social worker obtains only sufficient and appropriate data required to provide medical care, determine immediate safety, and assess whether a report is required. Directness about the nature of the inquiry, why the inquiry is being done, and what may follow for the child and caregiver is necessary at all times.

COUNSELING FOR CARE PLANNING AND DECISION-MAKING

When the medical care requirements have been determined, a safety plan formulated, and decisions made regarding the involvement of the CPS agency, the caregivers should be counseled as to what they can expect. Part of this intervention is designed to assist the caregiver in establishing some measure of active control by outlining how they can be constructive participants throughout the course of treatment. Counseling is also an opportunity to prepare them for post-hospital care participation, including care that might involve the CPS agency.

SOCIAL WORK TREATMENT

The healthcare social worker may be called upon to provide clinical treatment services for the family. This can include crisis intervention for situations that develop or grief counseling in anticipation of the possible loss of a child as a result of out-of-home placement or death. Such assessments may take several hours or several days. Should a CPS worker become involved, these services can be jointly offered.

INFORMATION AND RESOURCES

Throughout the course of the work with families in which maltreatment is suspected, it is impossible to provide clients with too much information. If one assumes that a sense of mastery, control, and compliance can be attained by clearly articulating what is to be expected, the importance of sharing information becomes self-evident. When the social worker aims to eliminate surprises and to establish clear expectations, caregivers are allowed the opportunity to practice competency in their roles.

◆ THE LAW

The role and responsibility of any mandated reporter and his or her organization are directed primarily by a clear understanding of jurisdictional laws. There is, however, significant variation in the legislative language about child maltreatment among states, which can lead to an unacceptable rate of either under-reporting or over-reporting of cases (Forman & Bernet, 2000).

In order to prevent these extremes in the identification and reporting of suspected cases of maltreatment, organizational plans must be established based on a clear understanding of the local legislation. This can be a challenge. For example, a review of state laws reveals wide variation regarding the degree of certainty required by a mandated reporter before a report is filed (Forman & Bernet, 2000). These state laws are also transformed into working protocols and definitions by the CPS agency that has been delegated authority for enforcement of the laws. The development of healthcare organizational plans should therefore be informed and guided by both sets of information. The intersection between the law and its operating definition as established by the CPS agency can be a significant point of contention for healthcare organizations. There can be no short cut for advanced, direct communication between representatives of the mandated health agencies and the CPS partner in understanding local standards.

Despite the most carefully described plans and practices, human dimensions will still be introduced into the management of suspected child maltreatment cases. As the severity of the medical situation causes a sense of urgency, there is an understandable desire to find a quick and permanent remedy to a complex set of needs. A variety of both personal and professional opinions can occur within the mandated reporting agency itself or between the mandated medical facility and the CPS agency. In either instance, swift problem-solving is required in order to reconcile differences regarding legal definitions, the interpretation of maltreatment, the duty to report, and care planning. These situations require a clear understanding of law, policy, and procedure. Further, they must be guided by professional assessment and interventions that remain focused on child safety and caregiver capacities to provide for that safety.

HEALTHCARE ORGANIZATION POLICIES AND PROCEDURES REQUIREMENTS

The following is a list of the requirements and policies needed in healthcare organizations:

1. A legal understanding of what constitutes child maltreatment within the organization's jurisdiction

2. An understanding of the working definitions of maltreatment that are established by the public agencies charged to investigate and intervene

3. Pre-established organizational criteria that differentiate the level of concern required for the involvement of child welfare services from the legal threshold to report child maltreatment

◆ PRACTICAL APPLICATIONS

The healthcare assessment objective in all cases of suspected child maltreatment is to provide needed medical care and treatment and a plan for the immediate safety of the child. Sometimes this outcome is possible within the child's family and sometimes it is not. The social worker is required to obtain sufficient data to allow the team to establish an appropriate care plan for the child and family. The plan must include information about events leading up to an injury as well as information about the family's overall psychosocial functioning. The social worker accomplishes this task by establishing an effective therapeutic rapport

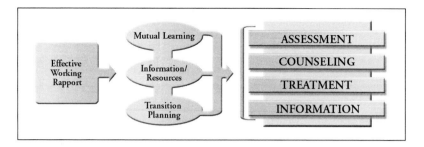

Figure 9-1. *Social work functions and services.*

and organizing the choice of services using the social work functions already outlined (Figure 9-1).

EFFECTIVE WORKING RAPPORT

The work of the healthcare social worker in child maltreatment is accomplished through the establishment and maintenance of an effective working rapport with the family. It is through this relationship that the professionals will best be able to make a reasonable and accurate determination about the medical and psychosocial needs of the child and caregiver(s).

Since the instrument of care is the social worker as an individual person and professional, it is important that the social worker has a firm grasp of his or her own capacity for empathetic understanding of families in which maltreatment has occurred. Without ever condoning acts of maltreatment, the social worker should be able to see through the eyes of the caregivers and work with them in a respectful and constructive manner.

Germain (1984) outlines essential elements in the initial phase of the helping process in the classic text *Social Work Practice in Health Care, An Ecological Perspective*. Germain starts with an emphasis on social worker interactions that will convey empathetic concern, respect, and hopefulness. In applying Germain's thinking to child maltreatment, the social worker is challenged to manage personal and client resistance while exploring and assessing only the factors that bear on the current situation. The relevance of Germain's work to child maltreatment is further demonstrated in her emphasis on balancing the need to collect data with responsiveness to the needs of the caregivers. Finally, rapport and relationship are built as the social worker and caregivers join in the mutual establishment of needs, goals, and actions.

Effective working rapport is maintained through attention to some fundamentals in professional interactions. Introductions of staff members, for example, are important, but so too is an understanding of the role that each will play while working with the family. Social workers in a healthcare organization must be particularly clear in establishing that their affiliation is with the medical facility and not the CPS agency. This is not to separate the potential partnership with the CPS colleague, but rather to be sure that the family knows that there are different roles and responsibilities. Introductions by name and title should be further supplemented by simple explanations about what the social worker is going to do and why he or she is doing it. For example, a caregiver might be told: "I am a social worker here at the hospital. I am part of the team of doctors and nurses who are working with your son today. Doctor Jones and a nurse, Sara, are examining Bobby right now. Our purpose is to take care of his injuries first, but we also need to learn how this happened so that we can help you in seeing that it doesn't happen again. You and I will have a conversation, and then I will ask Dr. Jones and Sara to join us and together we will make a recommendation to you."

Clients must have sufficient information and direction available in understandable terms to allow them to participate appropriately, especially at the early stages of the process. In a complicated child maltreatment assessment, there can be significant emotion among the team members concerning the circumstances of the injury, and this can fuel client anxiety. Providing information about who is involved, their roles and responsibilities, and an explanation of why they are doing certain things can often ameliorate client distress. Effective working rapport is established and maintained through an appreciation of the continuing need of the caregivers for dignity and respect despite any culpability for the injuries. Simple gestures to maintain rapport include providing a private place to talk and keeping the information about the assessment restricted to only those who need to know it. Effective working rapport is also developed when all professionals demonstrate the ability to competently handle the sad, angry, or contrary behaviors of a caregiver. When social workers can help clients maintain a constructive role in the assessment and care planning process, the clients are reassured that they are in competent professional hands. A client who is threatening or intimidating can be advised that his or her behavior is not acceptable and that there are consequences of such behavior. For example: "By raising your voice now and threatening to leave with your child, others might incorrectly conclude that you have something to hide. What I would like you to do is to stay with me and tell me more about what happened so that we can make a reasonable determination about how we will best be able to help you make your child safe." The level of success in meeting the child welfare and child protection goals of the assessment often depends on how well the initial rapport is established.

MUTUAL LEARNING

The exercise of evaluating a suspected case of maltreatment calls for mutual learning between the caregiver and the social worker. At its center is the balance of learning about what the client needs while displaying and reporting what the social worker can do in relation to those needs. Once the social worker has done an introduction and initial gestures have been made to establish an effective working rapport, the next step is to discover why the child has come or been brought to the facility. This task is accomplished not only by focusing on the facts but also by maintaining sensitivity to the caregiver's fears about what has happened to his or her child and the consequences of the events. This capacity for mutual learning requires the professional to be clear about his or her function and role in cases of suspected child maltreatment. It further requires that the professional has the interpersonal skills for advancing a dynamic situation confidently and empathetically without becoming overly identified or under-involved with the family.

The social worker should introduce the possibility that a mandatory report to a CPS agency could become necessary in the earliest phase of a serious child maltreatment assessment. Caregivers may already have anticipated this course of action, and their concern should be addressed directly. Asking a series of probing questions without adequate explanation can only lead to undue anxiety, resistance, or resentment. An appropriate response to an anxious question from a caregiver might be, for example: "Yes, I am a mandated reporter under state law and I am obligated under that law and our hospital procedures to notify the CPS agency when a situation warrants it. I don't know if that is the case with your family. I would like you to help me answer that question. Whether we make a report to CPS or not, our goals will be the same: the safety of your child and your ability to care for him appropriately."

If the initial presentation of the child makes a CPS report inevitable (as in the case of severe trauma or neglect), the obligation to report and its purpose and impact on the family should be addressed early and directly. For example: "As you know, your son has sustained severe injuries and you've told us that this wasn't an accident. By law, the hospital is required to report this matter to the CPS agency. The purpose of this reporting is to introduce services that will allow your child to be safe."

Healthcare social workers in this situation should be careful that they do not attempt to represent the decision-making of the public agency. Once an individual CPS social worker has been identified, the healthcare-based social worker should collaborate with this CPS colleague and plan communication about the post-hospital care with the caregivers.

Once there has been an interdisciplinary team decision about care plans and a decision to make a report to a CPS agency, that fact should be communicated to the caregiver in clear terms that he or she can understand. This can be done with any combination of individuals from the team as long as the focus is maintained on the effectiveness of the communication. As in other parts of the assessment and care-planning process, the caregiver should be given information about what will happen next and what will be expected of him or her.

The presentation of a suspected case of child maltreatment gives rise to many feelings and expectations for action by team members. Depending on the severity of the injuries and the patient's medical and social prognosis, the social worker and other healthcare providers may inadvertently display abruptness that may be offensive to the caregiver. Staff members who are adjacent to the situation but not directly involved in the case may unwittingly add to the emotional drama by inquiring about the situation or milling in the area where the assessment is taking place. The specifics of this scene vary, but all share the common opportunity to be reshaped by professionals who wish the caregiver to become actively engaged in the assessment and treatment functions embedded in this evaluation.

Caregivers who have brought a child for medical care after a possible act of maltreatment should be presumed to be asking for help. Professionals must avoid intentionally or unintentionally subjecting a caregiver to inappropriate interactions as punishment because their values and sensitivities have been offended. Indeed, professional codes of ethical conduct require a clear obligation to treat all clients with professional excellence and respect. While it may be a challenge to see a caregiver who has seriously injured a child as a needy individual in his or her own right, professional objectivity is essential. There is no justification for less than professional interactions with a suspected abuser.

The manner in which an assessment is conducted contributes positively or negatively to the goal of maintaining an effective working rapport. Treating a caregiver with an investigative authority but without concern for the person as an individual contributes to resistance and even contrary behavior. Positive interaction with caregivers predisposes the relationship toward mutually beneficial outcomes that ensure child safety and competent family functioning.

Transition Planning

The decision to make a report under the state laws is a point of transition because it introduces additional professionals into the situation. This transition to CPS can be made easier or more difficult by virtue of how the hospital and CPS staff describe each other to the caregiver and how they relate to each other over the course of their mutual work with the family. The healthcare professionals and the CPS professionals must have a true partnership in order to be most effective with these children and their caregivers.

There are several ways in which inter-organizational collaboration can be displayed so that effective working rapport can transcend hospital boundaries. Reports of suspected child maltreatment generally require that a mandated reporter place a telephone call to a statewide hotline and then follow up with a written report to the CPS agency. Once a decision has been made to file a report it is important for the caregiver to know what is actually being reported. Showing the caregiver the actual written document that will be filed with the state report and even having him or her present as the phone call is made to a hotline can be useful. While allowing the caregiver to witness these activities, the healthcare social worker has an opportunity to summarize for the state agent what has transpired at the hospital and what it is that the caregiver understands will be taking place with the CPS agency. The purpose of including the caregiver in this activity is two-fold. One is to diminish the caregiver fear that something more is being said or reported than was disclosed to him or her. The second is that, by witnessing the professional agency interaction, the caregiver can appreciate the professional collaboration between the private and public institutions, and their mutual confidence and common purpose. Obviously, the strength of the inter-organizational relationships should be well-established before this activity.

If the situation is such that a CPS worker will be coming to the hospital, the social worker at the hospital should first convey to the CPS worker the course of the interdisciplinary work to that point. It would be helpful to not only describe the challenges of working with the caregiver through the assessment but also to share what has proven an effective way to engage the caregiver. A social worker might report, for example, that despite initial concerns about talking to hospital staff, a caregiver responded to a particular staff member quite well. The social worker could then suggest that the individual be present as the CPS worker is introduced to the caregiver. The CPS worker should also be informed if the team discovers more caregiver compliance after overcoming a caregiver's cognitive limitations. After this information has been exchanged, the hospital team and the CPS worker should plan to meet the caregivers.

When meeting with the caregiver, the hospital social worker should introduce the CPS worker, and briefly describe once again why this individual was brought into the case and what he or she will be doing. The hospital social worker's ability to confidently introduce the public sector colleague and that agency's capabilities will help the caregiver through the transition to this new professional. As a way of building a connection with the CPS agency, the hospital social worker should summarize the assessment and the recommendations of the healthcare team and comment on the caregiver's understanding of this plan. There should be a frank discussion about how the caregiver participated in the process at the hospital and how that experience can be used as the CPS social worker begins to work. Finally, there should be an expressed goal to pass on the hospital staff's effective working rapport with the caregiver to the CPS worker.

This same process of transition should be maintained as a patient moves from an emergency department to an inpatient service and a new care team. It is also relevant at those times when a child may be discharged to a foster home. Whatever has been learned during the working relationship with a particular family should be thought of as a cumulative commodity that can be passed on to new parties who will be involved in the family's care.

◆ THE IMPOSSIBLE SITUATION

"Impossible situations" in child maltreatment seem to be innumerable. This description tends to be used when frustration on the part of the professionals is generated by the presentation of a severely injured child and a caregiver who is very contrary in behavior. A hopeful worldview would suggest that unpredictable behavior is understandable under the circumstances, and that it is a call for help. Social workers, and all health professionals, must answer the call with optimism that developing a caregiver's capacity to be competent in the care of children is more often than not an achievable goal. A first step toward this goal is an effective working relationship, established by professionally addressing ambivalence, passivity, or frank resistance on the part of the caregiver.

No matter what the presenting circumstance and behavior of a family, both the child and the caregivers have an unqualified right to a thorough evaluation of their medical and psychosocial needs that will result in professional recommendations best suited to meeting short- and long-term needs. The conclusions are derived from the professional assembly of information within compassionate and caring transactions that are designed to assure the safety of the child and the competence of the caregivers.

Team members should also treat each other thoughtfully. Stress that develops in the challenging situations of dealing with child maltreatment can invade otherwise collaborative interactions among professionals. Individuals should be alert for the inappropriate expression of this tension among team members and even with the family. It is not unreasonable for a difference of professional opinion or feeling to be present; it is, however, unacceptable to allow this to cause conflict that interferes with service delivery and team performance. Each professional's work must be valued and respected as a part of the treatment plan.

◆ REFERENCES

Bosak, M., & Tietjen, W. R. (1996). <u>Workshop: Continuous Career Improvement for the Reforming Health Care Environment.</u> Kansas City, MO: 31st Annual Meeting and Educational Conference of the Society for Social Work Leadership in Health Care.

Forman, T., & Bernet, W. (2000). A misunderstanding regarding the duty to report suspected abuse. <u>Child Maltreatment, 5</u>(2), 190-196.

Germain, C. B. (1984). <u>Social work practice in health care: An ecological perspective</u> (pp. 97-124). New York: The Free Press.

Giardino, A., Christian, C., & Giardino, E. (Eds.). (1997). <u>A practical guide to the evaluation of child physical abuse and neglect</u> (p. 24). Thousand Oaks, CA: SAGE Publications.

Helfer, R. E., & Kempe, R. S. (Eds.). (1987). <u>The battered child</u> (4th ed.). Chicago: University of Chicago Press.

Inglis, J.D. (1997). Psychosocial assessment. In A. Giardino, C. Christian, and E. Giardino (Eds.), <u>A practical guide to the evaluation of child physical abuse and neglect</u> (pp. 233-245). Thousand Oaks, CA: SAGE Publications.

Kerson, T. S. (1997). <u>Social work in health settings: Practice in context</u> (2nd ed.) (pp.15-39). New York: The Haworth Press.

Krugman, R. (1987).The assessment process of a child protection team. In R. E. Helfer and R. S. Kempe (Eds.), <u>The battered child</u> (4th ed.). Chicago: University of Chicago Press.

Monteleone, J.A. (Ed.). (1996). <u>Recognition of child abuse for the mandated reporter</u> (2nd ed.) (pp. 16-17). St. Louis, MO: G.W. Publishing, Inc.

National Association of Social Workers (NASW). (1996). <u>Code of Ethics.</u> Washington, DC: NASW Press.

NASW Task Force on Social Work Practice. (1981). <u>NASW Standards for Social Work Practice in Child Protection.</u> Washington, DC: NASW Press.

Turnell, A., & Edwards, S. (1999). <u>Signs of safety: A solution and safety oriented approach to child protection casework</u> (pp.29-83). New York: W.W. Norton & Company.

Chapter 10

THE ROLE OF THE SCHOOLS IN CHILD ABUSE

PEGGY S. PEARL, ED.D.

Schools have legal and ethical reasons to be involved in cases of child maltreatment. Whether the primary reporter of the maltreatment, the alleged perpetrator, or a collateral in an investigation, school personnel should know the legal issues pertaining to child maltreatment. For various reasons, teachers may be reluctant to report their concerns to child protective service agencies, but no reasoning removes the legal requirement for involvement. Beyond this legal requirement, schools have ethical obligations to participate in community efforts to improve the well-being of all children. Data consistently show that educational professionals take their role as mandated reporters very seriously and that they make a large percentage of the reports of child abuse and neglect (Sedlak & Broadhurst, 1996).

◆ REPORTING STATUTES

WHO REPORTS?

Currently, teachers in all fifty states, U.S. territories, and the District of Columbia are mandated by law to report any suspected child maltreatment to the state protective services child abuse hotline. In addition to fulfilling legal obligations, school personnel provide valuable assistance to families in crisis by filing these reports. Because child abuse is a symptom of a family needing help, schools can best aid parents in accessing assistance by alerting the child protective services of possible child maltreatment. Each state's statutes define child abuse, provide confidentiality to reporters, and specify who shall and who may report. For a list of the state protective services agencies, see Appendix I at the end of this chapter.

The law requires teachers to report immediately to the state protective services agency if they "suspect or have reason to believe" children are being mistreated. No state requires that individuals who make reports to the state child abuse hotline prove that the abuse has occurred before making the report, as that will be determined during the subsequent investigation (Kalichman, 1993; Romeo, 2000; Tower, 1992; U.S. Department of Health and Human Services [USDHHS], 1992; USDHHS, Children's Bureau, 1998).

CONTENTS OF THE REPORT

The information necessary for making the report commonly includes the following:

1. Name of the child who is the alleged victim

2. Age of the child

3. Home address or address where the child can be located

4. Parent(s) name(s), phone number(s), and address(es), if known

5. Type of abuse

6. Alleged perpetrator. (Some states will ask, but most of the time the reporter will not know the perpetrator and should not make unfounded allegations. If the child told the reporter, then this information should be included as part of the report.)

7. Specific indicators of the maltreatment (what exactly led the reporter to make the report)

8. Whether this is an emergency or if the child is in imminent danger

9. Name, phone number, and address of the reporter. (Some states allow anonymous reports, but knowing the name and phone number allows the state agency to obtain additional information if necessary.)

The determination of whether abuse occurred rests with the state protective services agency.

LEVEL OF PROOF REQUIRED TO REPORT

Because no state requires that those individuals who make reports in good faith to the state child abuse hotline prove that abuse has occurred before making the report, most child protective services agencies do some initial screening when they receive a report (Tower, 1992; USDHHS, Children's Bureau, 1998). Therefore, the individual taking the child abuse report will ask for as many details as the reporter can give. It is recommended that reporters write down specific facts before making the report. This will ensure that all the known details are reported to the child protective services. If left to memory, some important details may be inadvertently omitted.

PENALTY FOR NOT REPORTING

Nearly every state has a penalty for mandated reporters not reporting child maltreatment, ranging from a misdemeanor to a felony charge. In recent years, states have begun to prosecute individuals for noncompliance with reporting statutes. In some states, mandated reporters may be convicted whether or not they knew a report was required and regardless of whether the failure was deliberate or a case of negligence (Caulfield, 1979, 1981; Tower, 1992; USDHHS, Children's Bureau, 1998). Individuals and/or school districts may also be sued in civil court for not reporting suspected abuse. The civil action will not result in imprisonment of the negligent staff member but will result in a financial award to the individual filing the case. Considering the litigious nature of contemporary society, individuals and school districts should follow state statutes, district policy, and their own moral obligations when deciding whether or not to make a report of child maltreatment.

IMMUNITY FROM CRIMINAL PROSECUTION AND CIVIL LIABILITY

Every state, territory, and the District of Columbia provides immunity from civil liability and criminal penalty for mandated reporters who report in good faith. Good faith means that the individual understood the indicators of child abuse, observed those indicators, and/or was told by a child of maltreatment, and therefore had reason to suspect or believe that abuse had occurred and made the report without malice or specific intent to harm (Tower, 1992).

◆ SCHOOL POLICIES ON REPORTING

PURPOSE OF THE POLICY

All school districts should have a clear and specific written policy dealing with reporting child maltreatment. This should be distributed to all school district professional staff and parents. Having a specific written protocol ensures that every child is protected equally under state laws. Additionally, it gives school personnel, including teachers, nurses, counselors, social workers, and administrators, the guidance needed regarding specific steps to be taken and how to fulfill the state statute. The school district protocol supports teachers and reduces their feelings of vulnerability when they are reporting. The standardized policy prevents some children's needs from being ignored, some parents from being the victims of prejudice, and some personnel from becoming overzealous. Review of the policy must be part of regular in-service training for all staff. Topics for staff in-service training should include identification of symptoms indicating child abuse and neglect, protocol for reporting child abuse, and techniques for working with child abuse victims in the classroom.

CONTENTS OF THE POLICY

The statutes of each state will determine the specific requirements to be included in a child abuse reporting policy. The exact wording of these statutes varies from state to state. The policy should be written by an interdisciplinary task force that includes, among others, parents and teachers. A sample policy is in Appendix II at the end of this chapter. The policy should address all forms of child maltreatment, including alleged abuse by school district personnel. Also included are the written notations to be placed in the student's file documenting specifically what was observed, when, and by whom. Since most child abuse is a pattern of incidents rather than a single event, the student's file may have several entries. If a single incident does not clearly indicate abuse, a mandated reporter may choose to wait to make an official report until a developing pattern of incidents raises his or her suspicion. However, if the behavioral indicators are clear or the child tells an adult of the abuse, it should be reported immediately. Policies vary regarding who actually makes the phone call. Some school districts designate one person (counselor, nurse, principal, or teacher) to receive all the information and make all calls, usually with the individual who began the process present. Other school districts instruct the individual with the concern to make the hotline call, usually in the presence of the counselor or building principal, and then to write a summary of what was said for the student file. Some states send mandated reporters a form to complete and mail to the child abuse hotline following the phone report. The summary should include the date and time of the report, the name of the person accepting the call, the details given to the hotline personnel, and the name of any other school personnel consulted in making the decision to report the suspected abuse (Halperin, 1979; Kalichman, 1993; Tower, 1992; USDHHS, 1998).

After a case is reported to the child protective services agency, there should be a follow-up procedure. Some states automatically provide follow-up information to mandated reporters. In others, the reporter will need to inquire about the disposition of the case. In still other states, confidentiality requirements may prevent the sharing of information between child protective services and the public schools.

The Federal Family Educational Rights and Privacy Act of 1974 (FERPA), which governs the release of information from school records, does not bar the reporting of suspected child abuse and neglect by educators. In most cases, educators rely on their own knowledge and observations when reporting suspected child abuse and neglect, not school records. Therefore FERPA does not generally apply because no school records are involved. In a small number of cases it may be necessary for child protective services agencies to consult school records to determine whether a suspected child abuse and neglect report should be made. Ordinarily, parental consent is required before information contained in school records can be released. However, exceptions can be applied in cases of suspected abuse and neglect. Prior parental consent is not required when disclosing information from school records if a "health or safety emergency" exists. It is the position of the National Center on Child Abuse and Neglect (NCCAN) and the Fair Information Practice Staff (the federal unit that administers FERPA) that child abuse or neglect is generally considered a "health or safety emergency" if the state definition of child abuse and neglect is limited to situations in which a child's health or safety is endangered. NCCAN and the Fair Information Practice Staff agree that the responsibility for determining whether a "health or safety emergency" exists must be accepted by the school official involved on a case-by-case basis. Thus, if a school official determines that an emergency exists, information in records can be disclosed without parental consent and without violating the provisions of FERPA.

Another exception to the prior consent rule exists if the release of information in school records is made to particular officials to whom such disclosure is required by state statute, if the statute was adopted before November 19, 1974. The National Education Association 1984 study of legal regulations affecting teachers compiled all state child abuse and neglect reporting statutes that require reporting by educators to state or local authorities. Most were enacted before November 19, 1974, so in most states the release of information from school records to state or local child protective services agencies is permitted under FERPA. Educators and school districts should check with legal counsel to be certain whether a particular state enacted a reporting law before November 19, 1974, and to determine whether this exception to the FERPA provision applies in their jurisdiction (Caulfield, 1979; Tower, 1992).

REPORTING INSTITUTIONAL ABUSE

School districts should include in the child abuse reporting policy the protocol to be followed when a school employee is the alleged perpetrator. If the individual has direct supervision of children, the school district must determine if the school employee can continue with this assignment. Several options must be considered while the investigation is being conducted (Tower, 1992):

- Will the employee be moved to another position without contact with children?

- Will the employee be placed on unpaid leave?

- Will the employee be placed on paid leave?

- Will there be a change in the supervision of the employee?

- Will the employee retain access to children?

Most investigations take about 30 days, sometimes longer. When the individual's position does not require direct supervision of children, such as school district office personnel, financial officers, or maintenance staff, removal from the position during the investigation may not be warranted.

When a report is made, the principal or other school administrator should attempt to gather facts rather than defend the staff member or school system. It is inappropriate for the school official to become defensive. All findings must be documented. School officials must determine if or when legal counsel for the school and/or staff member should be involved in the process. As with any case of suspected child abuse and neglect, the interview of the child should be conducted by protective services and/or law enforcement investigators to prevent excessive hardship on the child. State law varies slightly as to what agency investigates cases of abuse and neglect outside of the child's home—protective services, the juvenile court, or law enforcement officials. Depending on the situation, the school system may be named as the alleged perpetrator.

When the parent comes to the school to report the instance, the principal should listen carefully and take notes concerning what is said. The principal should maintain an open attitude and listen without becoming defensive, accusing staff, or denying accusations. During the discussion, the principal should make it known to the parent that a report to the state child abuse and neglect hotline is the next appropriate action. The school must keep a record of the entire discussion. In most instances, the individual named in the allegation should not be told of the allegation until interviewed by the investigative worker. The school administrator should then meet with the staff member to hear his or her version of what happened. Next the administrator should meet with any other people named by the child or the alleged perpetrator to gather related information.

Children with special needs are at high risk for abuse from all child caregivers, including parents and teachers. Selection of teachers to work with these children is especially important. The in-service training of individuals who work with children with special needs should include the particular areas they must deal with, for example, restraint, personal hygiene care, or isolation. The teacher working with a team of professionals must regularly re-evaluate the developmental appropriateness of all classroom procedures and practices. The Individualized Education Plan (IEP) should be carefully monitored to ensure that all procedures, policies, and activities are consistent with the goals stated in it.

◆ ONCE A REPORT IS MADE

Once a report to the state child abuse and neglect hotline has been made, school staff should continue to be supportive of the child. By its very nature, disclosing child abuse, especially sexual abuse, becomes a crisis for the child and family. The following can be supportive responses to the child:

- Treat the child in the same way before and after the report. Many times a child is pitied or is treated as if he or she has been "broken" or "damaged."

- Treat the child with respect and understanding; be sensitive to the child's needs.

- Be sensitive to times when the child may need to be alone or to talk.

- Be aware of mood changes. Children often feel depressed or anxious after a report. Frequently, especially with sexual abuse, this rethinking and depression or anxiety lead the child to recant the story. When a child recants the story of abuse, the professional should not assume that the abuse did not occur.

- Help the sexual abuse victim avoid inappropriately touching others by defining appropriate behaviors.

- Listen when the child appears to want to talk, but do not quiz. Observe and respond to nonverbal communication.

- Praise the child for his or her courage in reporting and assure the child that it was not his or her fault.

- *DO NOT* promise the child that the abuse will never happen again (that cannot be guaranteed).

- Provide the child with opportunities to feel in control of self and the environment.

Maltreated children have been manipulated into silence. A powerful, often trusted, and assumed knowledgeable individual may convince the child to stay silent by making statements such as the following:

"It is OK not to tell this secret. No one else will understand."

"Your mother knows and approves."

"If you tell, it will break up your family."

"If you tell, I will kill your mother."

"If you tell, I will go to jail."

These are powerful statements. Children need permission and authority to tell their secret. After they share the secret, they need support. Whatever the secret, children fear what will happen next, that no one will believe them, or that they will be punished. Children need a nonpunitive, nonconfrontational environment in which they are valued and given control over their lives following the report.

DISCIPLINE IN SCHOOLS

Although corporal punishment is legal in many states, school districts should institute policies that prohibit corporal punishment of children. Research shows that corporal punishment is associated with the following effects (Straus, 1994; Wissow, 1990):

- Negative influence on learning

- Increased aggressive behavior in children

- Increased fearfulness and anxiety in children

- Failure to encourage children to learn self-discipline

Teachers should be taught alternative methods of discipline and positive guidance techniques. Schools can then serve as role models for nonviolent conflict resolution for this and future generations of parents (NCPCA, 1987; Straus, 1994).

All schools should have a written policy outlining appropriate discipline techniques that have been approved by parents, teachers, and other school personnel. This policy is provided to all parents when their children enroll in school. Some schools require that parents read the statement and sign it, indicating that they have read and understand the policy. Other districts allow parents to exercise other options if they disagree with the stated policy. For example, some districts state that corporal punishment will be used unless parents present a signed statement that they do not want it used. Others allow corporal punishment only for children whose parents have given specific written consent. Schools should establish clear rules and expectations of students and provide projected non-violent consequences for failure to comply with these rules. Written discipline policies should include at least the following information:

A statement of the program's philosophy regarding guiding children's behavior:

1. The goal of discipline is to help children learn self-control.

2. Discipline techniques reflect realistic expectations for children's behavior based on an understanding of child development.

3. Positive guidance techniques are individualized, based on the situation and the child's age and stage of development.

4. Corporal punishment and isolation of children are prohibited.

5. Children will not be subjected to verbal outbursts or remarks that are belittling or intimidating.

6. Discipline approaches will help children to develop problem-solving skills and learn the logical consequences of behavior.

7. Examples of positive guidance techniques appropriate for children of different ages.

8. Designation of who will discipline children and under what conditions.

9. Designated point at which parents will be asked to participate in planning strategies to help children overcome troublesome behaviors.

10. Methods for staff to assess the effectiveness of the discipline techniques being used.

Instituted policies that reduce the need for punishment, such as the following:

1. Provide students with choices and options for decision-making.

2. Make sure students know the school's expectations and the consequences for noncompliance.

3. Provide predictable routine in attractive, orderly, and effective classrooms.

4. Increase positive interactions with adults inside and outside the classroom.

5. Ensure developmentally appropriate curriculum.

6. Provide opportunities to assist others in meaningful ways.

7. Ensure that there are opportunities for students to feel pride in themselves in a cultural context.

8. Encourage all school personnel to be alert and observant of individual students as well as the total environment to ensure appropriateness of these policies.

More positive reinforcement for students also emphasizes what is right and prevents the assaults on the child's self-esteem commonly seen in the use of physical punishment (Green, 1988; NCPCA, 1987; Straus, 1994; Tite, 1993).

FALSE ALLEGATIONS

After an allegation has been made and an investigation carried out, the charge may be found to be false. False allegations come from various sources and reflect many different motivations. Children who falsely accuse do so for a variety of reasons. They may be disturbed, seeking attention, coached by someone else, or seeking revenge; alternatively, they may simply be misinterpreted. Determining the reason that a false report was made can often help both the child and the alleged perpetrator (Tite, 1993; Tower, 1992).

DEFENSE AGAINST ABUSE IN SCHOOL

The best defenses against both abuse and false allegations are education, supervision, and open communication. School personnel should be regularly educated on what is and is not a developmentally appropriate environment for children of various ages. Additionally, educating children about good touch and bad touch helps them understand the appropriate adult-child relationship and their rights in such situations (Anderson & Levine, 1999; Powers, Jaklitsch, & Eckenrode, 1989; Straus, 1994; Tite, 1993).

Supervision of school personnel can be an important prevention technique. Are all personnel appropriately qualified for their position? Do they have adequate in-service training and supervision? Do they have opportunities to discuss situations with a supportive individual before the situation becomes a crisis? Do personnel have opportunities to provide and receive peer support? Are all personnel treated with respect, given opportunities to make appropriate professional decisions, and valued as contributing members of the educational team? Staff need opportunities to collaborate with peers. The collaborative effort will allow sharing of expertise and building on strengths to improve professional practice. Staff members who support each other will be better able to support and respect the strengths of the children and families they work with.

Openness means that parents are encouraged to participate in the school and that there are few, if any, places where staff can be alone with children in the school. Window shades or curtains should be removed from windows or should be readily movable, except when needed for specific purposes (Anderson & Levine, 1999). Openness also means that children are only alone in a room or office with an adult when there is a specific reason, such as individual testing or counseling. Appropriate supervision of the rest rooms in elementary schools should ensure that no adults are routinely alone with one or two children. The openness of a school facilitates improved communication and support between staff and with parents.

In some instances, however, access to the school should be controlled. Individuals who are not staff should routinely sign in and out of the office so that the school administration is aware of who is in the building. Additionally, the requirement to sign in may deter some individuals who have no appropriate reason for being in the school. The routine sign-in policy should not deter parents from entry but should provide them with a feeling of safety for their children.

◆ SELECTION OF PERSONNEL

Prevention of child maltreatment in school is heavily based on the selection of appropriate school personnel. The process involves writing clear, detailed job descriptions and qualifications, conducting in-depth interviews, performing reference checks and background checks, observing candidates with children (if appropriate to the position), and doing an evaluation after a probationary period.

BACKGROUND RECORD CHECKS

All personnel who work with children must be carefully screened before employment. This screening should be complete and comprehensive. Some state statutes require both a criminal records background check and a child abuse and neglect hotline check of individuals who have the care, custody, and control of a child outside of the child's home. This requires asking the individual for permission to check with federal and state law enforcement officials, as well as the state child protective services agency. Requiring applicants to sign a form giving permission will itself screen or eliminate some who have a history of mistreating children.

The purpose of the background check is to determine if the applicant has a history of conviction or a conviction pending involving any of a variety of crimes, including child abduction, child pornography, child sexual assault, assault, murder, rape, kidnapping, and/or other violent crimes. If an individual's background checks reveal no record, however, it does not necessarily mean the individual has no criminal history. The check reports only the legal record in the specific geographic area checked for the specific crimes identified. Many abusers have never been reported, investigated, confirmed, or prosecuted. Therefore the check is only one piece of the process. The same screening process may be extended to include volunteers when the volunteer is not under the constant, direct supervision of a professional staff person.

INTERVIEWING

The interview should involve more than one interviewer. Each applicant should be interviewed in at least two situations and should be asked the same series of questions to determine appropriateness to work with children. A list of sample questions is given in Table 10-1. For record-keeping purposes, when many individuals are applying and being interviewed, applicants may be asked to respond to some questions in writing. For example, the applicant may be presented with two or three typical classroom situations and asked how he or she would handle each one. Because of the intensity of the position, working with children is naturally stressful. A sense of humor may help individuals deal with the routine job stress. Therefore evidence of a sense of humor may indicate that the individual could handle various stressful situations and not mistreat children.

Table 10-1. Sample Interview Questions

- What children's behaviors make you angry and how do you cope with that anger?

- What would you do if a child threw a rolled up paper at another child across the room? What would you do if a child hit another child?

- Give a couple of examples of situations in which you were successful in disciplining a child.

- How do you handle the routine stress of working with children?

- What have you done to increase parent involvement in your classroom?

- Describe a normal classroom appropriate to the grade level you are applying for. What type of routine would you follow? What would it look like? What would the children be doing? What would you be doing?

The screening process can involve interview questions relating to how the individual would handle a series of common discipline situations. These questions help determine the applicant's knowledge of child growth and development as well as methods of positive discipline. They can be especially helpful in screening for individuals who may be at risk to verbally or emotionally abuse children. Questions relating to normal expectations and classroom routine should provide insight into how age-appropriate the applicant's expectations are and how the applicant sees the adult-child relationship.

The interviewer is permitted to ask questions that are directly related to the job. Questions cannot relate to how the applicant was disciplined as a child nor to how the applicant disciplines his or her own children. It is not job related or appropriate to ask how the individual deals with stress, handles crises, or manages time and resources. It is not job related or appropriate to ask whether the applicant has a history of maltreatment, mental illness, or substance abuse.

REFERENCE CHECKS

Checking references from previous employers is also an important part of the screening process. Reference checks should be extended beyond written letters. Phone calls to persons given as references who have worked directly with and supervised the individual are important sources of information. Specifically, all previous employers should be asked if they would re-employ the individual. Questions should also be asked about what discipline techniques the individual used, and the answers should be compared to those given by the applicant. Other questions for professional references could include the following:

1. When and where was the applicant observed working with children?

2. Did the applicant routinely ask for support from supervisors or colleagues when needed?

3. Did the applicant appropriately use solicited information?

4. How does the applicant handle criticism and frustration on the job?

5. What skills does the applicant demonstrate in working with children?

6. How does the applicant communicate with students? with parents? with co-workers? with supervisors?

7. How does the applicant demonstrate knowledge of child growth and development?

8. How does the applicant build self-esteem in children?

If an applicant is employed at the time of the interview, permission to contact the current employer should be requested. It is important to listen carefully to what each reference says about the applicant; the interviewer should add a written summary of each interview to the information in the applicant's file. Although it may seem unnecessary, school personnel should always verify the college degree and teaching credentials of each applicant by examining official documents, not copies or a resume.

◆ OTHER POLICY CONSIDERATIONS

IN-SERVICE TRAINING OF STAFF AND VOLUNTEERS

Routine in-service education for teachers, counselors, social workers, nurses, librarians, and administrators should include such topics as indicators of child maltreatment (neglect or physical, emotional, and sexual abuse), the reporting process, and working with victims in the classroom. Other topics to be included should relate to special areas within these more global topics, such as the psychosocial needs of homeless children and the impact of media and community violence on children. Building self-esteem, reinforcing assertive behaviors, praising children, and teaching interpersonal communication skills are also important topics for teachers to explore in their own career development.

Some indicators of child abuse are physically obvious or directly stated, but most are not. In addition to recognizing non-specific behavioral indicators, teachers and school personnel need to know that there is a strong relationship between animal abuse and child abuse. Families that abuse or mistreat pets and other animals frequently mistreat children. When children tell of inappropriate violence and failure to care for animals at home, this is a "red flag" to indicate they also may have been abused. Children who mistreat pets and other animals may be victims of abuse themselves. When a child speaks of his or her own cruelty to animals, adults should realize the child is in desperate need of counseling and individual services. When one child bullies another, this too may be an indicator that something is wrong with the way he or she has been treated—another red flag and evidence that a referral to counseling is needed (Loar & White, 1998; Arkow, 1998).

SCREENING VOLUNTEERS

A specific screening process for volunteers should be developed for each school district by a committee of administrators, teachers, and parents. For the safety of the children, non-parents with an open protective services case, a case under investigation, or a conviction or pending criminal prosecution should not be allowed to volunteer in the school or at school-sponsored activities. Parents with open protective services cases should not be automatically screened out of volunteering in the child's school. These parents need to be a part of the school district's parent involvement program to improve their parenting skills, reduce social isolation, and learn more about the resources available to them and their children. Within the parent-friendly school, many opportunities should be available to learn positive parenting skills as well as improve the parents' self-esteem. The important issue is placement of all volunteers where they are appropriately supervised and never left alone with children.

SUPERVISION OF VOLUNTEERS

Volunteers add to the effectiveness of the schools. They assist the school in many valuable roles. Each volunteer needs to be specifically placed in the most appropriate role, then given a short but detailed job description and someone to periodically supervise him or her. Supervision in its most basic definition is observing the individual, anticipating any potential problems, then redirecting the individual before any problems occur. The supervision process also provides periodic feedback to the individual concerning his or her effectiveness, a very important component for volunteers. A smile and thank you helps them feel that they are needed and that their time and effort are appreciated.

The supervision of a volunteer involves a quick visual check of what he or she is doing. It should not be a time-consuming process. Replacing door panels with glass or plexiglass is an easy way to increase visual contact with volunteers. The more open and visible everything is in a school, the safer both children and adults are.

◆ BEYOND THE LEGAL MINIMUMS

Because of their special relationship with children and families, schools must work with the total community to support families. An African proverb states, "It takes a village to raise a child." Schools should send representatives to serve on community-based child protection teams, participate in local community councils on child abuse prevention, and initiate the formation of such groups if they are not present in the community. Schools should be community leaders in developing a wide range of prevention programs. Table 10-2 identifies some of the ways schools can support families. All parents should have access to parenting information and support services.

Schools must work with other human services agencies, child protective services, the juvenile court, and law enforcement to develop community-wide prevention and treatment services. The collaborative work will assist educators in staying current on topics related to child welfare in the broader sense (Tutty, 1997). The interaction will also facilitate an exchange of concerns and improve communication to build a better community for everyone.

Table 10-2. Some Ways in Which Schools Can Support Families

1. Provide accessible and affordable before-school, after-school, and "school's out" child care for working parents.

2. Provide parent education and support groups for parents with special concerns, including those who are divorcing, single, non-custodial, grandparents-as-primary-caregivers, foster parents, or parents of children with special needs.

3. Provide parent education classes to help parents learn age-appropriate expectations for their children.

4. Provide evening, day, and/or Saturday parent-teacher conferences for custodial and non-custodial working parents.

5. Implement family play nights to allow parents free or inexpensive opportunities to enjoy parenting more and to relieve routine life stresses. Open playgrounds to families on evenings and weekends.

6. Institute homework help lines to allow students and/or parents obtain assistance with homework.

7. Incorporate more parents into the school volunteer program. This builds the self-esteem of both children and parents.

8. Offer within the schools Alcoholics Anonymous (AA) and Narcotics Anonymous groups for parents and students, as well as Al Anon for the friends and families of alcoholics.

9. Allow community groups the use of school facilities in the evening and on weekends for art, drama, music, recreation, and sports groups for children and families.

In their role as change agents, schools are morally bound to offer prevention programs to facilitate the parenting process in this and future generations. Table 10-3 identifies some specific long-range prevention programs that schools should consider in the planning process. The total curriculum should include instruction on nonviolent conflict resolution, interpersonal communication, child development, resource management, and stress management. Schools must respond to the cultural, economic, and social changes within each community to assist the children and families in coping with these changes. School personnel are morally and ethically bound to assist in the prevention of child maltreatment and intervention on behalf of abused children (Daro, 1994; Tutty, 1997).

Table 10-3. Long-Range Prevention Programs

1. Teach non-violent conflict resolution skills beginning in early childhood classrooms and use peer playground monitors.

2. Involve parents and children in policy development.

3. Involve parents in lunchroom, library, and playground supervision.

4. Include a wellness curriculum that addresses both physical and emotional wellness for each grade, K-12.

5. Provide support groups to students experiencing similar life stresses, such as divorce, death of a family member or friend, family or community violence, substance abuse in the family, relocation, or peer problems.

6. Initiate volunteer programs that encourage each student to use his or her skills to help others in the community.

7. Provide work and play experiences for each child with individuals who are different from them.

8. Allow all children opportunities to achieve their dreams.

For every seven children in our schools, one child has experienced some type of child abuse. Of the approximately 41 million children in America's elementary and secondary school classrooms, nearly 6 million are victims of child maltreatment (USDHHS, Children's Bureau, 1998). As staggering as these statistics are, they are merely cold, impersonal numbers and don't tell the story of a child whose trust in human beings has been stripped or whose emotional stability is being destroyed by frequent verbal and physical assaults. How do we measure the damage to a child's potential by the actions of adults, often the child's caregivers? A tear is shed, a life is scarred before really living, or contributions are short-circuited before being made. These numbers must be thought of as human beings (USDHHS, Children's Bureau, 1998).

Because a maltreated child has predictable classroom behaviors, developmental abilities, and academic needs, the teacher can play a meaningful and pivotal role in providing a positive environment within which the child's maturational process can be enhanced. The rest of this chapter briefly describes the student with a history of maltreatment and discusses some teaching techniques that may optimize the learning environment for abused and maltreated children.

◆ CHARACTERISTICS OF CHILDREN WITH A HISTORY OF MALTREATMENT

The various types of abuse are associated with a variety of findings. Tables 10-4 and 10-5 list a variety of characteristics observed in a sample of runaway and homeless children who were maltreated, and the percentage of the victims demonstrating each characteristic by gender and type of maltreatment. The age of the child at the time of abuse, the duration of the abuse, and the relationship of the abuser to the child determine the consequences of the abuse and characteristics evident in the victim. More problematic behaviors develop as the

Table 10-4. Possible Behavioral Indicators of Maltreatment

Indicator	Overall (*n*=216)		Males (*n*=85)		Females (*n*=131)		Probability
	n	%	*n*	%	*n*	%	
Poor self-esteem	123	57.2	50	58.8	73	56.2	
Depression	122	56.5	45	52.9	77	58.8	
Adamant about not going home	83	38.4	24	28.2	59	45.0	*p* < .01
School/academic dysfunction	68	31.5	28	32.9	40	30.5	
Frequent control issues	53	24.5	17	20.0	36	27.5	
Overall runaway pattern	53	24.5	17	20.0	36	27.5	
Truancy	48	22.2	19	22.4	29	22.1	
Change in affect relating to certain adult	47	21.8	18	21.2	29	22.1	*p* < .05
Suicide attempt/ideation	38	18.1	10	11.8	29	22.1	*p* < .05
Drug/alcohol abuse	36	16.7	20	23.5	16	12.2	*p* < .03
Preoccupation	36	16.7	15	17.7	21	16.0	
Very secretive	32	14.8	10	11.8	22	16.8	
Assaultive/aggressive behavior	30	13.9	14	16.5	16	12.2	
Problems with hygiene	27	12.5	17	20.0	10	7.6	*p* < .01
Abnormal sleep patterns	26	12.0	9	10.6	17	13.0	
Sudden/chronic withdrawal	22	10.2	10	11.8	12	9.2	
Health complaints	22	10.2	6	7.1	16	12.2	
Gravitates toward abused and neglected youth	21	9.7	8	79.4	13	9.9	

Table 10-4. Possible Behavioral Indicators of Maltreatment—*continued*							
Indicator	**Overall** (*n*=216)		**Males** (*n*=85)		**Females** (*n*=131)		**Probability**
	n	%	*n*	%	*n*	%	
Petty stealing	20	9.3	15	17.7	5	3.8	*p* < .001
Excessive sexual acting out	16	7.4	4	4.7	12	9.2	
Sudden change in behavior	13	6.0	3	3.5	10	7.6	
Self-mutilation	12	5.6	4	4.7	8	6.1	
Abusive romantic partners	11	5.1	0	0.0	11	8.4	*p* < .01
Extreme modesty	11	5.1	4	4.7	7	5.3	
Criminal behavior	11	5.1	9	10.6	2	1.5	*p* < .01
Eating disorders	11	5.1	4	4.7	7	5.3	

Adapted and reprinted with permission from Powers, Jaklitsch, & Eckenrode, 1989.

child matures, but no one specific finding is consistently observed in all cases of child maltreatment (Anthony, 1974; Eckenrode, Laird, & Doris, 1993; Kendall-Tackett & Eckenrode, 1996; Kendall-Tackett, 1997; Lynch & Roberts, 1982; Pearl, 1990).

In learning to survive in their environment, child abuse victims have adapted in one of two ways: (1) with externalized and under-controlled behaviors or (2) with internalized and over-controlled behaviors. Most adults stereotypically see the child abuse victim as an aggressive, negative child who is incapable of playing or working acceptably with other children or adults. This is, in fact, an accurate description of only about one-fourth of the victims in any group. Because aggressive and hyperactive children demand attention, they are the children that adults must deal with. Both their language and behavior are assaultive, and these children do not listen to directions or instructions. They appear to be impervious to disapproval and attack other children physically and verbally. The inability to delay gratification, impulsivity, and distractibility of abused children prevents any relief from their demands on teacher attention. They may see themselves as bad, unlovable, and stupid. They expect punishment and will call attention to their own misbehavior, appearing to gain little or no pleasure from either activities or people. Without treatment, they grow more aggressive; however, they respond best to a very calm, highly structured environment (Eckenrode, Laird, & Doris, 1993; Kempe & Kempe 1978; Kendall-Tackett, 1997; Kendall-Tackett & Eckenrode, 1996; Pearl, 1988).

Indicator	Sexual Abuse (n=47)	Physical Abuse (PA) Only (n=37)	Neglect (n=59)	PA & Neglect (n=69)	Probability
Poor self-esteem	74.5	35.1	54.4	61.8	$p < .01$
Depression	70.2	43.2	40.4	66.7	$p < .01$
Adamant about not going home	40.4	37.8	35.1	42.0	
School/academic dysfunction	27.7	21.6	36.8	34.8	
Frequent control issues	17.0	21.6	29.8	26.1	
Overall runaway pattern	36.2	5.4	26.3	24.6	$p < .01$
Truancy	27.7	5.4	28.1	21.7	$p < .05$
Change in affect relating to certain adult	21.3	18.9	15.8	29.0	
Suicide	2.7	14.0	14.5		$p < .001$
Drug/alcohol abuse	25.5	13.5	19.3	11.6	
Preoccupation	10.6	8.1	21.1	21.7	
Very secretive	21.3	10.8	12.3	15.9	
Assaultive/aggressive behavior	12.8	10.8	17.5	14.5	
Problems with hygiene	12.7	5.4	10.5	17.4	
Abnormal sleep patterns	21.3	8.1	3.5	13.0	$p < .07$
Sudden or chronic withdrawal	12.8	2.7	12.3	10.1	

Table 10-5. Association of Type of Maltreatment with Behavioral Indicators

Table 10-5. Association of Type of Maltreatment with Behavioral Indicators—*continued*

Indicator	Sexual Abuse (n=47)	Physical Abuse (PA) Only (n=37)	Neglect (n=59)	PA & Neglect (n=69)	Probability
Health complaints	17.0	0.0	7.0	13.0	$p < .05$
Gravitates toward abused and neglected youth	12.8	5.4	8.8	10.1	
Petty stealing	10.6	5.4	7.0	13.0	
Excessive sexual acting out	19.5	0.0	7.0	4.4	$p < .01$
Sudden change in behavior	10.6	0.0	3.5	8.7	
Self-mutilation	10.6	0.0	5.3	5.8	
Abusive romantic partners	12.8	0.0	3.5	4.3	
Extreme modesty	4.3	2.7	7.0	5.8	
Criminal behavior	10.6	0.0	0.0	8.7	$p < .05$
Eating disorders	4.3	2.7	0.0	11.6	

Adapted and reprinted with permission from Powers et al., 1989.

The remaining three-fourths of all victims are overly compliant and appear to accept whatever happens to them. They are passive and obedient, stoic and unresponsive, withdrawn and shy, and easy to overlook. These behaviors reflect survival techniques. Abused children may feel guilty for misbehaving and responsible for upsetting parents or getting them in trouble. They are very sensitive to criticism by adults and need only mild suggestions to redirect their behavior. They need an environment that is accepting and encouraging. These children will respond best in a calm, predictable place in which to learn social skills and release their feelings. Often compulsively neat and overly desirous of meeting adult goals, they feel little joy or pleasure and have low self-esteem, but may show indiscriminate affection for adults (Kempe & Kempe, 1978; Sameroff et al., 1993; Starr & Wolfe, 1999; Trickett & McBride-Chang, 1995).

In their attempts to understand their world and avoid unpleasant experiences, abused children may "stare continually," never making eye contact with anyone. It is as if they think that by not looking someone in the eye, they make themselves invisible and therefore safe from attack. To teachers and observers, this child may appear dull or unresponsive or may be suspected to have hearing or sight deficits. This child is often reprimanded for daydreaming and not attending to classroom activities. In fact, the child is learning to "read" adult behavior. He or she is trying to avoid danger by carefully scanning the environment and making very detailed, accurate mental pictures of it. As these children become secure enough to talk (or later as adults), they often reveal an exceptional memory of their environment and the behaviors of those around them. Observers of child victims must be aware of this characteristic scanning behavior and not misread the behaviors or too quickly attempt to evaluate this child (Anthony, 1974; Belsky, 1993; Cicchetti & Carlson, 1989; Kendall-Tackett, Williams & Finkelhor, 1993; Rowe & Eckenrode, 1999).

EFFECTS ON DEVELOPMENT

Frequently, child victims have not developed a basic sense of trust, and subsequent psychosocial development is delayed. The child not only distrusts self and others but also lacks positive self-esteem, which is needed to try new experiences. As a result, the child fails to learn the age-appropriate behaviors for the family, peer culture, or classroom. The child's need to be safe and loved causes him to become excessively responsible for himself and the adults in his world. The child's own home environment is usually the only measure the child uses to determine the typical interaction of families in homes. Following the role models present in the home gives the child abuse victim few opportunities to learn positive coping, decision making, or interpersonal communication skills and provides little chance for enjoyment of life (Kendall-Tackett, Williams, & Finkelhor, 1993; Rowe & Eckenrode, 1999; Trickett & McBridge-Chang, 1995).

SEXUAL ABUSE

Sexual abuse victims share many of the characteristics just described but may exhibit some additional behaviors. They may exhibit an extreme external locus of control evident by attributing responsibility for their actions to others. They have experienced an exaggerated imbalance of power or control and may exploit other children. The child's sexual behaviors may be connected to feelings of anger, rage, frustration, humiliation, poor self-image, powerlessness, and/or lack of control and may be supported by irrational thinking. These children often have unresolved losses and exhibit boundary problems. They may be unable to identify or label feelings, so they lack the ability to express feelings. Since they may not have had their own feelings consistently validated, they may have difficulty in distinguishing their own feelings as being separate and different from the feelings expressed by others. Non-directed, compulsive, and aggressive behaviors are often exhibited as a reaction to the child's sense of helplessness and lack of control (Kendall-Tacket, Williams & Finkelhor, 1993).

Adolescents who act out may be victims of maltreatment. Because of their lack of maturity and mobility, they may be chronic runaways engaged in disruptive and criminal behavior, including prostitution and involvement in the drug trade to survive. These homeless children are at high risk for AIDS, drug overdose, suicide, and murder (de Charms, 1976; Kalichman, 1993; Kendall-Tackett, Williams, & Finkelhor, 1993; Powers, Jaklitsch, & Eckenrode, 1989). Sexually acting-out adolescents frequently may be victims of sexual abuse. Early pregnancy and prostitution also may be associated with sexual abuse (Kendall-Tackett, Williams, & Finkelhor, 1993; Ryan, 1989).

CONCLUSIONS

Child abuse negatively impacts normal development. Without intervention, the impact grows increasingly serious. The longer a child experiences abuse, the more serious the impact is on each area of development. Studies have demonstrated that neglected children perform more poorly on academic tasks than even other maltreated children; the decline is most drastic in junior high for males and high school for females. Recognizing behaviors manifested by children who have experienced child maltreatment is the first step the teacher must take in playing a meaningful role by providing the necessary learning environment for maltreated children. Although all abused children exhibit common patterns of behaviors and developmental delays, children who are abused and controlled through the maltreatment of a close family member demonstrate more problematic behaviors than children abused by acquaintances or strangers.

◆ CHARACTERISTICS OF THE TEACHER

Teachers' perceptions of themselves and their abilities to work with children may be related to their enthusiasm for their own childhood and sense of self-esteem about their early lives. Teachers rated as effective by students identify their own families as close, supportive, loving, and secure. Effective teachers commonly feel good about their own family's care and support of them. Research consistently identifies the effective teacher as a person with high self-esteem and the ability to nurture children (Curry & Johnson, 1990).

This should not imply that teachers who do not have this family background cannot be effective. However, it does imply that before any teacher can be effective in working with victimized children in the classroom, he or she must come to terms with emotions relating to child maltreatment. Likewise, a teacher who was a victim will need to work through his or her own problems before being able to be effective with students. The best solution is not to repress these feelings but to attempt to understand them. Local community mental health/support services may be valuable resources for the teacher. Self-help support groups, often patterned after the AA model, have a history of effectiveness with individuals who feel isolated by their problems. The group Adults Molested as Children was designed for past victims of incest. Writers' groups have also evolved for individuals with abusive histories. Support groups provide the victim with peer support that can lead to understanding and recovery. Additionally, there are numerous self-help books for people who have survived abusive childhoods. A teacher who has lived in or who is living in a chemically abusive family must also recognize the dangers of this situation and seek aid. As with any helping professional, a teacher must have good mental health to effectively work with or teach those who do not. Individuals who have been maltreated or lived in dysfunctional homes often fail to recognize indicators of abuse in children because of their own lack of understanding of what is normal (Pearl, 1990; Tower, 1992).

Teaching is nurturing. To be effective at nurturing, the individual must have had a wide range of positive experiences and a strong basic sense of trust

(Tower, 1992). Assuming the teacher is prepared to objectively and professionally work with maltreated children, the question arises, "What do I do when I suspect that a child has been maltreated?" All states have mandatory reporting laws. It is, therefore, incumbent upon the teacher to report any suspected child abuse or neglect.

◆ STRATEGIES FOR TEACHERS

Teachers need to make each classroom developmentally appropriate, with a curriculum guided both by their understanding of the developmental abilities of children within the age range being taught and by a responsiveness to individual differences in growth, individual personality traits, learning style, and family background (Bredekamp, 1987). The following strategies for teaching are most effective with victims of maltreatment while being appropriate for all children. The topics and techniques are divided into separate sections for ease of discussion only; in the developmentally appropriate classroom, they are integrated.

BUILD A SENSE OF TRUST

Children learn to trust themselves, and therefore others, when they have their needs met predictably by caring adults. When children have been maltreated in their own homes, where this basic trust normally develops, they frequently fail to develop trust. Trust can be learned later in life, however, when adults act in consistent, caring ways. The structure and routine of the classroom also provide predictability and facilitate the development of a sense of trust. Teachers help children develop a sense of trust when they keep their promises. By observing teachers plan, implement, and evaluate routine activities, children gain confidence that adults can meet their needs. Maltreated children are often unable to delay gratification because they have not been able to trust that the adults around them can or will carry out promises. Teachers should call each child by name, listen to what each child says both verbally and non-verbally, anticipate each child's needs, and then respond to these needs. Children who know that someone is listening begin to feel safe. To maintain the trust of children, teachers must maintain confidentiality and be someone children can always count on.

The adolescent is developmentally asking all adults, "Can I trust you to do what you say you will?" "Do your actions agree with my ideal concept of what should be?" "What do I believe, as compared to what you believe and what you think I should believe?" (Erikson, 1968). For the adolescent who was abused at an early age and lacks a basic sense of trust, this is an especially difficult task. Because the victim comes from a family where roles are non-distinct, the child is uncertain about what is "normal." The child needs to learn what is appropriate and positive. Because the basic sense of trust is lacking, the adolescent cannot rely on adults and therefore cannot sort out what he or she believes and values. To improve their sense of trust in themselves and others, children need adults who are consistent and dependable. The teacher also needs to respect privacy, protect confidentiality, and routinely "practice what he preaches" (Pearl, 1990).

EXPECT SUCCESS

As simple as it sounds, one of the most effective ways to build success is to expect success. Children who feel that others care about them doing well are more apt to achieve. To build success in children, teachers must say they care about each child and act like they care about each child. Many abused and especially neglected children have never known what it is to have others support their efforts and direct them toward achievement. Abused children commonly suffer from intellectual delays due to both the maltreatment and the general home environment. Even when the home provides materials and opportunities for intellectual development, stress and anxiety impede the normal acquisition and use of knowledge. However, the environment usually has lacked age-appropriate learning opportunities, guidance, and reinforcement of learning. The classroom must provide an environment in which intellectual skills can be learned when the child is emotionally ready.

Children who have been abused may initially lack the intrinsic motivation for learning and the joy from learning experienced by normal children. In an environment in which they are accepted as they are, allowed to succeed, and encouraged to meet their own needs rather than the needs of adults, these children eventually experience the joy of learning and develop curiosity (Forten & Chamberland, 1995).

Students should be placed in learning situations in which they are not valued or assessed according to their performance but rather as individuals—just for being. Academic performance or product of effort is evaluated as a separate issue by comparing performance to a predetermined standard of performance. The teacher should evaluate the product, not the producer. "Not all of the math problems are worked correctly" is an objective statement about the math problems. However, the statement "You failed to work all of your math problems correctly" devalues the student rather than evaluating the product.

When teachers require students to evaluate their own work against a predetermined evaluation scale, they are providing an environment that enhances the child's internal locus of control and allows the student to feel successful and self-determining (de Charms, 1976). Programmed instruction also places the student in control of progress and minimizes teacher evaluation. Students need a learning environment structured to build successes rather than directed toward correcting failures.

Teachers should provide a wide variety of opportunities for children to construct their own ideas. Children, regardless of background, need multiple opportunities to improve their knowledge base. Different learning styles as well as different emotional states influence the acquisition of knowledge.

TEACH SOCIAL SKILLS

Social skills allow maltreated children to reduce their isolation and to build a web of relationships. Children need to feel connected to others in a mutually supportive system. Abusive families may be isolated, untrusting, and fearful of the outside world. The children of such families may have no positive role models except those they see at school. The feelings of connectedness help build bonds of trust and reduce fear—another example of the interrelatedness of human development.

Teachers should encourage abused children to stand up for themselves and should support them when they do. Initially an aggressor may listen only because the teacher is literally standing behind the victim, but the notion that people have rights and can assert them appropriately and effectively is important. These are children whose personal rights have been violated. They need a place where this does not happen and a role model to show them how to prevent it in a non-violent manner. Efforts must be made toward helping the child develop assertiveness and resistance. Opportunities should be provided for the child to interact with a small group of age-mates. The adult working with this small group must defend and support each individual's rights while directly teaching skills that will assist each group member in successful group interaction. Mainstreaming the child who has been maltreated into a group of children who have not been maltreated allows the victimized child to see models of appropriate behavior. Due to the interrelatedness of development, the child's ability to learn social skills is directly related to emotional development (Forten & Chamberland, 1995; Lawrence, 1987; Tite, 1993).

TEACH LIFE SKILLS

Teachers should set realistic standards, not ideals, because students who have lived in dysfunctional homes already have difficulty with "what is" and "what should be." The curricular content of all classrooms should allow students to learn life skills without racial, ethnic, or gender bias. Self-esteem develops in the context of mastering changing life tasks and challenges.

The curriculum should include basic life skills such as health and physical education, money management, stress management, non-violent conflict resolution, nutritional competence, food preparation, and interpersonal communication. Students need to learn that all families have money management problems and that planning to prevent the problem is a better course of action than merely blaming other family members. Older students in math, business, and home economics classes can have classroom exercises based on case studies of individuals and families solving money management issues to offer opportunities to practice resource management, communication, and negotiation skills. By practicing problem-solving and decision-making in the classroom, the student experiences an alternative family lifestyle. Simple group projects in any discipline allow the student to construct knowledge relating to the subject matter as well as learn interpersonal communication and negotiation skills. Students should be allowed to make age-appropriate decisions and live with the consequences, for example, "Would you like to work with Erin or Sandy?" or "Which of these three books would you like to read for Monday?" All of the choices must be real and require students to accept the consequences of their decisions. All classroom activities must reflect various socioeconomic levels as well as cultural and ethnic backgrounds.

TEACH COMMUNICATION SKILLS

In most abusive homes, interpersonal communication is poor (Miller-Perrin & Perrin, 1999). The curriculum should include units on interpersonal communication, conflict resolution, and family/personal resource management. All of these units are especially important to young people who have no role model for appropriate interpersonal communication. In abusive families, the person in whom ultimate power is vested may communicate in vague terms or expect no two-way communication. The child may have been routinely punished for replying to adults even conversationally; therefore, the curriculum must begin with the basics. Additionally, the classroom must be structured to give all students opportunities for communication with peers as well as with the teacher.

In giving instructions, adults should make sure the directions are clear and simple. Because children feel that what is nearer to them is more important, adults should be physically near the child when giving directions. Teachers should use a clear, quiet voice, while looking directly at the child. Children who have lived with many commands and general uneasiness will not respond well to general directions given from across the room. As with all children, teachers should give some latitude when giving instructions to allow the child to make simple decisions. It is important that the adult's words and body language convey the same message. Child abuse victims are not easily fooled by people who say one thing and do another. Calm body language will placate and relax the child more than words. Voice tone is more important than what is said. The teacher should be careful to make sure that the voice says what is intended. "Time to begin writing now?" spoken with a questioning voice leads the child to disobey the spoken words. "It is time to begin writing now" spoken in a clear, calm manner will tell the child specifically what to do.

The adult should tell the child what specific behaviors or actions are appropriate and expected rather than what not to do. "Clean up your desk and get ready for lunch" is too vague. "Place the writing papers in your folder, place the folder in your desk and return all books to the shelf in alphabetical order, wash and dry your hands, and then go to the lunch table" provides the child with directions for appropriate action. The more concise and specific the directions, the better they define appropriate actions. After each appropriate action, teachers need to provide lots of praise, smiles, and hugs to the child. All staff should model calm behavior. Additionally, the staff should exhibit an appropriate sense of humor (Bredekampe, 1987; Honig, 1985, 1986).

Puppetry can be used to facilitate language development and communication skills. Puppets provide non-threatening opportunities to gain new experiences for students at various developmental levels. Young students may use them for storytelling, acting out stories, or free play. Secondary school students may be involved in the preparation of puppet shows or simple presentations to younger students. Puppets may also allow an avenue for children who have been maltreated to release feelings and gain relief from disclosure. Puppets are a versatile educational tool that facilitates development in many areas.

ALLOW STUDENTS TO BE STUDENTS
Because they have been reared in an environment in which they parented their parents as well as younger siblings, victimized children may be overly helpful to teachers and classmates. This may be the student who the teacher "loves to have in class" or the assistant he or she "so desperately needs." However, the teacher must not succumb to the temptation to accept the help this student seems to need to give and seems to enjoy giving. The student is demonstrating the only survival technique that has previously brought acceptance and praise. Because the child was praised and accepted for doing responsible helpful tasks, especially cleaning, he or she learned that the same helpful behavior will earn predictable and needed praise in school. As important as it is for children to learn helpfulness, they also need to develop skills in relating to peers as equals and adults as caregivers. When academic and social skills are lacking, this student tries to succeed by cleaning and helping. While this behavior gains approval and perhaps passing grades from the teacher because it is easy to reinforce, the pattern of repetition fails to teach appropriate communication or social skills and often allows the student to become further victimized by peers.

CASE STUDY

The fifth grade teacher describes Mary to her mother: "Mary is a great student. She always volunteers to help me put materials away, clean up, and is the best help at finding lost items. She always has a ready smile and a willing hand with whatever needs to be done. She seems to sense when I need something done and steps right in and does it. Sometimes, however, her homework is not completed, and her test scores should be higher." Her mother replies, "Well, she is usually helpful at home but she doesn't get things really clean and isn't organized enough when she puts the laundry away."

The teacher must be alert to the student who is "excessively" responsible and redirect that student to more appropriate behaviors. This often involves observing the group activity and assisting and encouraging the student to say, "I have done my assigned tasks. I'll help you complete yours, but I won't do them for you." This says to the victimized child, "You have rights and responsibilities just as each member of the group does." Since other students frequently recognize the vulnerability of the child, comments such as "Sandy didn't do her part . . . " may be a common response when the victimized child asserts herself. The teacher must verify what the assigned tasks were and what tasks were left uncompleted. Teachers must not automatically come to the aid of any child because they "feel sorry" for him or her. Defending the rights of the maltreated child shows that the teacher values the child and his or her rights, teaches assertive behavior, and allows the child to see appropriate means of resolving peer conflict that will be needed when he or she encounters sibling conflict as a parent (Pearl, 1990).

In working with this extremely helpful student, teachers must remember that this student needs positive interactions with adults; the teacher, librarian, coach, and principal are all appropriate for this role. However, special attention must be paid to the part the role model plays. The teacher must be careful not to become another adult that the child "cares for" or fall into the easy pattern of allowing the student to take care of her and pick up after her to the extent that she comes to treat the student like an adult, creating yet another situation of role reversal. Rather, the teacher should tell the student that she can use a "student assistant" during a specific hour of the day or before school. The student is then responsible for specific routine tasks, rather than for remembering what the teacher needs to do next or has forgotten to do. It is useful to carefully outline in writing and post in a specific place the appropriate tasks for the student assistant. Following each task, the teacher should identify the expected level of proficiency on which the "assistant" will be evaluated and periodically evaluate the level of proficiency exhibited in completing the tasks. Praising the student for specifically completing tasks is better than making general comments such as "You're working hard, that's good" or "You're super to have around and you do so much hard work." Specific praise allows the student to feel good about herself or himself, learn skills for the world of work, and gain additional insight into the "normal world." This type of "businesslike arrangement" is mutually beneficial to the student and the teacher.

TEACH POSITIVE COPING SKILLS

Behaviors such as empathy, understanding the points of view of others, good verbal skills, good attentional processes, reflectiveness, problem solving skills, inner locus of control, frustration tolerance, and appropriate responses to success appear to be possible to teach. Some other behaviors seem to be more complex and global and do not easily lend themselves to an instructional and training approach. Among these more complex behaviors are having the ability to detach from the dysfunctional behaviors of others, being personable and well-liked, being a creative thinker, practicing autonomous thinking, being optimistic, having a sense of humor, being aware of personal power, having a future orientation, and having a well-developed value system.

Students need instruction in good management and coping skills, including various opportunities to practice those skills. Students with a history of maltreatment have routinely developed dysfunctional coping skills that lead to additional victimization, self-defeating behaviors, and maltreatment. Such children and adolescents frequently follow poor role models. The resulting behavior is either inappropriately acting out or depression. Because of the number of hours teachers spend with children each day, they are ideal role models for positive coping skills. Appropriate coping skills can be taught by modeling, role-playing from scripts, or allowing students to view videotapes that set up a situation and then require the students to discuss the alternative solutions.

Resource management should be integrated into the curriculum. The individual can be taught how to avoid many stressful situations with good management techniques. Many resource management and stress management programs are available in a variety of formats. Some interactive computer programs may be especially helpful for students who lack the language skills necessary for verbal role-playing.

When alcoholism is present in the family, confrontation skills are essential to each child's ability to learn positive coping strategies. However, this requires more involvement than the classroom teacher can provide and these situations are best handled by referral to community resources, including mental health professionals or support groups, such as Alateen. The classroom teacher can educate students about the resources available to individuals and families with chemical addiction problems but cannot cure or treat the student. The teacher should provide a role model of positive responses to stress and ensure that the classroom environment does not cause additional stress for the child. Good coping skills are perceiving yourself in control of your life and having good self-esteem.

PROVIDE PLEASANT EXPERIENCES

There is educational merit to making learning fun or at least pleasant and enjoyable. Children who have been maltreated have had few, if any, experiences of pleasurable activities, and often when they do have fun they are not allowed to appropriately enjoy it. The school is an important place for the student to develop new interests, hobbies, and skills. All students, but especially maltreated students, need to hear the teacher speak about the pleasant odors, flavors, and touches in the world around them. Students who have been maltreated often have not had their senses stimulated in common and pleasant ways (Helfer, 1991). These children or adolescents need opportunities to have these experiences and see an adult enjoying or appreciating them. The physical education, art, music, science, and family and consumer sciences classrooms routinely provide a wide variety of these experiences. Firsthand exploration of the world through the senses is necessary for any individual who is going to be able to nurture the next generation (Helfer, 1991). The teacher must continually offer extra attention to ways of adding pleasant sensory experiences to the curriculum.

CASE STUDY

The students in English class are asked to write about one of their favorite activities. Several minutes later the teacher notices that Sammi is just sitting, staring out the window. The teacher asks, "Why haven't you started to write about what you enjoy doing, Sammi?" Slowly, the reply is, "I guess I don't have anything I enjoy doing."

The child with a history of maltreatment has for so long been made to feel guilty for enjoying even the simplest of activities that he or she may no longer be able to feel or express joy. When a teacher observes that a student enjoys an activity, it should be acknowledged along with a brief discussion of similar experiences that the student might enjoy. The teacher must give the student permission to feel good about the things he enjoys. By providing a wide variety of learning experiences, the teacher gives students more opportunities for success as well as more opportunities for having pleasant sensory experiences. It should be recognized that what one student enjoys may not be at all pleasant for other students. Many students find pleasure in tasks that other students may see as very distasteful, for example, dissecting a frog, doing math, performing messy art activities, doing research in the library, or writing poetry. The teacher should acknowledge student enjoyment, praise successes, and encourage students to feel pride and pleasure even when it involves doing what is "different." (As an encouragement, classrooms should have, as standard equipment, colorful posters stating, "It's OK to be different.") An environment in which students are encouraged to enjoy learning will always be an environment in which more learning takes place.

All students need the role model of an adult who enjoys the everyday world. Children who have grown up in a dysfunctional family urgently need to see adults who can laugh when things are funny and who love to care for special plants, play the guitar or piano, go fishing or running, make cookies, sew with the latest fabric, listen to the rain on the roof, or enjoy the songs of the birds. They need role models who take pride and pleasure in the things they do well, who willingly try new activities, who read and enjoy learning, and who demonstrate pleasure in their interactions with people of all ages, genders, races, and ethnic backgrounds. Teachers can be that role model for their students.

BUILD SELF-ESTEEM

Self-esteem is a complex, multifaceted phenomenon related to the development of values, moral character, and personality. It includes feelings about the social, cognitive, moral, and physical/motor aspects of the individual. The four major aspects of self-evaluation are acceptance, power/control, competence, and moral virtue (Lawrence, 1987; Pearl, 1990).

All teachers should be aware of the importance of student self-esteem and include in the curriculum ways for children to improve their self-images. To children who have been victimized and who have experienced extreme external control and manipulation, these activities are especially important. The activities included should encourage students to focus on their positive abilities and actions, to learn positive behaviors, and to seek methods for self-improvement. Fugitt (1983) provides a variety of activities for inclusion in lesson plans to build student self-esteem and to help students progress from victim to survivor. Improving their knowledge of the world around them also provides students with information on community resources and how to access those resources for personal growth in areas such as athletics, dance, physical education, art, and music. For all students, knowledge brings with it the feelings of power and being in control, which are essential to building positive self-esteem (Lawrence, 1987).

As children gain mastery over their bodies, their feelings about themselves as unique individuals improve. Physical education, recreation, drama, and movement/dance provide valuable opportunities to gain greater body awareness, define personal boundaries, and improve self-concept. Additionally, physical activities allow the individual to stimulate the senses, release feelings and anxiety, engage in communication, experience physical and emotional joy, and know feelings of both control and freedom. When these activities are done with others, there are additional opportunities for developing decision-making, problem-solving, coping, and communication skills as well as a sense of trust. Programs such as Outward Bound that involve survival training are especially helpful to participants in developing trust, cooperation, impulse control, self-confidence, and self-sufficiency. If properly structured, physical activities may also allow individuals to feel the joy of success.

To build their sense of worth, all children need opportunities to be responsible, caring members of society. Children of all ages need opportunities to feel that they are capable of helping others: for example, by listening to younger students read, acting as a student librarian, volunteering at the recycling center, or working as a stage hand for the school or community theater. Teachers need to empower children to understand that they can choose to make a difference through public service. Choosing to care is different from perpetuating the role reversal and overly responsible behavior learned as a survival technique in the child's home. If it is done out of choice, service to others allows the individual to feel personal value.

IMPROVE ACADEMIC SKILLS

Because of prior experiences, victimized children often lack dispositions for learning, such as curiosity, resourcefulness, independence, initiative, responsibility, and goal-directed behaviors. One third of all abused and neglected children repeat at least one grade in elementary school (Tower, 1992). Ideally, the school experience allows children to slowly develop these abilities. Early maltreatment interrupts the normal growth of trust, autonomy, independence, and initiative; child abuse robs children of their childhood. The child must go back and work through each of these psychosocial stages and construct the knowledge necessary for academic competency. Teachers must structure the environment to allow children with varied backgrounds and dispositions to learn.

As already noted, abused children need a learning environment that is calm, structured, and predictable. An individual study area may assist some children in focusing on the academic tasks before them. The classroom environment may overly stimulate children who have spent much of their lives in chaos. Other children may have or may develop learning disorders and need to be evaluated for special services. Teachers must structure the environment for success. Instructions may need to be written and clearly divided into simpler tasks to allow the child to complete parts of the total assignment and then move to the next one, rather than be overwhelmed by complex tasks. Clearly, children who have not lived in calm, ordered environments need special attention.

PROVIDE AVENUES TO GAIN INSIGHT

Bibliotherapy is one way to help children who are the victims of abuse gain personal insight; bibliotherapy literally means to treat through the reading of books. The goals of bibliotherapy are to teach students to think constructively and positively, to encourage them to talk freely about their problems, to help them analyze their attitudes and modes of behavior, to point out that there is more than one solution to a problem, to stimulate an eagerness to find an adjustment to problems that will lessen conflict with society, and to assist them in comparing their problems with those of others. Although the teacher is not a therapist or a counselor, he or she can request that books about children who have dealt positively in adverse circumstances be available in school libraries and can include some readings as part of required and optional assignments (Table 10-6). High school students can gain insight into their own lives by reading or acting out with puppets such books with younger children in child development laboratories, as teacher assistants, or by working in the school or community library. In addition to providing therapeutic value to students who have been maltreated, these books teach all students what is appropriate treatment of children and become part of a child abuse prevention program (Pearl, 1990).

◆ RESILIENCY OF CHILDREN

Despite the devastating consequences of maltreatment, some children overcome these obstacles and succeed in school and in life. Researchers have called these children invulnerable, stress resistant, or vulnerable but invincible (Osofsky, 1999). These children share the following four characteristics:

1. An active, evocative approach to solving life's problems, enabling them to negotiate successfully an abundance of emotionally hazardous experiences

2. A tendency to perceive their experiences constructively, even if the experiences caused them pain or suffering

3. The ability to gain other people's positive attention

4. A strong ability to use faith in order to maintain a positive vision of a meaningful life

Teachers can assist these resilient children in turning their vulnerability into resiliency by actions such as the following:

1. Encouraging children to reach out to friends, teachers, and others

2. Accepting the children and assisting them in building on their strengths, rather than expecting failure and allowing them to become overwhelmed with their problems

3. Conveying to the children a sense of responsibility and caring and rewarding them for helpfulness and cooperation

4. Encouraging the children to develop a special interest, hobby, or activity that can serve as a source of gratification and self-esteem

5.   Modeling coping skills

6.   Providing dependability

"Beating the odds" occurs when someone cares enough to reach out to the child, providing an alternative to giving up (Osofsky, 1999).

◆ TRAINING AND SUPPORT FOR ALL EDUCATIONAL STAFF MEMBERS

Teachers working with child abuse victims require additional specific training in the special needs of abuse victims. Teachers also need support and encouragement as they attempt to meet the needs of child abuse victims. Teachers not specifically trained to work with these special needs children can quickly become frustrated because the traditional methods of working with children do not produce the desired changes. The progress is slow and the behaviors of these children are extreme. To prevent becoming overly frustrated, teachers must be aware that although abused children respond negatively to friendly overtures, teachers need to continue to be warm, encouraging, and accepting, with lots of hugs and smiles. An adult model of sharing, helping, and comforting is important in assisting children to develop trust and empathy.

All staff members require training specifically for interactions with child abuse victims. When special needs children are mainstreamed into the classroom, the teacher-child ratios must be lowered to allow staff to individualize instruction and to prevent their being overwhelmed by the demands placed on them. Volunteers and aides are vital to making the classroom more effective.

Teachers need principals, school nurses, and counselors to provide evaluation of techniques being used and to provide input into each child's developmental record and/or individualized educational plans. Further, this process allows the teacher an appropriate release for feelings of anxiety and frustration. The ability to verbalize frustrations and laugh with accepting co-workers helps relieve stress.

Maintenance of short, daily logs on each child provides the needed data for preparing progress reports and also serves to document for the teacher the progress that each child is making. To be effective, teachers should be provided with a work environment in which everyone can feel good about themselves and valued for their contributions to the program, in which they have the opportunity for meaningful input, and in which there is evidence of progress toward definable goals.

◆ SUMMARY

By statute in all fifty states, U.S. territories, and the District of Columbia, school personnel are mandated to report to the protective services child abuse and neglect hotline when they have reason to believe that children are being abused or neglected. The requirement is not that they prove abuse or neglect occurred but that they report their reasons to believe that it has. School districts should, therefore, adopt policies for preventing and reporting abuse and neglect, and for working with students in the classroom. In addition, they should provide all personnel and parents of children in the district with copies of the policies relating to child abuse and neglect reporting and discipline. Although classroom teachers are not therapists, they can guide the victimized student to facilitate personal growth and insight through specific classroom assignments and make referrals to other sources of assistance in the school

Table 10-6. Examples of Books for Bibliotherapy

Alphin, E. M. (2000). <u>Conterfeit son.</u> New York: Harcourt Brace.

Behm, B. J. (1999). <u>Tears of joy.</u> Thiensville, WI: Wayword Publishing Co.

Benedict, H. (1985). <u>Recovery: How to survive sexual assault for women, men, teenagers, their friends and family.</u> New York: Doubleday. Ages 11-18; RL Gr 5.

Cole, B. S. (1987). <u>Don't tell a soul.</u> New York: Marian.

Crutcher, C. (1986) <u>Stotan.</u> London: Greenwood.

Declements, B. (1987). <u>No place for me.</u> New York: Viking.

Grosshandler, J. (1989). <u>Coping with verbal abuse.</u> New York: Rosen Publishing Group.

Harvest, V. (1988). <u>Growing up abused.</u> Cheney, WA: High Impact Press.

Havelin, K. (2000). <u>Incest: "Why am I afraid to tell?" (Perspectives on relationships).</u> Mankato, MN: Lifematters Press.

Hayden, T. L. (1987). <u>One child.</u> New York: Putman.

Hoban, J. (1998). <u>Acting normal.</u> New York: HarperCollins Juvenile.

Jocoby, A. (1987). <u>My mother's boyfriend and me.</u> New York: Dial Books.

Klassen, H. (1999). <u>I don't want to go to Justin's house anymore.</u> Washington, DC: Child Welfare League of America.

Klein, V. (1986). <u>Bad-mad boy, honey bear and the magic waterfall.</u> Somerville, NJ: Hage Publications.

Klein, V. (1986). <u>I-am, pa-pah and ma-me.</u> Somerville, NJ: Hage Publications.

Kropp, P. (1987). <u>Take off.</u> St. Paul, MN: EMC Publications.

Leite, E., & Espeland, P. (1989). <u>Different like me: A book for teens who worry about their parent's use of alcohol/drugs.</u> Minneapolis, MN: Johnson Institute.

Loftis, C. (1995). <u>The words hurt.</u> Far Hills, NJ: New Horizon Press.

MacHovec, F. J. (1990). <u>Hitting and hurting: A children's guide to prevent physical abuse.</u> Dobbes Ferry, NY: Oceana Educational Communications.

MacLean, J. (1987). <u>Mac.</u> Boston: Houghton.

Madison, A. (1979). <u>Runaway teens.</u> New York: Elsevier/Nelson Books.

Michener, A. J. (1998). <u>Becoming Anna: Autobiography of a sixteen-year-old.</u> Chicago: University of Chicago Press.

Miklowitz, G. D. (1987). <u>Secrets not meant to be kept.</u> New York: Delacorte Press.

Table 10-6. Examples of Books for Bibliotherapy—*continued*

Miller-Lachman, L. (1987). <u>Hiding places.</u> Madison, WI: Square One Publishers.

Mufson, S., & Kranz, R. (1991). <u>Straight talk about child abuse.</u> New York: Facts on File.

Page, C. G. (1987). <u>Hallie's secret.</u> Chicago: Moody Press.

Posner, R. (1987). <u>Sweet pain.</u> New York: M. Evans.

Quinn, P. E. (1986). <u>Renegade saint: A story of hope, a child abuse survivor.</u> Nashville: Abingdon Press.

Rosa, G. (1978). <u>Edith Jackson.</u> London: Viking.

Seixas, J. S., & Youcha, G. (1985). <u>Children of alcoholism: A survivor's manual.</u> New York: Harper & Row. Ages 11-14; RL Gr 6.

Spelman, C., & Weidner, T. (1997). <u>Your body belongs to you.</u> Morton Grove, IL: Albert Whitman & Co.

Swan, H. & Mackey, G., (1983). <u>Dear Elizabeth: Diary of a survivor of sexual abuse.</u> Leawood, KS: Children's Institute of Kansas. Ages 11-18; RL Gr 6.

Trottier, M. (1997). <u>A safe place.</u> Morton Grove, IL: Albert Whitman & Co.

Turner, A. W. (2000). <u>Learning to swim: A memoir.</u> New York: Scholastic Trade Books.

Woolverton, L. (1987). <u>Running before the wind.</u> Boston: Houghton.

system and/or community. Teachers and all school personnel can be all-important role models of predictability, trustworthiness, and joy in living and learning for the maltreated child. Beyond their legal requirements, schools have ethical requirements to support families in fostering the optimal development of each child. Ready to learn means many things, including freedom from community and family violence, intolerance, and prejudice. It does indeed take a village to raise a child.

◆ REFERENCES

American Association for Protecting Children. (AAPC). (1986). <u>Highlights of official child neglect and abuse reporting 1984.</u> Denver, CO: The American Humane Association.

Anderson, E. M., & Levine, M. (1999). Concerns about allegations of child sexual abuse against teachers and the teaching environment. <u>Child Abuse and Neglect, 23</u>(8), 833-843.

Anthony, E. J. (1974). The syndrome of the psychologically invulnerable child. In E. J. Anthony and C. Koupernick, (Eds.), <u>The child in his family: Children at psychiatric risk.</u> New York: Wiley.

Arkow, P. (1998). Correlations between cruelty to animals and child abuse and the implications for veterinary medicine. In R. Lockwood and F. R. Ascione (Eds.), Cruelty to animals and interpersonal violence: Reading in research and application. West Lafayette, IN: Purdue University Press.

Belsky, J. (1993). Etiology of child maltreatment: A developmental-ecological analysis. Psychological Bulletin, 114, 413-434.

Bredekamp, S. (Ed.) (1987). Developmentally appropriate practice in early childhood programs serving children birth through 8. Washington, DC: National Association for the Education of Young Children.

Caulfield, B. A. (1979). Child abuse and the law. Chicago: National Committee for the Prevention of Child Abuse.

Caulfield, B. A. (1981). Child abuse and the law: A legal primer for social workers. Chicago: National Committee for the Prevention of Child Abuse.

Cicchetti, D., & Carlson, V. (Eds.). (1989). Child maltreatment: Theory and research on the causes and consequences of child abuse and neglect. New York: Cambridge University Press.

Curry, N. E., & Johnson, C. N. (1990). Beyond self-esteem: Developing a genuine sense of human value. Washington, DC: National Association for the Education of Young Children.

Daro, D. (1994). Prevention of child sexual abuse. Future Child, 4(2), 198-223.

De Charms, R. (1976). Enhancing motivation in the classroom. New York: Irvington.

Eckenrode, J., Laird, M., & Doris J. (1993). School performance and disciplinary problems among abused and neglected children. Developmental Psychology, 29, 53-62.

Erikson, E. H. (1968). Identity: Youth and crisis. New York: Norton.

Forten, A., & Chamberland, C. (1995). Preventing the psychological maltreatment of children. Journal of Interpersonal Violence, 10(3), 275-295.

Fugitt, E. D. (1983). "He hit me back first": Creative visualization activities for parenting and teaching. Rolling Hills Estates, CA: Jalmar Press.

Green, F. (1988). Corporal punishment and child abuse. The Humanist, 48(6), 9-10, 32.

Halperin, M. (1979). Helping maltreated children: School and community involvement. St. Louis, MO: Mosby Press.

Helfer, R. E. (1991). Childhood comes first: A crash course in childhood for adults (3rd ed.). East Lansing, MI: Author.

Helfer, R. E., & Kempe, R. S. (1987). The battered child (4th ed.). Chicago: University of Chicago Press.

Honig, A. S. (1985). Compliance, control and discipline. Young Children, 40, 47-52.

Honig, A. S. (1986). Stress and coping in children. Young Childen, 41, 47-59.

Kalichman, S. C. (1993). <u>Mandated reporting of suspected child abuse: Ethics, law and policy.</u> Washington, DC: American Psychological Association.

Kempe, R. S., & Kempe, C. H. (1987). <u>Child abuse.</u> Cambridge, MA: Harvard University Press.

Kendall-Tackett, K., & Eckenrode, J. (1996). The effect of neglect on academic achievement and disciplinary problems: A developmental perspective. <u>Child Abuse and Neglect, 20,</u> 161-169.

Kendall-Tackett, K. (1997). Timing of academic difficulties for neglected and nonmaltreated males and females. <u>Child Abuse and Neglect, 21</u>(9), 885-887.

Kendall-Tackett, K. A., Williams, L. M., & Finkelhor, D. (1993). Impact of sexual abuse on children: A review and synthesis of recent empirical studies. <u>Psychological Bulletin, 113,</u> 164-180.

Koraleck, D. (1992). <u>Caregiving of young children: Preventing and responding to child maltreatment.</u> McLean, VA: The Circle, Inc.

Lawrence, D. (1987). <u>Enhancing self-esteem in the classroom.</u> London: Paul Chapman Publishing, Ltd.

Loar, L., & White, K. (1998). Connections drawn between child and animal victims of violence. In R. Lockwood and F. R. Ascione (Eds.). <u>Cruelty to animals and interpersonal violence: Reading in research and application.</u> West Lafayette, IN: Purdue University Press.

Lynch, M. A., & Roberts, J. (1982). <u>Consequences of child abuse.</u> New York: Academic Press.

National Committee for the Prevention of Child Abuse (NCPCA). (1987). <u>Policy statement on corporal punishment in schools and custodial settings, Working Paper No. 17.</u> Chicago: Author.

Miller-Perrin, C. L., & Perrin, R. D. (1999). <u>Child maltreatment: An introduction.</u> Thousand Oaks, CA: Sage Publications.

Osofsky, J. D. (1999). The impact of violence on children. <u>The Future of Children, 9</u>(3), 33-49.

Pearl, P. (1990). Working with child abuse victims. <u>Illinois Teacher, 34</u>(2), 70-74.

Pearl, P. (1988). Working with preschool-aged child abuse victims in group settings. <u>Child & Youth Care Quarterly, 17</u>(3), 185-194.

Powers, J. L., Jaklitsch, B., & Eckenrode, J. (1989). Behavioral characteristics of maltreatment among runaway and homeless youth. In J. T. Pardeck (Ed.), <u>Child abuse and neglect.</u> Washington, DC: U.S. Department of Health and Human Services.

Romeo, F. F. (2000). The educator's role in reporting the emotional abuse of children. <u>Journal of Instructional Psychology, 27</u>(3), 183-184.

Rowe, E., & Eckenrode, J. (1999). The timing of academic difficulties among maltreated and non-maltreated children. <u>Child Abuse and Neglect, 23</u>(8), 813-832.

Ryan, G. (1989). Victim to victimizer: Re-thinking victim treatment. <u>Journal of Interpersonal Violence, 4</u>(3), 325-341.

Sameroff, A. J., Seifer, R., Ballwin, A., & Ballwin, C. (1993). Stability of intelligence from preschool to adolescence: The influence of social and family risk factors. Child Development, 64, 80-97.

Sedlak, A. J., & Broadhurst, D. D. (1996). The third national incidence study of child abuse and neglect. Washington, DC: U.S. Department of Health and Human Services, U.S. Government Printing Office.

Starr, R. H., Jr., & Wolfe, D. A. (1999). The effects of child abuse and neglect: Issues and research. New York: Guilford Press.

Straus, M. A. (1994). Beating the devil out of them: Corporal punishment in American families. New York: Lexington Books.

Tite, R. (1993). How teachers define and respond to child abuse: The distinction between theoretical and reportable cases. Child Abuse and Neglect, 17, 591-603.

Tower, C. C. (1992). The role of educators in the protection and treatment of child abuse and neglect, DHHS Publication No. (ACF) 92-30172. Washington, DC: U.S. Department of Health and Human Services.

Trickett, P. K., & McBride-Chang, C. (1995). The developmental impact of different forms of child abuse and neglect. Developmental Review, 15, 311-337.

Tutty, L. M. (1997). Child sexual abuse prevention programs: Evaluating. Who Do You Tell, 21(9), 869-881.

U.S. Department of Health and Human Services (USDHHS). (1992, March). Administration for children and families; administration on children, youth and families; National Center on Child Abuse and Neglect. Child abuse and neglect: A shared community concern. Washington, DC: U.S. Government Printing Office.

U.S. Department of Health and Human Services, Children's Bureau. (1998). Child maltreatment 1996: Reports from the states to the National Child Abuse and Neglect Data System. Washington, DC: U.S. Government Printing Office.

Wissow, L. S. (1990). Child advocacy for the clinician: An approach to child abuse and neglect. Baltimore, MD: Williams & Wilkins.

◆ APPENDIX I: LIST OF STATE PROTECTIVE SERVICES

Alabama
Bureau of Family and Children's Services
64 N. Union Street
Montgomery, AL 36130
Phone: (205) 261-3409

Alaska
Division of Family and Youth Services
Department of Health and Social Services
Alaska Office Building, Rm. 204
Pouch H-01
Juneau, AK 99811
Phone: (907) 465-3170

Arizona
Administration for Children, Youth and Families
1717 W. Jefferson Street
P.O. Box 6123
Phoenix, AZ 85005
Phone: (602) 255-3981

Arkansas
Department of Human Services
Division of Social Services
Donaghey Building, Suite 317
7th and Main Streets, P.O. Box 1437
Little Rock, AR 72203
Phone: (501) 371-2521
Statewide Child Abuse Hotline: (800) 482-5946

California
Office of Child Abuse Prevention
Adult and Family Services Division
Department of Social Services
744 P Street
Sacramento, CA 95814
Phone: (916) 323-2888
Central Registry of Child Abuse: (916) 445-7586

Colorado
Division of Family and Children's Services
Department of Social Services
1575 Sherman Street
Denver, CO 80203
Phone: (303) 866-2551
Statewide Hotline (other than metro Denver) (800) 842-2288

Connecticut
Division of Children's and Protective Services
Department of Children and Youth Services
170 Sigourney Street
Hartford, CT 06105
Phone: (203) 566-5506
Statewide Child Abuse Reporting Hotline: (800) 842-2228

Delaware
Division of Child Protective Services
Department of Services for Children, Youth and Their Families
824 Market Street, 7th Floor
Wilmington, DE 19801
Phone: (302) 571-6140
Statewide Child Abuse Reporting Hotline: (800) 292-9582

District of Columbia
Family Services Administration
Commission on Social Services
Randall Building
1st and Eye Streets, S.W.
Washington, DC 20024
Phone: (202) 727-5947
Child Abuse and Neglect Reporting: (202) 727-0995

Florida
Children, Youth and Family Services Programs Office
Department of Health and Rehabilitation Services
1317 Winewood Blvd.
Building 8, Room 317
Tallahassee, FL 33609
Phone: (904) 488-8762
Statewide Child Abuse Reporting Hotline: (800) 342-9152

Georgia
Office of Child Protective Services
Division of Family and Children Services
Department of Human Resources
47 Trinity Avenue, S.W.
Atlanta, GA 30334
Phone: (404) 894-2287

Hawaii
Family and Children's Services
Public Welfare Division
Department of Social Services and Housing
P.O. Box 339
Honolulu, HI 96809
Phone: (808) 548-5846

Idaho
Division of Welfare, Child Protection
Department of Health and Welfare
Statehouse
Boise, ID 83720
Phone: (208) 384-3340

Illinois
Division of Child Protection
Department of Children and Family Services
1 N. Old State Capitol Plaza
Springfield, IL 62706
Phone: (217) 785-2513
Statewide Child Abuse Reporting Hotline: (800) 252-2873

Indiana
Division of Child Welfare-Social Services
Field Services (Child Abuse)
141 South Meridian Street
Indianapolis, IN 46225
Phone: (317) 232-4431
Statewide Child Abuse Reporting Hotline: (800) 562-2407

Iowa
Protection Services
Division of Social Services
Department of Human Services
Hoover State Office Building
Des Moines, IA 50319
Phone: (515) 281-6802
Statewide Child Abuse Reporting Hotline: (800) 362-2178

Kansas
Family Services Section
Youth Services
Department of Social and Rehabilitation Services
2700 W. 6th
Smith-Wilson Building
Topeka, KS 66606
Phone: (913) 296-4657

Kentucky
Department of Social Services
Cabinet of Human Resources
275 E. Main Street
Frankfort, KY 40204
Phone: (502) 564-4650

Louisiana
Protective Services
Office of Human Development
Department of Health and Human Resources
P.O. Box 44367
Baton Rouge, LA 70804
Phone: (504) 342-4049

Maine
Protective Services for Children
Office of Social and Rehabilitation Services
State House
Augusta, ME 04333
Phone: (207) 289-2971
Statewide Child Abuse Reporting Hotline: (800) 452-1999

Maryland
Protective Services
Office of Child Welfare Services
300 W. Preston Street
Baltimore, MD 21202
Phone: (301) 576-5242
H.E.L.P./Resource Project
Office of Child Welfare Services
300 W. Preston Street
Baltimore, MD 21202
Phone: (301) 576-5245

Massachusetts
Department of Social Services
24 Farnsworth Street
Boston, MA 02210
Phone: (617) 727-0900
Statewide Child Abuse Reporting Hotline: (800) 792-5200

Michigan
Children's Protective Services
Office of Children and Youth Services
Department of Social Services
300 S. Capitol Avenue, P.O. Box 30037
Lansing, MI 48909
Phone: (517) 373-7580

Minnesota
Child Abuse and Neglect
Social Services Division
Department of Human Services
Centennial Office Building, 4th Floor
St. Paul, MN 55155
Phone: (612) 296-8337

Mississippi
Adult and Child Protective Services
Division of Social Services
Department of Public Welfare
P.O. Box 352
Jackson, MS 39205
Phone: (601) 354-0341
Statewide Child Abuse Reporting Hotline: (800) 222-8000

Missouri
Division of Family Services
Department of Social Services
Broadway State Office Building
P.O. Box 1527
Jefferson City, MO 65102
Phone: (573) 751-4247
Statewide Child Abuse Reporting Hotline: (800) 392-3738

Montana
Community Services Division
Department of Social and Rehabilitation Services
P.O. Box 4210
Helena, MT 59604
Phone: (406) 444-5622

Nebraska
Child Protective Services
Human Services
Department of Social Services
301 Centennial Mall South
5th Floor, P.O. Box 95026
Lincoln, NE 68509-5026
Phone: (402) 471-3121

Nevada
Welfare Division, Protective Services
Department of Human Resources
Capitol Complex, 251 Jeanell Drive
Carson City, NV 89710
Phone: (702) 885-4730
Youth Services Division
Department of Human Resources
505 E. King Street, Room 603
Carson City, NV 89710
Phone: (702) 885-5982

New Hampshire
Protective Services
Bureau of Child and Family Services
Department of Health and Welfare
Hazen Drive
Concord, NH 03301
Phone: (603) 271-4405
Child Abuse Reporting, Info-Line: (800) 852-3311

New Jersey
Division of Youth and Family Services
Department of Human Services
CN 717, P.O. Box 510
Trenton, NJ 08625
Phone: (609) 292-6920
Office of Child Abuse Control/Hotline
1230 Whitehouse-Mercerville Road
Trenton, NJ 08625
Phone: (800) 792-8610

New Mexico
Family Protective Services
Social Services Division
Human Services Department
P.O. Box 2348
Santa Fe, NM 87503-2348
Phone: (505) 827-4372
Statewide Child Abuse Reporting Hotline: (800) 432-6217

New York
Division of Children and Family Services
Department of Social Services
40 N. Pearl Street
Albany, NY 12243
Phone: (518) 474-9428
State Operations/Child Protective Services Hotline: (518) 474-9607
Statewide Child Abuse Reporting Hotline: (800) 342-3720

North Carolina
Protective Services Unit
Family Services Section
Department of Human Resources
325 N. Salisbury Street
Raleigh, NC 27611
Phone: (919) 733-2580

North Dakota
Children and Family Services
Department of Human Services
State Capitol
Bismarck, ND 58505
Phone: (701) 224-2316

Ohio
Bureau of Children's Protective Services
Division of Family and Children's Services
Department of Human Services
30 E. Broad Street
Columbus, OH 43215
Phone: (614) 466-2146

Oklahoma
Child Welfare Services
Department of Human Services
P.O. Box 25352
Oklahoma City, OK 73125
Phone: (405) 521-3778
Statewide Child Abuse Reporting Hotline: (800) 522-3511

Oregon
Children's Services Division
Department of Human Resources
318 Public Service Building
Salem, OR 97310
Phone: (503) 378-4374 or (503) 378-3016

Pennsylvania
Office of Children, Youth and Families
Department of Public Welfare
P.O. Box 2675
Harrisburg, PA 17120
Phone: (717) 787-4756
Statewide Child Abuse Reporting Hotline: (800) 932-0313

Rhode Island
Child Protective Services
Department of Children and Their Families
610 Mount Pleasant Avenue
Providence, RI 02908
Phone: (401) 861-6000 Ext 2332
Statewide Child Abuse Reporting Hotline: (800) RI-CHILD

South Carolina
Child Protective and Preventative Services Division
Department of Social Services
P.O. Box 1520
Columbia, SC 29202-1520
Phone: (803) 758-8593

South Dakota
Child Protection Services
Department of Social Services
Richard F. Kneip Building
700 N. Illinois Street
Pierre, SD 57501
Phone: (605) 773-3227

Tennessee
Child Protective Services
Office of Social Services
Department of Human Services
111-7th Avenue, N.
Nashville, TN 37203
Phone: (615) 741-5929

Texas
Office of Services to Families and Children
Department of Human Services
P.O. Box 2960
Austin, TX 78769
Phone: (512) 450-3448
Statewide Child Abuse Reporting Hotline: (800) 252-5400

Utah
Protective Services
Child Abuse Registry
Division of Family Services
Department of Social Services
150 W. North Temple Street
Salt Lake City, UT 84110
Phone: (801) 533-7128

Vermont
Protective Services
Department of Social and Rehabilitation Services
Agency of Human Services
103 S. Main Street
Waterbury, VT 05676
Phone: (802) 241-2142

Virginia
Child Protective Services
Bureau of Child Welfare Services
Department of Social Services
8007 Discovery Drive
Richmond, VA 23288
Phone: (804) 281-9081
Statewide Child Abuse Reporting Hotline: (800) 552-7096

Washington
Child Protection Services
Division of Community Program Development
Department of Social and Health Services
State Office Building 2
Olympia, WA 98504
Phone: (206) 753-0206

West Virginia
Children's Protective Services
Division of Social Services
Department of Human Services
1900 Washington Street, E.
Charleston, WV 25305
Phone: (304) 348-7980
Statewide Child Abuse Reporting Hotline: (800) 352-6313

Wisconsin
Protective Services
Office for Children, Youth and Families
Department of Health and Social Services
State Office Building
1 W. Wilson Street, P.O. Box 7850
Madison, WI 53707
Phone: (608) 267-2245

Wyoming
Child Protective Services
Division of Public Assistance and Social Services
Department of Health and Social Services
Hathaway Building
Cheyenne, WY 82002
Phone: (307) 777-7892

◆ APPENDIX II: SAMPLE CHILD ABUSE AND NEGLECT POLICY FOR SCHOOLS
Policy Component Narrative

Purpose

Family Law Article, Title 5, Subtitle 7

To inform all employees and volunteers in the local school systems of the statutory requirement to report suspected child physical abuse, sexual abuse, or neglect, and to inform employees and volunteers of their immunity from civil liability or criminal penalty for reporting.

To establish procedures to be used by all employees and volunteers of the local school system in making oral and written reports to the local department of social services/law enforcement agency for suspected cases of child physical abuse, sexual abuse, or neglect.

Who Must Report

Family Law Article 5-704, 5-705

Maryland law requires that every health practitioner, educator, human services worker, or law enforcement officer who has reason to believe that a child has been subjected to physical abuse or sexual abuse shall immediately report to the local department of social services or appropriate law enforcement agency. The report, in both oral and written form, shall be made as soon as reasonably possible, but in any case the written report must be made within 48 hours of the suspicion of possible abuse to the local department of social services and the local State's attorney. Maryland law also requires that every health practitioner, educator, human services worker, or law enforcement officer who has reason to believe that a child has been a victim of neglect shall immediately report to the local department of social services. The report, in both oral and written form, shall be made as soon as reasonably possible, but in any case the written report must be made within 48 hours of the suspicion of possible neglect to the local department of social services.

Further, any person other than a health practitioner, educator, human service worker, or law enforcement officer, including any other employee of the local school system and volunteers in the local school system who has reason to believe that a child has been subjected to physical abuse, sexual abuse, or neglect, shall immediately report to the local department of social services or the appropriate law enforcement agency as prescribed in the above paragraph.

Where school personnel or volunteers are unsure whether abuse or neglect has taken place, the situation should be discussed with the local department of social services.

Sanctions for Failure to Report

Education Article 6-202, Education COMAR 13A.07.01.10

On the recommendation of the county superintendent, a county board may suspend or dismiss a teacher, principal, supervisor, assistant superintendent, or other professional assistant for misconduct in office, including knowingly failing to report suspected child abuse in violation of Family Law Article, Title 5, Subtitle 7 (Child Abuse/Neglect), Annotated Code of Maryland.

Upon the recommendation of a local board of education or the Assistant State Superintendent in Certification and Accreditation when the individual is not employed by a local board of education in Maryland, any certificate issued under the State Board of Education's regulations may be suspended or revoked by the State Superintendent if the certificate holder is convicted of a crime involving child abuse or neglect or is dismissed by a local board for knowingly failing to report suspected child abuse in violation of the Family Law Article.

Definitions

Family Law Article 5-701 to 5-715, Education Article 6-107

A. Educator or Human Service Worker: Any professional employee of any correctional, public, parochial or private educational, health, juvenile service, social or social service agency, institution, or licensed facility. Educator or Human Service Worker includes: any teacher, counselor, social worker, caseworker, and any probation or parole officer. However, a child may not be considered to be abused solely because he is receiving nonmedical religious remedial care and treatment recognized by State law.

Family Law Article

14-101 et seq.

B. Child: Any person under the age of eighteen (18) years. Persons eighteen (18) years of age or older who are believed to lack the capacity to care for their daily needs ("vulnerable adults") are protected by the Adult Protective Services Program. A health practitioner, police officer, or human service worker who suspects that a vulnerable adult has been subject to abuse, neglect, self-neglect, or exploitation is required to report such a situation orally and in writing to the adult protective services division of the local department of social services. Any other person may make a report. Any person who makes a report under these provisions is entitled to confidentiality and immunity from civil liability.

C. Abuse: (1) The physical injury of a child by any parent or other person who has permanent or temporary care or custody or responsibility for supervision of a child or by any household or family member under circumstances that indicate that the child's health or welfare is significantly harmed or at risk of being significantly harmed or (2) sexual abuse of a child, whether physical injuries are sustained or not.

D. Sexual Abuse: Any act or acts involving sexual molestation or exploitation, including but not limited to incest, rape, or sexual offense in any degree, sodomy, or unnatural or perverted sexual practices, on a child by any family or household member or by any other person who has the permanent or temporary care or custody or responsibility for supervision of a minor child. Sexual molestation or exploitation includes, but is not limited to contact or conduct with a child for the purpose of sexual gratification, and may range from sexual advances, kissing, or fondling to sexual crime in any degree, rape, sodomy, prostitution, or allowing, permitting, encouraging, or engaging in the obscene or pornographic display, photographing, filming or depiction of a child as prohibited by law.

E. Neglect: Child neglect means the leaving of a child unattended or other failure to give proper care and attention to a child by the child's parents, guardian, or custodian under circumstances that indicate that the child's health or welfare is significantly harmed or placed at risk of significant harm. However, a child may not be considered to be neglected solely because the child is receiving nonmedical religious remedial care and treatment recognized by State law.

Examples of Child Neglect

DHR-SSA Child Protective Services Policy Manual .01.04.04

A neglected child is one who is:

- left unattended or inadequately supervised for long periods of time.

- showing signs of failure to thrive, or psycho-social dwarfism that has not been explained by a medical condition. There may be other evidence that the child is receiving insufficient food.

- receiving inadequate medical or dental treatment.

- significantly harmed or at risk of harm as a result of being denied an adequate education due to parental action or inaction.

- wearing inadequate or weather-inappropriate clothing.

- significantly harmed due to a lack of minimal health care and/or fire safety.

- ignored or badgered by the caretaker.

- forced to engage in criminal behavior at the direction of the caretaker.

Immunity

Family Law Article

Any person who makes or participates in the making of a good-faith report of abuse or neglect or participates in the investigation or in a judicial proceeding resulting therefrom shall in so doing be immune from any civil liability or criminal penalty that might otherwise be incurred or imposed as a result thereof.

Possible Abuser

Family Law Article 5-701

Any parent, guardian, adoptive parent, or other person who has the permanent or temporary care or custody, or who has the permanent or temporary care or custody or responsibility for the supervision of a child or any household or family member, may be considered an abuser under the statute. Educators and other school employees having temporary care or custody or responsibility for the supervision of a child during the school day may also be deemed abusers under the statute and, when suspected of child physical or sexual abuse or neglect, must be reported immediately to the local social services agency or the appropriate law enforcement agency, orally and in writing as prescribed by law, by the person who has reason to believe that abuse or neglect has occurred.

Reporting Procedures

(Oral Report) Family Law Article 5-704, 5-705

Any employee of the local school system or volunteer in the local school system who suspects a case of child physical or sexual abuse has occurred shall make an oral report to the local department of social services or to the appropriate law enforcement agency. In a case of suspected neglect, the oral report should only be made to the local department of social services. The responsibility of an employee or volunteer of the local school system to report suspected cases of child abuse or neglect is mandatory. The oral report must be made as soon as possible, not-withstanding any provision of law, including any law on privileged communications. In addition to making an oral report, the school employee or volunteer shall also inform the local school principal that a case of suspected child abuse and/or neglect has been reported to the department of social services or law enforcement agency. It is the obligation of the principal to insure that cases of suspected child abuse or neglect brought to his/her attention by any school employee or volunteer are fully reported by the employee or volunteer if this has not already been done.

(Written Report) Family Law Article 5-704, 5-705

The person making the oral report to the department of social services or appropriate law enforcement agency is also responsible for submitting a written report.

The written report must follow the oral report and be made within forty-eight (48) hours of the contact which disclosed the existence of possible abuse and/or neglect.

Contents of Written Report

Family Law Article 5-704, 5-705

An oral or written report shall contain as much of the following information as the person making the report is able to furnish in suspected cases of child abuse and/or neglect:

Abuse/Neglect Report Contents:

1. The name, age, and home address of the child;

2. The name and home address of the child's parent or other person who is responsible for the child's care;

3. The whereabouts of the child;

4. The nature and extent of the abuse/neglect of the child, including any evidence or information available to the reporter concerning previous injury possibly resulting from abuse or neglect; and

5. Any other information that would help to determine the cause of the suspected abuse or neglect; and the identity of any individual responsible for the abuse.

Report Distribution

Family Law Article 5-704

Copies of the written report for abuse or neglect shall be sent to the local department of social services. Copies of the written report for abuse also shall be sent to the local State's attorney office. Additional distribution shall be determined by the local school system but shall be limited to persons who have a true need-to-know and shall not violate the confidentiality requirements discussed below. The local school system shall not maintain copies of written child abuse or neglect reports.

Confidentiality

Family Law Article 5-707, Article 88A Section 6(b)

DHR COMAR 07.02.07.05E

Department of Human Resources (DHR) regulations require that the identity of the person reporting a case of suspected child abuse and/or neglect shall not be revealed. Protective services staff must protect the identity of the reporter unless required by court order to reveal the source. Educators are encouraged to share information about the reported family, but protective services staff may not identify any reporting source to a reported family unless the educator has given written permission to protective services to reveal his/her identity.

Family Educational Rights and Privacy Act of 1974 (FERPA)

All records and reports concerning protective services investigations of child abuse and/or neglect and their outcomes are protected by the confidentiality statute Article 88A, Section 6(b). Unauthorized disclosure of such records is a criminal offense subject to a fine of up to $500.00 or imprisonment for up to 90 days, or both. Under this statute, information contained in reports or records concerning child abuse and/or neglect may be disclosed only:

1. Under a court order;

2. To personnel of local or State departments of social services, law enforcement personnel, and members of multidisciplinary case consultation teams who are investigating a report of known or suspected child abuse or neglect or who are providing services to a child or family that is the subject of the report;

3. To local or State officials responsible for the administration of the child protective service as necessary to carry out their official functions;

4. To a person who is the alleged child abuser, or to the person who is suspected of child neglect if that person is responsible for the child's welfare and provisions are made for the protection of the identity of the reporter or

any other person whose life or safety is likely to be endangered by disclosing the information;

5. To a licensed practitioner who, or any agency, institution, or program which is providing treatment or care to a child who is the subject of a report of child abuse or neglect; or

6. To a parent or other person who has permanent or temporary care and custody of a child, if provisions are made for the protection of the identity of the reporter or any other person whose life or safety is likely to be endangered by disclosing the information.

Investigative Procedure

Validation of suspected child abuse is the responsibility of the department of social services, assisted by the police. School personnel shall not attempt to conduct any internal investigation or an independent review of the facts.

School Procedure

A school employee may briefly question a child to determine if there is reason to believe that the child's injuries resulted from physical or sexual abuse, or by the child's caretaker and/or household member (e.g., What happened to you? How did this happen?). However, in no case should the child be subjected to undue pressure in order to validate the suspicion of abuse and/or neglect. Any doubt about reporting a suspected situation is to be resolved in favor of protecting the child and the report made immediately.

Third Party Presence During Investigative Questioning

Education COMAR 13A.08.01.08

In the event that a child is questioned by the protective services worker and/or police during the school day on school premises in an investigation of either child abuse and/or child neglect, whether the child is the alleged victim or a nonvictim witness, "the superintendent or the superintendent's designated representative shall determine after consultation with the individual from the local department of social services or the police officer whether a school official shall be present during the questioning of a pupil." The school official should be selected on a case basis for the purpose of providing support and comfort to the student who will be questioned. The regulations express a preference for having a third party present during questioning except in circumstances where the superintendent or the superintendent's designee, in consultation with the protective service worker determines that a third party should not be present during the interview. This may occur, for example, where the presence of a third party may inhibit the child's responses.

Article 88A Section 6(b) DHR COMAR 07.02.07.05D

DHR COMAR 07.02.07.17

The local department of social services shall notify school reporting sources of the receipt of the report. School personnel may request the local department of social services to call a multidisciplinary team meeting to share information and concerns to the extent permitted by the confidentiality statute and to coordinate planning for services to the child. Appropriate school personnel are expected to participate in the team meetings in accordance with the procedure established between the local department of social services and local school system.

Parental Notification

Education COMAR 13A.08.01.08

Although the regulations express a preference for parental notification, the school principal or the principal's designee is not required to notify parents or guardians of investigations on school premises involving suspected child abuse or neglect. The principal, in consultation with the protective service caseworker, may decide whether the parents should be informed of the investigative questioning. It may be determined, for example, that disclosure to the parents would create a threat to the well-being of the child (COMAR 13A.08.01.04B).

Emergency Medical Treatment; Access to Medical Records

Family Law Article 5-709, 5-711, 5-712

In the event that a child is in need of emergency medical treatment as a result of suspected abuse or neglect, the school principal, in collaboration with the school nurse or other health professional when available, shall arrange for the child to be taken immediately to the nearest hospital. The protective services worker or law enforcement officer should be consulted before taking the child to the hospital when feasible; in cases where the emergency conditions prevent such consultation, the protective services worker should be notified as soon thereafter as possible. In all other instances, it is the role of the protective services worker and/or law enforcement officer to seek medical treatment for the child.

Information contained in school health records needed during the existence of a health and safety emergency may be disclosed without parental consent and without violating the provisions of Federal Educational Rights and Privacy Act (FERPA) of 1974.

Educators are required to provide copies of a child's medical/health records information, upon request to the local department of social services as needed as part of a child abuse/neglect investigation or to provide appropriate services in the best interest of a child who is the subject of a report of child abuse or neglect.

Removal of Child from School Premises

Family Law Article 5-709, 5-710, 5-712 DHR-SSA

Child Protective Services Policy Manual .01.03.04, and Education COMAR 13A.08.01.08E

The child may be removed from the school premises by a protective services worker or police officer only if:

1. Local social services has guardianship of the child;

2. Local social services has a shelter order or a court order to remove the child. (Verification of shelter care order by school personnel can be made by calling the local juvenile services agency intake officer.) A joint decision by the principal and the protective services worker should be made regarding

who will notify the parents of the action to remove the child from school. Usually this notification will occur as part of the social worker's initial family visit, or as part of the contact made to arrange the initial family interview. However, in the absence of a joint decision, the superintendent or the superintendent's designated representative shall insure that prompt notification of removal from school is made to the pupil's parent or guardian.

Parental Awareness

Parents should be advised of the legal responsibility of school staff to report suspected cases of abuse and/or neglect. In order to facilitate positive interactions between the school and home/community, it is often helpful to inform parents of this before a problem arises. A letter should be sent to all parents at the beginning of the school year.

Information Dissemination

Information on child abuse and neglect should be disseminated as follows:

1. Provide annual training sessions to all school employees on child abuse/neglect policies and procedures, symptoms, programs and services, and prevention curriculum.

2. Implement, as a part of the curriculum, an awareness and prevention education program for all students.

3. Initiate a public awareness program for students, parents, and the community at large. Information may be disseminated in school newsletters or with report cards. Presentations may be conducted at PTA meetings and at meetings of other community organizations.

Chapter 11

ART THERAPY

MARCIA SUE COHEN-LIEBMAN, M.A., M.C.A.T., A.T.R.-B.C.

♦ OVERVIEW AND DEVELOPMENT OF THE PROFESSION

The therapeutic use of art and the inherent therapeutic properties associated with the creative process coalesced in the early twentieth century. Artwork created by mentally ill patients was studied in an effort to ascertain the connection between art and illness. At the same time, educators began to study the symbolic and emotional communications conveyed in the spontaneous art created by children. The ideas of "art in therapy" and "art as therapy" ultimately converged, resulting in art therapy being recognized as a national mental health profession. Rubin (1979) states, "Whether art is creative or responsive, the therapeutic value is not limited to the clinic or hospital or to deviant populations. It is a way of working with experiences which are difficult to understand or assimilate" (p. 12).

Art therapy has evolved into a recognized profession that offers a wide variety of applications, including assessment, treatment, prevention, intervention, and investigation. The practical application of art therapy and its inherent potential continue to extend into nontraditional arenas, including forensic investigations (Cohen-Liebman, 1999). Subspecializations continue to develop and flourish, including educational art therapy, medical art therapy, and forensic art therapy.

FORENSIC ART THERAPY

Forensic art therapy (FAT) extends the practical application of art beyond the traditional realms of evaluation and treatment (Cohen-Liebman, in press; Cohen-Liebman & Gussak, 1998). In FAT, art therapy practice and theory are integrated within a legal context to assist in investigations. FAT is investigative in nature but has clinical overtones. It is for fact-finding purposes and is used in investigation rather than intervention. When employed within the confines of a forensic process, this method of investigation assists in achieving specified goals and objectives.

DEFINITION OF THE PROFESSION

Art therapy is a human service profession that uses art media, images, the creative process, and client responses to art productions as reflections of an individual's development, abilities, personality, interests, concerns, and conflicts (American Art Therapy Association [AATA], 1999). Art therapists use drawing, painting, sculpture, and other art forms as means of both verbal and non-verbal communication. Clients gain insight through participation in their own art-making process. The expression of thoughts and feelings is encouraged within a safe and supportive context. The art therapist works with the client to comprehend what the client describes both visually and verbally. The goals of art therapy depend on the client's therapeutic needs. Intrinsically, art therapy is used to foster personal growth and promote self-awareness.

Art therapy practice is based on the knowledge of human developmental and psychological theories, which are implemented in the full spectrum of assessment and treatment (AATA, 1999). Within a therapeutic application, art therapy may provide a means of reconciling emotional conflicts, developing social skills, managing behavior, solving problems, reducing anxiety, aiding reality testing, and increasing self-esteem (AATA, 1999). The theoretical orientation of art therapy includes psychoanalytic theory as well as art education.

Art therapists use their backgrounds as artists and their knowledge of art materials in conjunction with clinical skills and training in psychotherapeutic principles and methods. The art therapist integrates media, images, personal dynamics, and the creative process. Art therapy theory, philosophy, and methods are also central to the practice.

Art therapy is an effective treatment for those who are developmentally, medically, educationally, socially, or psychologically impaired. It is practiced in mental health, rehabilitation, medical, educational, and forensic institutions. Art therapists serve populations of all ages, races, and ethnic backgrounds. Art therapists provide services to individuals, couples, families, and groups (AATA, 1999).

Art therapists serve in many capacities, including clinical, administrative, educational, and supervisory. Traditionally, art therapists have served as primary therapists or as adjunct members of treatment or educational teams. Within these capacities, art therapists collaborate with physicians, psychologists, nurses, social workers, counselors, and teachers. Art therapists provide a range of services encompassing prevention, assessment, and treatment of emotional, social, and physical problems. Increasingly, art therapists interface with and participate as members of multidisciplinary child protection teams (Cohen-Liebman, 1999).

THE AMERICAN ART THERAPY ASSOCIATION
The profession of art therapy is regulated by a professional national organization, the American Art Therapy Association (AATA). AATA has developed guidelines for the education, training, and practice of art therapists. Standards of excellence for educational programs and for professional and ethical practice have been established by AATA.

AATA is a non-profit organization that was founded in 1969. It is governed and directed by a nine-member board elected by the membership, which exceeds 5,000 members in five membership categories. Affiliate chapters of AATA have been established throughout the United States to promote art therapy on a local level. Chapters assist local and regional communities by providing information about the profession.

AATA has established goals that govern the organization, including "the progressive development of the therapeutic use of art, the advancement of research, the improvement of standards of practice, the development of criteria for training art therapists, and the exchange of information and experience through publications, meetings and seminars" (Rubin, 1979, p. 14). Professional qualifications for entry into the field include a master's degree from an accredited academic institution or a certificate of completion from an accredited institute or clinical program (Levick, 1983; Lusebrink, 1989). Graduate training programs include practicum experience in addition to classroom training. Professional literature includes *The American Journal of Art Therapy, The Arts in Psychotherapy,* and *Art Therapy: Journal of the American Art Therapy Association.*

Conceptually, AATA's philosophy, goals, and objectives endeavor to ensure that credentialed art therapists deliver the highest standard of care possible to the general public. AATA's vision for the 21st century is the recognition of art therapy as an integral part of all healthcare delivery systems. The Mission Statement of the American Art Therapy Association (1999) is as follows:

> The American Art Therapy Association, Inc. (AATA) is an organization of professionals dedicated to the belief that the creative process involved in the making of art is healing and life enhancing. Its mission is to serve its members and the general public by providing standards of professional competence, and developing and promoting knowledge in, and of, the field of art therapy.

Information regarding art therapy as a profession, as well as the professional association, is available from AATA. A recent publication by AATA (2000) entitled *Ethical Considerations Regarding the Therapeutic Use of Art by Disciplines Outside the Field of Art Therapy* provides guidance for mental health practitioners. The healing that is associated with the creative process is not exclusive to art therapy and is not owned by art therapists; rather, the therapeutic use of art is the discriminating factor that distinguishes art therapy from other professions (AATA, 2000). AATA (2000) has established recommendations for the use of art by non-art therapists, including guidelines for when consultation with an art therapist or a referral to one is merited.

ART THERAPY CREDENTIALS BOARD

The AATA regulates educational, professional, and ethical standards for art therapists. The Art Therapy Credentials Board (ATCB) is an independent organization that grants postgraduate registration and board certification. The designation Art Therapist Registered (ATR) is granted by the ATCB to individuals who have successfully completed educational and professional requirements. The designation of Board Certified (BC), a credential requiring maintenance through continuing education credits, is granted by the ATCB to individuals who have successfully passed the national certification examination. Re-certification is required every five years by re-examination or by documentation of designated activities. The latter can be achieved through continuing education credits, publications, presentations, exhibitions, and other activities that demonstrate professional competence.

Psychiatrist Michael Vaccaro (1973), proposed soon after the establishment of the AATA that art therapy be understood as a branch of psychiatry. He wrote, "Art therapy is steeped in a long and rich tradition of sound theoretical principles and therapeutic practices" (Vaccaro, 1973, p. 253). He acknowledged that "The American Art Therapy Association has recognized and accepted its role of formulating guidelines for accredited education and training; validating research; and promulgating an ethical code of professional conduct for its members" (Vaccaro, 1973, p. 253). Vaccaro (1973) defined the education and training of the art therapist in the following manner:

> The art therapist undergoes a specialized training graduate program affiliated with a medical college or a university where he is offered sound theoretical principles and therapeutic techniques, which have been tested by time and scientific experiment. Concomitant with his academic training he is gradually exposed to the vicissitudes of a supervised clinical experience (p. 255).

ART PSYCHOTHERAPY OR ART AS THERAPY

Two schools of thought are fundamental to the profession. Identified as *Art Psychotherapy* and *Art as Therapy*, both have contributed to the progressive development of the field. Often basic tenets associated with both schools of thought are integrated in the practice of art therapy. Psychoanalytic tenets provide the basis for both.

ART PSYCHOTHERAPY

Margaret Naumburg was the first person credited with using art expression as a therapeutic modality. She began encouraging her patients to draw spontaneously and to free associate to their drawings in the 1940s. Her use of art was based upon psychoanalytic theory and practice. She believed that art therapy was dynamically oriented and was dependent upon the transference relationship between patient and therapist (Naumburg, 1987). She integrated psychoanalytic theory and techniques with her own ideas regarding drawing and personal symbolism (Junge & Asawa, 1994; Rubin, 1984). Art psychotherapy is a process-oriented approach that involves the use of media (art materials), clinical behavior, and the associations of the client.

ART AS THERAPY

In contrast, Edith Kramer concentrated on the integrative and healing properties of the creative process itself. Her theories evolved out of her work with children in the 1950s. For Kramer, the healing quality inherent in the creative process was analogous to the usefulness of art in therapy. In the creative act, conflict is re-experienced, resolved, and integrated (Rubin, 1984). A key factor in Kramer's work is the concept of sublimation. For Kramer art provided "a way of integrating conflicting feelings and impulses in an aesthetically satisfying form, helping the ego to control, manage, and synthesize via the creative process itself" (Rubin, 1984, p. 12). Kramer stressed the power of the creative process. She sought to understand a child's psychological functioning and to offer interventions accordingly (Junge & Asawa, 1994). In art as therapy, the therapist functions as an auxiliary ego and assumes a more supportive role. The integrative and healing properties of the creative process are central to this theoretical construct.

Both Naumburg and Kramer formed their theoretical orientations from their respective experiences and backgrounds in psychoanalysis. Although both were psychoanalytic in their orientation, each incorporated different aspects of psychoanalytic theory in her respective formulation of the therapeutic use of art (Junge & Asawa, 1994; Rubin, 1984). Kramer subscribed more fully to Freudian principles, but it was Naumburg who emulated Freud's techniques

(Ulman, 1986). For Naumburg, therapeutic art expression allowed for symbolic communication, which bypasses difficulties encountered with verbal communication. Within the therapeutic relationship, the therapist seeks to uncover insights into the conflictual areas of the client's psyche. If the client is unwilling or afraid to lift traumatic material into consciousness, the use of art media can allow for expression of this material in a safe and nonthreatening manner. As a result, a client may be able to express conflicts without becoming fully conscious or aware of them. The patient is encouraged to discover for himself or herself the meaning of the artwork.

ART AND DREAM WORK

Art and dream work are analogous in that material exists on two different levels. That which we see or remember and that which is not visible or is symbolic are the two parameters associated with both art and dreams. The manifest content in dreams is what we remember when we are awake. In art the manifest content is the collection of lines, shapes, forms, and colors that comprise the surface of an artistic creation. The manifest content is not necessarily recognizable or representational. The latent content is the underlying material, including issues, thoughts, feelings, and concerns, that gives rise to the manifest content in both art and dreams. To comprehend the symbolic imagery that gave rise to the manifest content, the visible manifestation is addressed in art therapy through the drawing out of the client's associations. Art therapy engages the client on different levels. The process of understanding the underlying issues invokes a verbal response from the client. Artwork is the process of the latent material becoming manifest. The manifest content does not have to be recognizable; rather, it is a reflection of the latent material that produced it. The patient's associations are significant in the comprehension of the symbolic imagery behind the manifest content.

MATERIALS/MEDIA

Media is a referential term used to describe art materials. Media may encompass a variety of items, including two- and three-dimensional materials. An art therapist is familiar with the inherent properties and resulting qualities of the media as well as what may be evoked by the introduction of certain materials. The art therapist assesses the stimulus potential of the media in conjunction with the coping skills of the client in an effort to introduce materials and tasks designed to meet the client's needs.

Art materials exist on a continuum from structured to less structured. Structured media have a definitive shape and form, and make a definitive mark. Two-dimensional art materials are representative of structured media, including pencils, Craypas, markers, and pastels. Unstructured media, such as clay or paint, require the user to give them shape and form. Unstructured media do not make consistent lines and are more subject to gravity. Different media evoke different responses and convey different messages. For example, media can be used to cover or uncover, let go or contain. It is the responsibility of the art therapist to know the inherent properties of the media in an effort to support the client. The choice of media affects the structure of the session and possible outcomes.

Knowledge of materials and the subtle and creative use of the media help facilitate the process. Elements to consider in selecting media for tasks and with regard to population include touch, texture, color, movement, rhythm, and space requirements. Other components to consider in the selection of media include concrete or abstract qualities, as well as the levels of risk-taking, mastery, and competence required. The art therapist can comprehend and interpret what is being expressed with regard to the media. This information provides the art therapist with knowledge regarding underlying issues, conflicts, and concerns associated with the client. Knowledge of materials and the subtle and creative use of the media help facilitate the process.

◆ ARTISTIC DEVELOPMENTAL LEVELS

A phase-specific developmental sequence is associated with children's drawings. A child can be advanced or regressed within the phases, but development is sequential and contingent upon mastery of skills (Levick, 1998; Malchiodi, 1998). Rhoda Kellogg collected drawings from all over the world and discovered that children begin to draw at the same age and in the same manner (Kellogg, 1970). In 1952, art educator Victor Lowenfeld determined that artistic development occurs in combination with a child's emotional, physical, and cognitive development. In his textbook for art teachers, Lowenfeld placed artistic development into a stage theory, recognizing sequential artistic development (Lowenfeld & Brittain, 1987). He determined that there is a correlation between intellectual, emotional, and artistic development.

Modifications of Lowenfeld's stage theory have evolved as art therapy has become more sophisticated and the machinations associated with children's artistic development have been refined. Lowenfeld's work remains seminal to art therapy and provides a basis for understanding artistic development. Lowenfeld's work is analogous to Piaget's stage theory of cognitive or intellectual development (Malchiodi, 1998). Although divided into different phases or stages, children's artistic development essentially encompasses three distinct sequences: scribbling (beginning of self expression); schematic (child's perception of his environment—people, things, objects); and naturalistic, realistic interpretation (Malchiodi, 1998). There are graphic expectations associated with each of the artistic developmental levels (Levick, 1998). Knowledge of typical developmental variants is essential to understanding the graphic productions created by children. Many factors and influences contribute to maturation in developmental spheres, including the artistic.

Lowenfeld placed artistic development into a stage theory that encompasses the developing child between the ages of 2 and 17 years. Lowenfeld's stages are identified as scribbling (2 to 4 years), preschematic (4 to 7 years), schematic (7 to 9 years), dawning realism (9 to 11 years), pseudo-naturalistic (12 to 14 years), and adolescent (14 to 17 years). Specified elements and artistic features are associated with each stage of development. Drawing and representational characteristics commonly associated with the developmental phases articulated by Lowenfeld are shown in Table 11-1. Figures 11-1 to 11-10 are examples of the different phases demarcated by Lowenfeld. The drawings illustrate artistic characteristics typically associated with the various phases.

Myra Levick, a pioneer in art therapy education, correlated the relationship between cognitive, psychosexual, and artistic development (Levick, 1983). This theoretical construct provides a foundation for the art therapist and a context for understanding drawings. The correlation between emotional development, intellectual development, and creative expression is fundamental to art therapy. Levick (1983) also developed criteria for the identification of defense

Table 11-1. Characteristics Associated with Artistic Developmental Stages

Drawing characteristics, space representation, and human figure representation are denoted for each phase.

Scribbling Stage (2-4 years)

    three phases

- Disorganized scribble
  - No control of movement
  - No connection between eyes and paper
  - No hand-eye coordination
  - Does not attend to activity
  - Marks not confined to paper
  - Kinesthetic feedback—activity feels good
- Controlled scribble
  - Realizes he or she can control marks
  - Connects eye to hand movements
  - Starts and stops
  - Immediate feedback
  - Repeats movements
  - Keeps marks on paper or drawing surface
  - Makes prefigural marks
- Naming
  - Kinesthetic to imaginative
  - Names marks
  - Relates marks to things
  - Changes subject identification
  - Makes intentional marks

Transitional or Design Stage (4-5 years)

- Phase between scribbling and preschematic
- Marks do not look representative
- Marks are more controlled than a scribble
- Scribbles begin to get organized

Some material is modified/adapted from Lowenfeld's stage theory (Lowenfeld & Brittain, 1987).

Table 11-1. Characteristics Associated with Artistic Developmental Stages—*continued*

- Geometric shapes and letters
- Designs
- Mandalas and tadpoles—head/body fusion
- Size determines importance

Preschematic Phase (4-7 years)

- Experiments with different ways of drawing something
- Draws what he or she knows
- Draws what is important to the child
- Not drawing what they see
- Space looks haphazard but is related to self
- Exaggerations and omissions
- By the end of this phase, draws a whole body
- Size determines importance
- Human figures not fixed forms
- Schema varies
- Subjectivity
- Elements not interrelated

Schematic Phase (7-9 years)

- Base line
- Skyline
- Proportion becomes more real
- Detail begins to demarcate what is important
- Space is linear—horizontally and vertically
- Use of space is subjective
- Marks are ordered
- Color is realistic
- Schema is flexible
- Still exaggerations and omissions
- Story-telling and time sequences
- X-ray of subject (can see through elements)

Table 11-1. Characteristics Associated with Artistic Developmental Stages—*continued*

Dawning Realism (9-12 years)

- Draw what they see and how they see
- Schemas do not vary
- Realistic representation
- No exaggerations or omissions
- Pencil and eraser
- Detail indicates importance
- Multiple base lines
- Depth is implied
- Perspective is not yet rendered
- Overlapping
- Base line becomes a plane
- Color is realistic
- Elements are interrelated

Pseudo-Naturalism (12-14 years)

- Realism
- Shading, shadows
- Perspective
- Foreshortening
- Three dimensional tricks
- Secondary sexual characteristics
- Exactness
- Details
- Action
- Stylizing
- Cartooning
- Infusion of elements with personal meaning

Table 11-1. Characteristics Associated with Artistic Developmental Stages —*continued*

Adolescent Art (14-17 years)

- Continued development of artistic skills
- Subjective interpretations
- Artistic elements
- Naturalism
- Perspective
- Abstraction
- Affect/mood
- Intentional distortion
- Exaggeration of detail

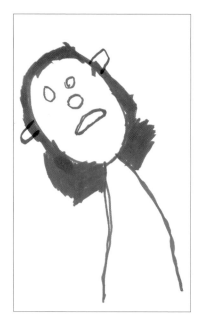

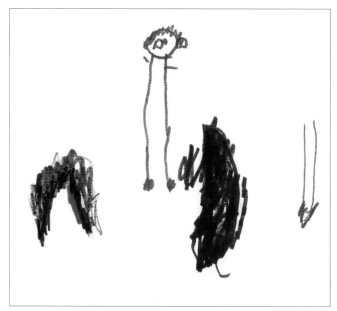

Figure 11-1. Preschematic Phase
Drawing by a 4-year-old girl depicts a developmentally congruent drawing of a figure. The figure is representative of head-foot fusion.

Figure 11-2. Preschematic Phase *Drawing by a 6-year-old female who is experimenting with colors, lines, and shapes, as well as attempts at figural representation.*

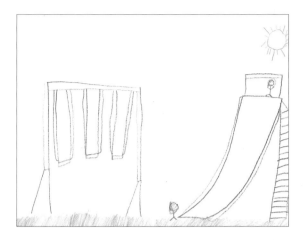

Figure 11-3. Schematic Phase *Drawing by an 8-year-old female. Elements are lined up on a base line, and spatially, the picture is organized linearly and vertically.*

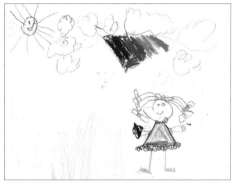

Figure 11-4. Schematic Phase *Drawing by a child who was almost six years old. Drawing has features associated with the schematic phase, including implied base line, spatial organization, skyline. Despite being somewhat advanced, the drawing shares characteristics with younger developmental stages.*

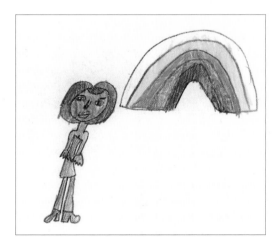

Figure 11-5. Dawning Realism *An 11-year-old child made this drawing. Despite the paucity of design, the features and details included in the depiction of the figure are indicative of the higher level of development that is associated with this phase.*

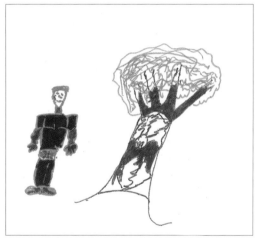

Figure 11-6. Dawning Realism *An 11-year-old boy made this drawing of a super hero. The manner in which the figure is drawn with shading is characteristic of this developmental phase.*

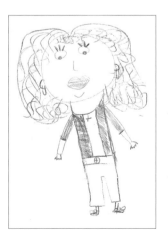

Figure 11-7. Pseudo-Naturalistic
This drawing was made by a 12-year-old who was allegedly molested by her father. The attention to detail and the inclusion of specific features, as seen in the face and the clothing, are aspects of this developmental phase.

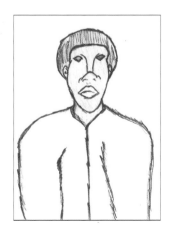

Figure 11-8. Pseudo-Naturalistic
This drawing by a 13-year-old includes stylization, exactness, and attempts at perspective. The drawing is indicative of a realistic representation.

mechanisms of the ego in graphic productions. Defense mechanisms exist on a continuum and are indicative of a client's level of functioning. Conflictual and nonconflictual aspects of ego development and function are exposed through graphic expression. This knowledge aids in the identification of areas of fixation, conflicts, and issues that are central to the individual. These theoretical constructs, in conjunction with the client's associations, provide art therapists with a foundation for understanding artwork as well as a framework for communicating this information.

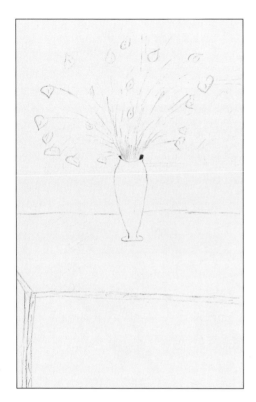

Figure 11-9. Adolescent This drawing by a 14-year-old shows artistic elements, natural artistic skills, perspective, and a real attention to detail.

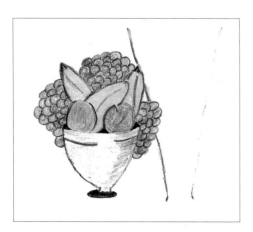

Figure 11-10. Adolescent This drawing is also by a 14-year-old. It is characteristic of this stage.

♦ INHERENT ADVANTAGES

The use of art expression as a therapeutic tool has inherent advantages. These advantages have been innate to the practice of art therapy since its inception. Although semantics may vary, the intrinsic advantages have been categorically identified by Wadeson (1980). She has identified six advantages, as follows:

1. *Imagery.* We think in images, rather than in words, and images are less threatening than words.

2. *Decreased defenses.* Visual expression provides distance and allows for uncovering of material that may be repressed.

3. *Objectification.* Artwork is a tangible or concrete product that is generated by the client. Since the artwork is created by the client, it is an objective expression. Drawings provide information that concretely reflect the victim's experience in an objective manner.

4. *Permanence.* Artwork makes concrete the behavior, thoughts, and feelings of a client at a particular point in time. The tangible nature of the artwork allows for review of the material as needed.

5. *Spatial matrix.* Graphic representation allows for information to be given on several levels. Unlike verbal communication, artwork is not limited to a linear configuration.

6. *Creative and physical energy.* The very act of creating allows for a release of physical and creative energy. Participation is invoked by the process.

♦ CHILD ABUSE INVESTIGATIONS

Forensic science and social science traditionally champion different principles and practices that appear mutually exclusive. Law and the social sciences have differing roles in the justice system (Perry & Wrightsman, 1991). In recent years, a symbiosis of sorts has developed between the two disciplines as a result of societal issues. As investigation and intervention become more of a team effort, the legal and social science disciplines can interact creatively. One area in which this is acutely apparent is in the investigation of child maltreatment. Child abuse is not an entity that can be investigated by an isolated profession. Child maltreatment is a societal problem that invokes a multidisciplinary response.

The field of child abuse prevention and treatment comprises representatives from a host of disciplines who work together when confronted with an allegation. Individuals who investigate and intervene in response to child abuse allegations work collaboratively by commingling their respective skills, resources, knowledge, and abilities to formulate an effective course of action. The central component of a child abuse investigation is an interview of the alleged victim by a specialized and highly skilled child interview specialist or law enforcement agent. Frequently, child abuse interviews are conducted at multidisciplinary interviewing centers that promote interagency collaboration and team cooperation. Fundamentally, multidisciplinary interview centers advocate a collaborative response intended to minimize secondary trauma associated with the investigative process while maximizing an integrated and comprehensive response. The Children's Advocacy Center is a centralized model that originated in Huntsville, Alabama, in 1985. The model has spawned over 300 specialized interview centers nationwide (Myers, 1998). A joint interview of the child is one of the most significant aspects associated with this concept. Investigative interviews are conducted according to investigative guidelines comprising distinct but not disparate phases.

In the investigation of allegations of child abuse, the interviewer gathers information in a non-threatening manner that is developmentally sensitive, comprehensive, and legally defensible. Additional goals of the interview include corroboration of the data collected, the exploration of alternate hypotheses, and credibility assessment while adhering to forensic practice. Interview objectives include the gathering of information, the corroboration of facts, and the assessment of competency. Myers (1998) stated that there is no single correct way to interview children, and there is no gold standard or singular protocol that investigators must follow. Faller (1990) favored general guidelines for evaluators and the capability of addressing the allegations in a variety of ways rather than a protocol. Poole and Lamb (1998) noted that there is "remarkable overlap in the interview guidelines from various research groups and professional panels" (p. 120).

DRAWINGS AND INVESTIGATIVE INTERVIEWS

Investigative interviews foster practices and procedures that require specially trained and highly skilled interviewers. Drawings can assist interviewers in achieving the goals and objectives associated with investigative interviews. Commensurate with a child's skill level and interactive patterns, drawings supplement and complement the format in a manner that is forensically sound, child-friendly, and non-threatening. Drawings afford benefits for a child victim engaged in an investigative process. The integration of drawings within an investigative interview offers advantages not only for the child but also for the team and the process (Cohen-Liebman, 1999).

Proponents of multidisciplinary investigations have supported the use of drawings within an investigative interview format for different reasons (Myers, 1998). Drawings have been identified as tools that may assist interviewers in eliciting information from children within an investigative interview process (Faller, 1996; Haralambie, 1999). The benefits of the participation of art therapists within the forensic arena have also been noted, and interview guidelines include discussion of the potency of drawings (Cohen-Liebman, 1999; Cohen-Liebman, in press; CornerHouse, 2000; Farley, 1987).

In an investigative interview directed at assessing allegations of child maltreatment, drawings provide insight into a child's skill level, the traumatic response, and often abuse-specific information. Many authors cite the relevance of drawings in the development of rapport and assessing a child's developmental level (Bourg et al., 1999; Cohen-Liebman, 1999; Davies et al., 1996; Poole & Lamb, 1998). Material that is initially presented through drawings may serve as a catalyst for eventual verbal disclosure of information. Details salient to the investigation may be depicted. Drawings can clarify and supplement verbalizations, as well as corroborate information. A child's experience can often be expressed pictorially through a drawing, which can later serve as evidentiary material (Burgess, Hartman, Wolpert, & Grant, 1987; Cohen-Liebman, 1995; Faller, 1993).

Children respond to the use of art materials in a forensic process in a variety of ways. Drawings allow children to express information in a non-direct manner, thus alleviating a traumatic response. The use of media allows for an alternate means of expression of underlying thoughts and feelings, thus allaying fears and anxiety that may inhibit interaction. Drawings provide children with a means for self-expression that is safe, non-threatening, and developmentally congruent. Although forensic implies an investigative application, the intrinsic therapeutic value of the use of drawings within a forensic process should not be underestimated.

Drawings in Forensic Investigations

The role of drawings within forensic investigations has been the subject of recent study (Cohen-Liebman, in press). Within a forensic context, drawings may function in one of three ways. First, they can be used in a supportive capacity as *interviewing tools or aids* in an effort to explain or clarify a child's experience. As an investigative implement, drawings are used to support the investigation of a matter that is often disputed in a courtroom. Second, drawings can be construed as *charge enhancements,* providing information that can help determine charges and identify additional elements to investigate. Charge enhancements include situational and contextual information that is relevant to the child's experience. For example, drawings may depict information pertaining to the perpetrator, the incident, the setting, or any combination of the three. Children may make disclosure drawings in which the abuse is depicted. Charge enhancements may provide support for the goals of investigation and prosecution. Third, drawings may contain material that is evidentiary in nature and serve as *judiciary aids.*

Case Examples
Drawings as Interviewing Aids and Tools

Figure 11-11 was drawn by a 7-year-old girl who was allegedly molested by a 15-year-old male cousin. The drawing reveals elements of her traumatic response to the alleged activity and contains material that spawned a discussion pertaining to the allegations. The child disclosed that she was afraid to discuss the allegations because she was having nightmares about the alleged perpetrator. Her picture depicted the faces that she saw in her dreams, and she articulated that she hears the alleged perpetrator saying he is going to get her. She reported that once she told her mother about the abuse, she began to hear and see things. She discussed the allegations and included in her drawing a depiction of her and her cousin on the couch while her mother was sleeping. She provided details about the abuse that were situational and contextual in nature. The drawing provided her with a means of exploring the allegations in a nonthreatening manner. The subject matter she depicted provided a bridge to eventual discussion of the allegations.

In Figure 11-12, a 4-year-old child utilized a drawing as a demonstrative tool within the interview process. The drawing enabled the child to identify body parts in a developmentally congruent manner. It also helped to establish rapport and aided in developmental assessment of the child.

Drawings as Charge Enhancements

Figure 11-13 was made by a 9-year-old boy who demonstrated some cognitive delays. He exhibited advanced sexual knowledge that was developmentally incongruent. He was referred for the exploration of sexualized behavior. The child had previously disclosed that his older brother, who was in his early twenties, made him watch pornographic movies. The victim was also forced to watch the older brother and his girlfriend engage in sexual activity. The younger child was made to perform a sex act on a female child at the direction of this older sibling. The allegations came to light when the 9-year-old was found, on more than one occasion, engaging in sexualized behavior with younger children. In discussing the allegations and his brother, the child expressed that he could not say anything. He proceeded to make a drawing of what he was unable to verbalize. He described his picture by saying that "he tied it around my neck." He reported and promptly recanted that his brother hanged him. Upon drawing the picture, the child disclosed that his brother tied a belt around his neck to make him comply with the demands to engage in sexual activity. The drawing provided the child with an alternate means of expressing what he was afraid to say. It also depicted situational material and associated details including the use of threats and force.

While in foster care, an 8-year-old female was molested by the biological son of her foster parents. The child disclosed that the 16-year-old boy sodomized her on multiple occasions. The child provided salient and detailed information pertaining to the abuse, including contextual and situational material. She demonstrated advanced sexual knowledge that was unusual for her developmental level. She displayed difficulty discussing the alleged abuse and she resorted

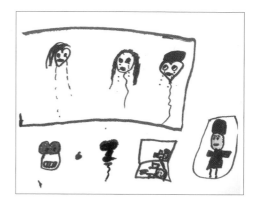

Figure 11-11. Drawing by a 7-year-old girl molested by a 15-year-old cousin.

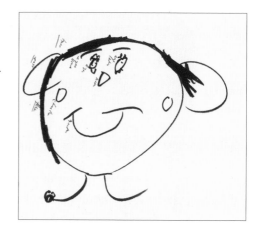

Figure 11-12. Drawing by a 4-year-old child.

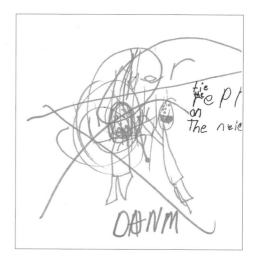

Figure 11-13. Drawing made by a 9-year-old boy forced to watch his older brother engage in sexual activity. The older brother also forced the child to engage in similar activity by tying a belt around the boy's neck to make him comply.

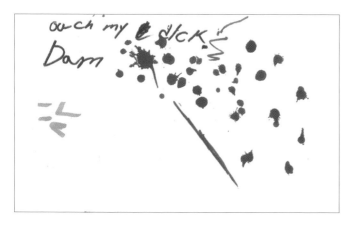

Figure 11-14. *Drawing by an 8-year-old girl molested by her 16-year-old foster brother, the biological son of the foster parents. He would say "ouch, damn" when he sodomized her. She depicted this graphically because she was unable to verbalize it.*

to the use of two-dimensional media to provide additional information as well as clarification. The child became increasingly agitated and expressed concern that she would get into trouble for verbalizing things said to her during the abuse by the alleged perpetrator. She utilized drawings to help her communicate what the boy said. The use of drawings appeared to provide her with a less threatening means of expression as well as distance. She expressed underlying feelings associated with guilt, shame, and betrayal. The child also conveyed her perception that the foster parents did not believe her as a result of her status as a foster child. She was also conflicted about statements made to her by the alleged perpetrator. She reported that he would say he loved her and then he would say "ouch." She explained that he would pull his pants down and place his private part in her butt and then he would say "ouch." The child indicated that he would say other things; however, she expressed that she could not say them. The child made several drawings in an effort to communicate what she was afraid and ashamed to say. She proceeded to depict what the 16-year-old would say to her (Fig. 11-14) when he molested her. She offered as explanation, "I guess he hurt himself or something." She then expressed that she was glad he hurt himself. In the process of creating this drawing, the child was able to release underlying anger in an acceptable manner, which is evident in the splotches made by her use of the media. The idiosyncratic nature of the drawing lends credence to the child's experience.

Drawings as Judiciary Aids

Figure 11-15 was drawn by a 7-year-old boy who was sexually abused by his mother's former paramour. The child's drawing provides detailed information that is developmentally congruent. The emotionally charged drawing captures the child's traumatic and emotional response. The child drew the picture in an effort to clarify his verbal description of the alleged activity. The alleged perpetrator is depicted in a jail cell with bars. The child identified body parts that were involved in the activity, including his and those of the alleged perpetrator. He drew extensions to indicate where body parts were placed. The 7-year-old expressed his anger by incorporating his thoughts and

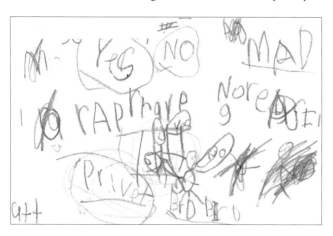

Figure 11-15. *Drawing by a 7-year-old boy raped by his mother's former paramour. The drawing captures the child's emotional response and depicts the alleged activity.*

feelings in the drawing. The child rendered himself saying "no" to the perpetrator who is saying "yes." The child attempted to express what happened to him through verbal associations and by writing the word "rape." He explained that "rape is touching people in a bad way that they do not like." As he discussed rape, he encircled the private parts on the figure identified as him and indicated where he was touched.

A 9-year-old female who was sexually molested by her stepfather depicted the alleged activity in Figure 11-16. The child disclosed that the alleged perpetrator would touch her and her sister while they were watching television in the living room. The faces on the children were originally drawn with smiles; however, as the child related information pertaining to the allegations and how her stepfather touched her and her sister, she altered the smiles and made them into frowns. She explained that the smile on the perpetrator's face remained because he liked what he was doing.

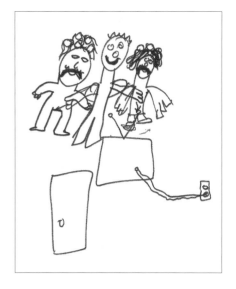

Figure 11-16. *A 9-year-old female molested by her stepfather depicted the alleged perpetrator molesting her and her sister while they watched television. She overwrote the expressions on the girls' faces and changed them from smiles into frowns as she spoke about the alleged activity.*

COMMON INTERVIEW GUIDELINE

The integration of drawings within an investigative interview format was examined in combination with the Common Interview Guideline (CIG) developed by Cohen-Liebman for the investigation of child sexual abuse allegations in the city of Philadelphia (Cohen-Liebman, 1999). The impetus to develop an interview guideline came from the need for a common language for the investigating agencies. The CIG promotes collaboration with the underlying premise that representatives from the agencies that intervene in the initial stages of an investigation work together as a team. The premise of collaborative investigative protocols or guidelines is to streamline and improve the investigative and judicial process. Investigative measures are directed at minimizing the need for repetitive interviews and multiple interviewers, while maximizing the information provided by a child. The resulting CIG had to incorporate distinct goals and purposes while meeting specified criteria associated with the identified investigating agencies. The CIG had to satisfy the investigative objectives associated with the respective disciplines, maintain forensic integrity, and allow for optimum elicitation of information. Fundamental to achieving these goals and objectives was the concept of a developmental framework that included a basic understanding of maturational spheres associated with children, as well as best practice with regard to interviewing children.

Five key components were identified as inherent to the creation of the CIG. Throughout the conceptual and developmental phases, it became increasingly apparent that these components were integral to a successful product. These elements were defined as follows:

1. Forensic interview, component phases

2. Interview techniques

3. Training curriculum, competency based modules

4. Cross-discipline and interagency issues

5. Team building and the issue of teaming

A 2-day workshop was designed to introduce the core components of the CIG through the explanation of the five underlying principles that comprise it. The workshop was intended to promote an appreciation for a CIG, as well as awareness of a collective process. The format was designed to incorporate the five key components in an effort to familiarize participants with the CIG. Thus, the agenda included experiential exercises to emphasize team-building and interagency collaboration, as well as specific exercises focusing on the component phases of the interview process and interviewing best practices.

INTEGRATION OF DRAWINGS INTO THE CIG

Drawings assist in attaining the specified goals and objectives affiliated with the interview process. Drawings complement and supplement the CIG and offer inherent advantages. They can be used in a parallel manner to the guidelines and serve as a bridge between the respective phases. They may serve as a stimulus for both the interviewer and the child to explore material that is manifest as well as latent.

The five phases of the CIG are Rapport Building, Developmental Assessment, Anatomy Identification, Fact-Finding, and Closure. Table 11-2 highlights the discriminating features associated with each phase of the guideline, as well as the corresponding attributes associated with the integration of drawings. The goals and objectives of the five phases of the investigative interview, as well as the integration of drawings with the guideline, are comprehensive and far more extensive than space permits. Highlights of essential criteria associated with each phase are included here. Note that the guideline is not a protocol and allows for fluidity and flexibility with regard to the phases. The phases are not intended to be rigid, and they may occur in any order, as well as overlap. They are presented sequentially for discussion purposes.

Rapport Building

In the rapport building phase, children are engaged, empowered, and encouraged to participate. Comfort is promoted, and the standard operating procedure is addressed, including the setting, task, expectations, and methods of both remembering and recording the memories. Accuracy is emphasized and children are encouraged to challenge authority, acknowledge confusion, and clarify misperceptions. Resistance to suggestion is also assessed.

Integration of Drawings

The very nature of the media makes the process child-friendly. Through the integration of drawings, a child can be engaged verbally or non-verbally. The selection of media promotes choice, which is empowering for a child, given that most children lack control in abusive situations or in the presence of authoritative figures. A drawing task can stimulate conversation and help establish trust with the child. Material that is initially presented may serve as a catalyst for eventual disclosure of information that may be salient to the investigation. Drawings can help bridge to the fact-finding phase. They may serve as a stimulus to explore additional material.

Case Examples

A 6-year-old boy made a spontaneous depiction of his family upon entering the interviewing room. The graphic composition led to a discussion of the family

Table 11-2. Integrating Drawings into the Common Interview Guideline (CIG)

CIG Component Phases	Integration of Drawings with CIG Component Phases
Rapport Building	
Engage Promote comfort, trust Active participation	**Develop comfort** Icebreaker **Promote trust**
Empower Provide choice = control	**Engagement** Verbally and non-verbally establish rapport
Encourage Challenge authority Correct, disagree	**Media** Stimulates participation Connotes child-friendly process Stimulates conversation
Address standard operating procedure	
Clarify misperceptions	Choice = empowerment/control
Emphasize accuracy Acknowledge confusion rather than guess	**Stimulus to explore topics** **Bridge to fact-finding**
Assess suggestibility	**Assess suggestibility**
Developmental Screening/Skills Assessment	
Assess skill level in various spheres Cognitive, social, emotional Linguistic, concepts Ability to interact	**Assessment of skill levels** Cognitive, social, emotional **Assess strengths/weaknesses**
Modify and adapt communication Language, tasks, style	**Assess ability to follow directives, remain on task** Ability to attend, focus
Evaluate Comprehension Assess type of questions	**Artistic Development** Assists in comprehension of developmental capabilities
Concepts Spatial relationships Prepositions Colors Numbers Developmentally congruent Tasks	**Mastery of developmentally congruent tasks** Letters Numbers Spatial relationships Prepositions
Assess congruency of concepts Truth/lie, real/pretend, right/wrong, good/bad	**Congruency of concepts** **Adaptation of communication**
Assess competency	**Assess competency**
Practice and role play	**Practice and role play**
Issue of mistake	**Information is utilized to adapt/modify communication style**

Table 11-2. Integrating Drawings into the Common Interview Guideline (CIG)—*continued*

CIG Component Phases	Integration of Drawings with CIG Component Phases
Anatomy Identification	
Identification of body parts Sexual and non-sexual	**Demonstration aid**
	Client generated product
Location, function of parts	**Externalization**
Sensory reference See, smell, hear, taste, touch	**Distance**
	Evidentiary material
Explore different touches	**Confirm verbal statements**
	Objectification
Fact-Finding	
Question continuum Open-ended to more focused and directed	**Disclosure drawings**
	Corroboration of facts
Reverse continuum of questions	**Details** Situational and contextual Idiosyncratic details
Non-leading questions General to specific	
	Facts
Details Contextual and situational Who, what, when, where, how	**Charge enhancements** Threats, force, bribes, coercion, rewards, use of media, pornography, photography
Specific facts	**Facilitate disclosure**
Details/information	**Pictorial clarification**
Corroboration of information	**Collateral material**
Collateral material	**Confirmation of verbal statements**
Charge enhancements	**Depict what child cannot say**
Explore alternate hypothesis	
Credibility assessment	

dynamics, which ultimately resulted in discussion pertaining to the alleged perpetrator. The drawing provided a means to explore related material in a nondirected manner that was appropriate for the child's developmental level (Fig. 11-17).

Figure 11-18 is a drawing made by a 7-year-old boy. The subject of a dinosaur eating a plant provided an opportunity for the child to become comfortable with the interviewer and the process. The child later disclosed that his 13-year-old uncle had "tried to do [him] in the butt."

	Integration of Drawings with CIG
CIG Component Phases	**Component Phases**
Closure	
Thank child for participation	Review
Leave door open for possible re-interview	Revisit
Address concerns and questions	Clarify
Avoid false hopes	Memory stimulus/trigger
Address personal safety	Bridge
Bridge to what happens next	Re-constitution
End positively	End positively

Table 11-2. Integrating Drawings into the Common Interview Guideline (CIG)—*continued*

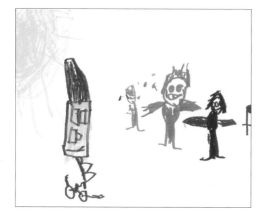

Figure 11-17. *A 6-year-old boy made a picture of his family that stimulated conversation and led to a conversation regarding the alleged perpetrator.*

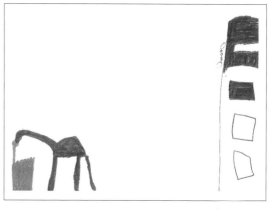

Figure 11-18. *This drawing was made by a 7-year-old male who was molested by his 13-year-old uncle, who "tried to do [him] in the butt."*

Developmental Assessment

The developmental assessment phase provides the interviewer with information pertaining to a child's skills and level of functioning. Developmental spheres that are assessed include cognitive, linguistic, social, and emotional. How the child processes information and the child's expressive-receptive capabilities are considered. Concept formation is also pertinent to determining the child's knowledge with regard to basic concepts and relationships. This information is important for the interviewer to assess in an effort to comprehend how a child communicates and interacts. The interviewer modifies and adapts language and concepts to communicate in a developmentally sensitive manner with the child.

Integration of Drawings

Assessment of a child's artistic developmental level assists the interviewer in comprehending the child's level of functioning. Drawings and the use of the

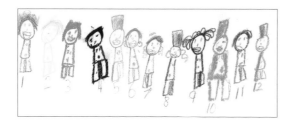

Figure 11-19. *A 6-year-old child depicted his knowledge of color identification, counting, and gender differences in this drawing to assist in the assessment of developmental functioning.*

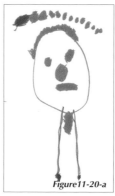 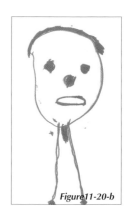

Figure 11-20-a   Figure 11-20-b

Figure 11-20. *(a) and (b) Both these drawings of figures with private parts were made by a 4-year-old female who denied sexual abuse despite medical findings consistent with such abuse.*

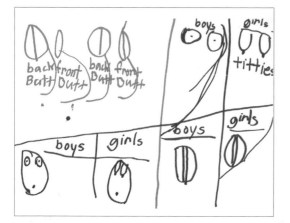

Figure 11-21. *In response to identification of body parts, this 7-year-old depicted her knowledge of male and female sexual body parts through this diagram. The child was highly sexualized and verbalized her knowledge. She made a series of drawings to depict the alleged activity.*

media provide information including skill level, mastery of developmentally congruent tasks, strengths, weaknesses, spatial relationships, and congruency of concepts. The child may be given specific tasks designed to provide information relevant to the process, including the ability to comprehend and follow directives, stay on task, and make identifications.

Case Examples
A 6-year-old boy illustrated how he responded to developmental assessment tasks in Figure 11-19. He demonstrated his knowledge of basic concepts, including color identification and gender differences, through his depiction of multiple figures. Artistically, his drawing is somewhat advanced for his developmental level.

Both drawings in Figure 11-20 were made by a 4-year-old female. The child depicted an age-appropriate rendering of a figure in each drawing. She included a private part in each drawing. The child had physical findings on her medical examination that were consistent with sexual abuse, yet she denied being touched by anyone.

Anatomy Identification
The anatomy identification phase provides information pertaining to a child's perception of body parts, different types of touches, and sensory reference. Information is obtained not to educate the child, but rather to evaluate the child's language, knowledge, and understanding.

Integration of Drawings
Drawings provide a child with a more comfortable method of depicting body parts and demonstrating knowledge about them. The use of a template, a diagram, or a client-generated product provides a less threatening means of identifying sexual body parts. The use of a drawing may distill apprehension associated with this phase because a drawing is an external object. As a result, the discussion of a picture is less threatening. Drawings can serve as demonstration tools.

Case Examples

A 7-year-old girl drew Figure 11-21. She disclosed that she learned nasty stuff from two cousins who were 8 and 9 years old. She reported that the boys taught her to "suck their dicks." She provided graphic and detailed accounts of the alleged activity that ensued between the children. The child was highly sexualized, and she was observed exhibiting sexually reactive behavior with a younger nephew. She made several drawings that were graphic in nature. The drawing functioned as a demonstration aid in addition to providing the child with a means of discharge for associated thoughts and feelings.

A 5-year-old boy who was diagnosed with ocular gonorrhea drew Figure 11-22. He identified the figure as a girl. He was initially reluctant to identify body parts. At the end of the interview, he identified the mark between the legs as a private part. The drawing provided a less threatening means of communication for the child, who demonstrated advanced sexual knowledge in his associations.

A 9-year-old female referred for allegations of sexual abuse by a 14-year-old cousin made the picture in Figure 11-23 in an effort to distinguish between boys and girls. Although she did not depict genitalia on the drawing, she was able to provide information pertaining to the differences between boys and girls, which provided a stimulus for disclosing information relevant to the allegations. Through this drawing, many of the tasks associated with the first three phases of the guideline were accomplished, including rapport building, developmental assessment, and anatomy identification.

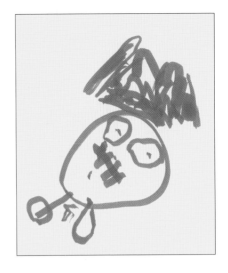

Figure 11-22. This drawing was done by a 5-year-old boy who was diagnosed with ocular gonorrhea. He depicted a figure that he identified as a girl. In response to identifying private parts, he placed a mark between the legs, which he stated was a private part. He indicated that a girl's private part is different from a boy's.

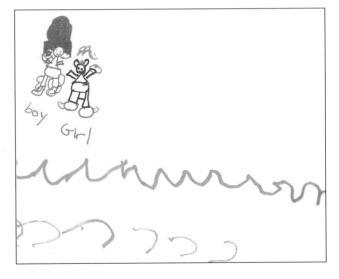

Figure 11-23. A 9-year-old female demonstrates age-appropriate understanding of gender differences.

Fact-Finding

In the fact-finding phase, information pertaining to the allegations is addressed. The previous three phases provide a foundation for the information that is gathered in this phase. By defeating the argument of suggestibility from the onset of the process, as well as demonstrating the child's developmental capabilities, the interviewer can explain and, if necessary, defend in court the type of questions and the tasks incorporated in the process. In the fact-finding phase, abuse-specific information is explored, including situational and contextual material, charge enhancements, and forensic elements. The latter refer to the use of threats, bribes, rewards, and punishment, as well as sexual aids, pornography, and media. Alternate explanations are explored as well.

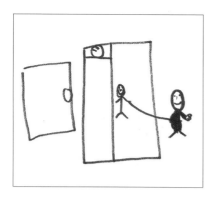

Figure 11-24. *A 7-year-old boy who disclosed being raped at school in the elevator drew this picture in an effort to clarify his verbal statements.*

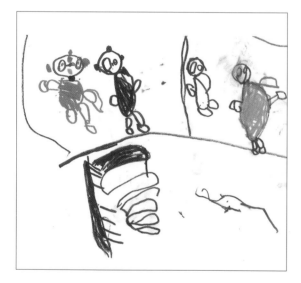

Figure 11-25. *A 6-year-old boy made a map of the scene he witnessed (the molestation of his 4-year-old brother by a babysitter) in an effort to provide details, including the location of the event.*

Integration of Drawings

In the fact-finding phase, drawings may yield information that is significant for prosecutorial and investigative purposes, including contextual and situational information. Children may lack the cognitive capability or the verbal capacity to articulate their abusive experiences (Burgess, McCausland, & Wolbert, 1981). Many times they will ask to draw rather than say what happened. Research indicates that children who are reticent to discuss their abusive experiences may become more willing to talk after they have visually depicted the abuse or salient details associated with the event (Kelley, 1984). Often children provide additional or supplemental information because the drawing serves as a trigger or stimulus. Disclosure drawings are pictures in which the child depicts the activity. Collateral material and corroboration of details and facts may surface in a graphic representation. A drawing may contain contextual information such as who, what, when, or where. Charge enhancements may be drawn that identify additional arenas to pursue. Drawings may provide clarification or confirmation of verbal statements in a concrete and objective fashion.

Case Examples

A 7-year-old male was found engaging in sexualized behavior with a younger male cousin. When questioned by his mother as to where he learned the activity, the child related that someone at school had done something to him. He disclosed that a man pulled him into an elevator, shut it off and pulled his pants down. The man then placed his penis in the child's buttocks. The child reported that the man had something white on his penis. The incident happened quickly and the man let him out of the elevator, according to the child. Figure 11-24 is a depiction made by the child to explain what happened. He reported that a "dude" at school pulled him into an elevator. He provided a narrative as he drew. He reported, "I was walking. He pulled me in—the dude and I got raped. He pressed this button and the doors were locked and closed and he raped me." The child continued to provide a graphic and detailed description of the incident. He described physical features of the alleged perpetrator including skin tone, physical build, and hair color. He also provided a description of the alleged perpetrator's clothing. He stated that the individual used force when he grabbed him and held him. The child also reported that the man covered his mouth with one hand. The picture, although sparse in detail, provided the child with a means of verbal elaboration. It also provided confirmation of his verbal associations. As a result of the picture, the child provided situational and contextual information, including forensic elements. He provided details that were idiosyncratic and descriptive.

Figure 11-25 is a map scene in which a 6-year-old boy depicted the scene he and a cousin observed from the hallway. Both he and the cousin were witnesses to the molestation of his 4-year-old brother by their baby sitter. The drawing provided corroboratory material that proved to be significant to the investigating agents. They confirmed that the stairs were dirty and blue as depicted.

A 5-year-old girl allegedly molested by her 11-year-old brother depicted an age-appropriate rendering (Fig. 11-26) in an effort to provide clarification to her verbalizations. She disclosed that her brother rubbed her vagina. The child attempted to depict the alleged activity. She explained that her brother said they were playing mommy and daddy. The child's picture is a scene of the bedroom where the activity took place.

Closure

The closure phase is critical to the process and has ramifications for future interactions with the child. It is imperative that the interview conclude positively rather than negatively. Several tasks are addressed in this phase, including establishing a context for a possible re-interview, bridging to what happens next, and addressing the child's issues, fears, and concerns. The child's participation is acknowledged, and information may be reviewed, revisited, or clarified.

Integration of Drawings

In the closure phase, drawings can be used to review or clarify information. They may also provide a positive means of concluding the process and help a child reconstitute, if necessary. They may be utilized as a memory trigger, as a bridge to what happens next, or as a transitional object. The latter reaffirms the child-friendly nature of the process and contributes to goodwill in the event a re-interview is necessary.

Case Examples

Figure 11-27 was drawn by a 6-year-old child who was molested by her 16-year-old half-brother. He reportedly made the youngster perform oral sex on him. During the interview, the child displayed difficulty relating information pertaining to the allegations. She became increasingly non-verbal, and exhibited embarrassment and shame. The drawing she depicted provided her with a means of reconstituting before the interview was concluded. The picture is somewhat advanced for her developmental level.

Figure 11-28 was the final picture made by the child discussed previously who was molested by a 16-year-old foster brother

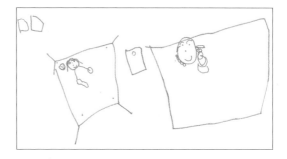

Figure 11-26. This drawing was made by a 5-year-old girl who attempted to show how she and her brother played mommy and daddy. The child's brother was 11.

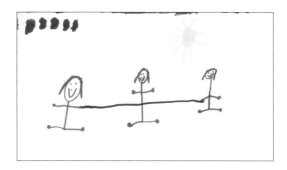

*Figure 11-27. A 6-year-old molested by her 16-year-old half-brother, who made her perform oral sex on him, made this drawing at the end of the interview.
The child displayed difficulty discussing the allegations. The drawing allowed her to conclude the process on a positive note.*

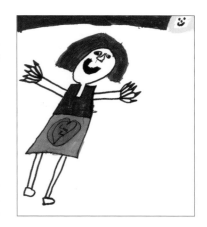

Figure 11-28. This is the final drawing made by the 8-year-old child who drew Figure 11-14. The drawing depicts her emotional response to the process and reflects the empowerment associated with the use of drawings, which allowed her to communicate previously undisclosed thoughts and feelings relating to both the abuse and her foster care placement.

(see Fig. 11-14). The child experienced a range of emotions as she related information relevant to her experience. Despite her reticence to discuss the allegations and her fear associated with disclosing information, she was able to communicate information through the use of drawings in a manner that was less threatening. The difficulty associated with the process was compounded by her emotional response; however, she was able to complete the interview and provide detailed information. The disclosure of information through the use of drawings and in conjunction with her associations enabled her to manage underlying thoughts and feelings. The ability to disclose information in a safe and supportive fact-finding environment contributed to feelings of empowerment as she communicated for the first time her feelings of ostracism associated with her placement into foster care, as well as her fears associated with the alleged perpetrator. Her drawing reflects her response to the process.

Final Note

Many authors concur that care should be taken in the interpretation of drawings (American Academy of Child and Adolescent Psychiatry [AACAP], 1990; Burgess & Hartman, 1993; Cohen-Liebman, 1995, 1999; Farley, 1987; Friedrich, 1990; Malchiodi, 1998; Schetky & Benedek, 1992; Sorenson, Bottoms, & Perona, 1997). Interviewers are cautioned not to interpret drawings in an effort to determine the likelihood of sexual abuse and not to over-interpret drawings. Burgess and Hartman (1993) advocate that those interpreting drawings should be professionals trained in interpreting artwork.

In recent years, researchers have sought to determine if the graphic productions created by sexually abused children differ from those of non-abused children. Cohen-Liebman (1995) compiled a composite list of indicators from the psychological and art therapy literature and research. The literature indicates that sole reliance upon a child's drawing as confirmation of sexual abuse is not plausible at this time (Cohen-Liebman, 1995; Hibbard, Roghmann, & Hoekelman, 1987; Malchiodi, 1990; Malchiodi, 1998; Sidun & Rosenthal, 1987). No single graphic indicator or cluster of indicators can conclusively support a finding of sexual abuse. In isolation, the presence of graphic indicators can neither prove nor disprove sexual abuse, but the presence of graphic indicators is indicative of the need for further investigation. The American Academy of Child and Adolescent Psychiatry (AACAP, 1990) guidelines state that the usefulness of drawings lies in the affect (emotion) and information they elicit and certain characteristics that may be suggestive of sexual abuse. The guidelines indicate that both spontaneous and directed drawings are helpful in forensic assessments.

♦ GENERAL CASE EXAMPLE 1

An 8-year-old female was referred for the exploration of allegations of sexual abuse. The alleged perpetrator was identified as her mother's paramour. The child allegedly disclosed to her maternal grandmother that her daddy (as she referred to the alleged perpetrator) "sticks his fingers up there." The child reportedly demonstrated the alleged activity. The child presented as verbal, interactive, and highly anxious. The child reported that she was there to get help because of what her step-dad did to her. She reported that her father put his hand up her private. She reported that she witnessed her father do the same thing to her younger sister. She began to draw the alleged activity in a non-directed and spontaneous manner. She provided a narrative as she drew. Initially, the child depicted the scene she witnessed as she observed it through the keyhole. Her underlying anxiety began to overwhelm her and she shaded in the view (Fig. 11-29-a). She wrote "door" to indicate where she was looking. She began to discuss an unrelated topic in an effort to manage underlying anxiety. She proceeded to draw on the same sheet of paper where she had previously begun to depict the abuse she witnessed involving her sister. On the paper she made a picture of a sleepover party with her friends.

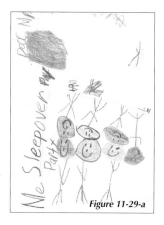

Figure 11-29-a

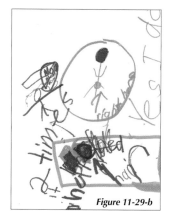

Figure 11-29-b

Figures 11-29. *(a) and (b) Both drawings were made by an 8-year-old who witnessed the molestation of her half-sister, the biological child of the alleged perpetrator. The first drawing began with the depiction of an abuse scene witnessed by the child. She drew the door to explain how she looked through the keyhole and watched her step-father touching her younger sister. She became overwhelmed as she spoke and she began to talk about less stress-provoking topics. The rest of the picture was devoted to a depiction of a sleep-over party that took place at her home. Her second drawing is a disclosure drawing in which she depicts what happened. She includes information pertinent to her experience in an effort to clarify and emphasize her verbalizations.*

The child returned to the topic of abuse and reported that she saw her sister sleeping on the bed. The alleged perpetrator, the biological father of the younger child, placed his finger in the younger child's private. The child provided information pertaining to the situation, including the location of the event, and contextual material, including details regarding the clothing of her sister and the alleged perpetrator. The child defined a private part and she disclosed that this activity also had happened to her. She became increasingly agitated and acted out the abuse with dolls. She then proceeded to have the sister doll yell at the father doll, which appeared to be a cathartic experience for her. After additional conversation, the child began to decompensate and the interview was terminated.

The child returned for a second interview. The child presented as distracted, and she demonstrated a tendency to shift between topics. Although she expressed a desire not to discuss the allegations, she began to write information pertaining to her experience, which she then verbalized (Fig. 11-29-b). In an effort to clarify her written information, she depicted a stick figure and highlighted the genital area by placing an arrow to indicate the location of the private part. She continued to draw. She drew what she described as a bed. She related that she was on the bed and her foot was sticking off of it. She

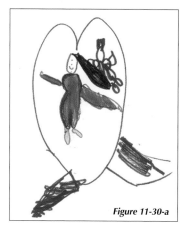

Figure 11-30-a

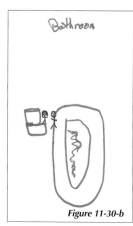

Figure 11-30-b

Figure 11-30. *(a) and (b) A 6-year-old girl was molested by her maternal grandfather. Her 9-year-old brother witnessed the activity. Both children were able to communicate verbally and pictorially what had happened. Both children were traumatized by the activity. They both exhibited betrayal issues with regard to the grandfather. The brother exhibited issues associated with guilt.*

indicated that she did not wish to continue the discussion. She then wrote on the drawing that it happened two times. She began to provide additional information pertaining to the alleged abuse. She included in her drawing a figure calling out to her mother. The drawing is quite complex as the child attempted to depict several elements associated with her own experience, as well as that of her sister. The spatial matrix quality allows for the expression of multiple events and salient situational and contextual details in the same drawing.

The drawings provided the child with a way of disclosing her abusive experience in a manner that was appropriate for her overall level of functioning. They provided her with an alternate means of communication that was cathartic. They complemented her ability to disclose information and provided support for her in relation to the process, as well as her mental well-being. They also served as interviewing aids and may in the future prove to be essential as judiciary or evidentiary material.

◆ GENERAL CASE EXAMPLE 2

A 6-year-old female and her 9-year-old brother were interviewed independently to explore allegations of sexual abuse involving the maternal grandfather. Both children disclosed that the grandfather abused the girl while she was in the bathtub. The brother reportedly witnessed the alleged abuse of his sister. Each child drew the activity as they experienced it. Figures 11-30-a (the sister's drawing) and 11-30-b (the brother's drawing) essentially depict the same scene. The sister's drawing shows her in the bathtub with the grandfather touching her. The brother's drawing reflects what he saw and is rendered in a fashion that is developmentally congruent, as is the sister's graphic depiction. The drawings proved to be salient with regard to situational details. The children were both traumatized by the experience. The brother appeared to be having a vicarious response and both children were referred for therapeutic intervention. The drawings provided clarification and confirmation of verbalizations made by both children. Their statements and their drawings were parallel and may at some point in the future prove to be salient in a judicial context.

◆ SUMMARY

For more information regarding the profession of Art Therapy and the American Art Therapy Association contact:

The American Art Therapy Association, Inc. (AATA)
1202 Allanson Road
Mundelein, IL, 60060-3803
1-888-290-0878 (toll free)
847-949-6064
847-566-4580 (fax)
e-mail—arttherapy@ntr.net
Web site—www.arttherapy.org

For more information regarding registration and certification of Art Therapists contact:
The Art Therapy Credentials Board, Inc. (ATCB)
3 Terrace Way, Suite B
Greensboro, NC 27403
1-877-213-2822 (toll free)
336-547-0017 (fax)
e-mail—info@atcb.com

◆ REFERENCES

American Art Therapy Association, Inc. (1999). <u>Art therapy: The profession.</u> Mundelein, IL: Author.

American Art Therapy Association, Inc. (2000). <u>Ethical considerations regarding the therapeutic use of art by disciplines outside the field of art therapy.</u> Mundelein, IL: Author.

American Academy of Child and Adolescent Psychiatry. (1990). <u>Guidelines for the evaluation of child and adolescent sexual abuse.</u> (Originally approved June 1988; modified December 14, 1990.) Washington, DC: Author.

Bourg, W., Broderick, R., Flagor, R., Kelly, D. M., Ervin, D. L., & Butler, J. (1999). <u>A child interviewer's guidebook.</u> Thousand Oaks, CA: Sage Publications.

Burgess, A. W., & Hartman, C. R. (1993). Children's drawings. <u>Child Abuse & Neglect, 17,</u> 161-168.

Burgess, A. W., Hartman, C. R., Wolbert, W. A., & Grant, C. A. (1987). Child molestation: Assessing impact in multiple victims. <u>Archives of Psychiatric Nursing, 1</u>(1), 33-39.

Burgess, A. W., McCausland, M. P., & Wolbert, W. A. (1981). Children's drawings as indicators of sexual trauma. <u>Perspectives in Psychiatric Care, 19</u>(2), 50-57.

Cohen-Liebman, M. S. (1995). Drawings as judiciary aids in child sexual abuse litigation: A composite list of indicators. <u>The Arts in Psychotherapy, 22</u>(5), 475-483.

Cohen-Liebman, M. S. (1997, November). <u>Forensic art therapy.</u> Preconference course presented at the annual conference of the American Art Therapy Association. Milwaukee, WI: AATA.

Cohen-Liebman, M. S. (1999). Draw and tell: Drawings within the context of child sexual abuse investigations. <u>The Arts in Psychotherapy, 26</u>(3), 185-194.

Cohen-Liebman, M.S. (in press). Using drawings in forensic investigations of child sexual abuse. In C. Malchiodi (Ed.), <u>Handbook of clinical art therapy.</u> New York: Guilford Publications, Inc.

Cohen-Liebman, M. S., & Gussak, D. (1998). <u>Investigation versus intervention: Forensic art therapy versus art therapy in forensic settings.</u> Paper presented at the annual conference of the American Art Therapy Association. Portland, OR: AATA.

CornerHouse. (2000). <u>Child sexual abuse forensic interview training manual.</u> Minneapolis, MN: Author.

Davies, D., Cole, J., Albertella, G., McCulloch, Allen, K., & Kekevian, H. (1996). A model for conducting forensic interviews with child victims of abuse. <u>Child Maltreatment, 1</u>(3), 189-199.

Faller, K. (1990). <u>Understanding child sexual maltreatment.</u> Newbury Park, CA: Sage Publications.

Faller, K. (1993). <u>Child sexual abuse: Assessment and intervention issues.</u> Washington, DC: U.S. Department of Health and Human Services, National Center on Child Abuse and Neglect.

Faller, K. (1996). <u>Evaluating children suspected of having been sexually abused: The APSAC study guides 2.</u> Thousand Oaks, CA: Sage Publications.

Farley, R. H. (1987, April). Drawing interviews: An alternative technique. <u>The Police Chief, 54</u>(4), 37-38.

Friedrich, W. N. (1990). <u>Psychotherapy of sexually abused children and their families.</u> New York: W.W. Norton & Company.

Haralambie, A. M. (1999). <u>Child sexual abuse in civil cases: A guide to custody and tort actions.</u> Chicago: American Bar Association.

Hibbard, R. A., Roghmann, K., & Hoekelman, R. A. (1987). Genitalia in children's drawings: An association with sexual abuse. <u>Pediatrics, 79</u>(1), 129-137.

Junge, M. B., & Asawa, P. P. (1994). <u>A history of art therapy in the United States.</u> Mundelein, IL: AATA.

Kelley, S. J. (1984). The use of art therapy with sexually abused children. <u>Journal of Psychosocial Nursing, 22</u>(12), 12-18.

Kellogg, R. (1970). <u>Analyzing children's art.</u> Mountain View, CA: Mayfield Publishing Company.

Levick, M. F. (1983). <u>They could not talk and so they drew.</u> Springfield, IL: Charles C. Thomas.

Levick, M. F. (1998). <u>See what I'm saying: What children tell us through their art.</u> Dubuque, IA: Islewest Publishing.

Lowenfeld, V., & Brittain, W. L. (1987). <u>Creative and mental growth.</u> New York: MacMillan Publishing Company.

Lusebrink, V. B. (1989). Education in creative arts therapies: Accomplishments and challenges. <u>The Arts in Psychotherapy, 16,</u> 5-10.

Malchiodi, C. (1990). <u>Breaking the silence: Art therapy with children from violent homes.</u> New York: Brunner/Mazel.

Malchiodi, C. (1998). <u>Understanding children's drawings.</u> New York: The Guilford Press.

Myers, J. E. B. (1998). <u>Legal issues in child abuse and neglect practice.</u> Thousand Oaks, CA: Sage Publications.

Naumburg, M. (1987). <u>Dynamically oriented art therapy.</u> Chicago: Magnolia Street Publishers.

Perry, N. W., & Wrightsman, L. S. (1991). <u>The child witness: Legal issues and dilemmas.</u> Newbury Park, CA: Sage Publications.

Poole, D.A., & Lamb, M.E. (1998). <u>Investigative interviews of children: A guide for helping professionals.</u> Washington, DC: American Psychological Association.

Rubin, J. (1979). Art therapy: An introduction. In <u>Conference on creative arts therapies</u> [monograph] (pp. 12-14). Washington, DC: American Psychiatric Association.

Rubin, J. (1984). <u>Child art therapy: Understanding and helping children grow through art</u> (2nd ed.). New York: Van Nostrand Reinhold.

Schetky, D. H., & Benedek, E. (1992). <u>Clinical handbook of child psychiatry and the law.</u> Baltimore, MD: Williams & Wilkins.

Sidun, N. M., & Rosenthal, R. H. (1987). Graphic indicators of sexual abuse in Draw-A-Person tests of psychiatrically hospitalized adolescents. <u>The Arts in Psychotherapy, 14,</u> 25-33.

Sorenson, E., Bottoms, B., & Perona, A. (1997). <u>Handbook on intake and forensic interviewing in the children's advocacy center setting.</u> Washington, DC: Office of Juvenile Justice and Delinquency Prevention.

Ulman, E. (1986). Variations on a Freudian theme: Three art therapy theorists. <u>The American Journal of Art Therapy, 24</u>(4), 125-134.

Vaccaro, M. (1973). The responsibility of the art therapist. <u>Philadelphia Medicine, 69,</u> 253-256.

Wadeson, H. (1980). <u>Art psychotherapy.</u> New York: John Wiley & Sons.

Chapter 12

THE INTERNET AND THE RISK FOR MALTREATMENT

DET. SGT. JOSEPH BOVA CONTI
ANGELO GIARDINO, M.D., PH.D.

In the coming years more and more children will have access to the Internet. Whether at home, the library, or school, the Internet has become a tool that children and teens use at all levels of education and communication. Professionals who work on behalf of children and teens must realize that this tool is also an area where seduction, *corruption, exploitation, and abuse can occur (Jezycki, 1998). Children may be at risk even while in the confines of school, daycare, or their own homes. This chapter deals with the challenge of keeping children safe while they take advantage of the vast potential that the Internet offers them.*

◆ WHAT IS THE INTERNET?

Our society has passed from the Industrial Age into the Information Age. Microchips, tiny as they are, have revolutionized the manner in which information is shared and have made society truly a global community. The information age has had a tremendous impact on children. Today many children are very familiar with computers and face an increasingly technology-driven world in the future. Even though some families do not own a personal computer, access is relatively easy. Many children have at least one friend whose family owns a computer. Children also have access to computers at school and in public libraries, where the computer is often used as a research and teaching tool and as a portal to access the World Wide Web (WWW) via the Internet. For a young person in today's world, being without computer skills is akin to being illiterate in years past.

The Internet is rapidly becoming a part of everyone's daily life. As the name implies, the Internet refers to a huge network of computers that are electronically linked via telephone lines, cable lines, and satellites so that users can communicate and access information while "online." The Internet began as a defense project in the 1960s. When universities discovered how useful the Internet was for sharing research and advanced knowledge, they became involved. Public and corporate applications soon followed. Today, anyone can access the Internet provided they have a modem; the right software, known as a web browser; and a connection point, such as an online service or Internet service provider (ISP). Millions of people around the world access the Internet and go online each day.

The WWW is perhaps the most well-known component of the Internet. Because of its sensory appeal, the WWW is the part most often accessed. Sites on the web contain colorful graphics, audio and video clips, and real-time communication. One can listen to music, see a historical tape, find out what is new at a museum or library, look at art, talk via the keyboard to other people with similar interests or hobbies, watch a live feed of current news, tour the White House, and do countless other worthwhile activities. Little regulation exists on the WWW, and the Internet's global character prevents any single company or government from exerting overall control of the content available online.

The Internet and WWW are very flexible and have appeal for almost every age group. For the very young child, the Internet offers learning games, clubs, and publications. For teens, there are chat groups, online magazines, games, and teen clubs. Students can access organization and government sites, academic resources, virtual exploration sites, and commercial education sites.

The Internet runs the gamut of human knowledge. Its electronic structure allows it to be updated more frequently than printed material could ever be. Children and teens benefit greatly from the self-directed learning experiences the Internet provides and especially from the boost of confidence that comes when they have successfully navigated the Internet to find information. Today the Internet is widely considered a critical component of a child's education, but it also gives children access to content of questionable value.

Unfortunately, there are web sites that children can access which contain material that is hateful, violent, or otherwise inappropriate for children. Children may stumble across these sites when doing a search because the methods used to complete a search are not designed to screen out material that might be inappropriate for children. For example, sites exist on the WWW for adults who want to post, view, or read sexually explicit material. While some of these adult-oriented sites make the effort to verify the visitor's age, usually by requesting a credit card number (assuming that children do not have credit cards), others make no effort in this direction. Software does exist that may help keep children away from such inappropriate sites, but these programs are not failsafe. On average, common software solutions used to keep children away from adult-oriented sites fail to block approximately 20% of objectionable sites (Consumer Reports, 2001).

While it is true that the Internet and computers have dangers, the benefits of their usage would seem to far outweigh the risks. To restrict access to computers is unrealistic and would be analogous to asking teens not to drive because accidents sometimes happen. As with all technological advances, such as television and cars, parents, teachers, and caregivers must be aware of the risks and take common sense steps to protect children. It is important to recognize the dangers and know what to do when they are encountered. The Pew Internet Tracking Report found that Americans are deeply worried about criminal activity on the Internet, with 92% of Americans saying they are concerned about child pornography on the Internet, and 50% saying that it is the most heinous crime that occurs on the Internet (Fox & Lewis, 2001).

KNOWING THE INTERNET

The best way to protect children as they use the Internet is for parents, caregivers, and teachers to guide and monitor computer use. Those adults and professionals who are responsible for children and their care should become familiar with computer use, including "surfing the 'Net," and be aware of the types of sites and services available online.

Before safety concerns can be addressed, it is important to have a basic knowledge of online terminology. Appendix I contains a glossary of various terms and online structures commonly associated with computer usage.

♦ RISKS ASSOCIATED WITH USING THE INTERNET

The major risks facing children on the Internet fall into the following categories (Magid, 1998):

1. Exposure to material that is inappropriate or encourages dangerous or illegal activity.

2. Exposure to harassment through demeaning or threatening e-mail chat or messages.

3. Revealing financial information (e.g., credit card numbers) that produces negative consequences.

4. Engaging in activity that has legal ramifications, possibly violating the rights of others (e.g., knowingly posting inaccurate information that causes others to act).

5. Safety issues, including physical molestation or other injury, resulting from sharing personal information or meeting a stranger in person.

Some of the more than 60 million people accessing the Internet will do so for inappropriate or illegal reasons (Armagh, Battaglia, & Lanning, 2000). Some will disguise themselves and use chat rooms, bulletin boards, or instant messaging services to communicate with a child and inappropriately gain his or her confidence. Using this type of manipulation, the perpetrator may ask for and receive personal information. Unfortunately, some of these people then use this information to arrange a face-to-face meeting with the child for the purposes of sexual abuse. One technique to note is when sexual predators create an online site that has the allure of a commercial enterprise and then use a "marketing strategy" to gain information about a child. By placing a banner ad on a site, advertisers can insert a tag or "cookie" on the child's computer that tracks where he or she clicks the mouse. Cookies can keep track of how often and when an individual visits a site, and where the visitor clicks the mouse while there. The term *digital profiling* refers to developing a portrait of the person gleaned from information gathered online. For example, if the banner advertises a contest or sweepstakes and offers the visitor a chance to register by filling in a name and address, the cookie can be linked to an actual person's online activity (Turow & Nir, 2000).

Visitors also may be manipulated into giving information when they are asked to register to use a site. Advocates for privacy protection on the WWW express concerns about the gathering of information. The principal problem presented by the WWW that is not seen with other customer records is its ability to easily connect information within and across databases and to apply the data immediately. Lawmakers have focused on the possibility of children giving out information without their parents' knowledge or consent. The majority of parents appear to be concerned about the information their teenagers may provide online. In the Annenberg study, 96% of the parents interviewed felt parental consent should be required before teenagers can provide any information online. Children do have concerns about protecting their privacy and are nervous about web sites having information about them. However, they are more vulnerable than adults to strategies that offer them opportunities to obtain a free gift in exchange for personal or family data (Turow & Nir, 2000).

The Internet offers anonymity impossible to achieve with any other form of communication. This anonymity often removes inhibitions. People not predisposed to speak intimately in person may do so over the Internet. It also allows a person to adopt a disguise. If a child says he or she knows an Internet friend very well, caregivers should remind the child that all he or she really knows is what the friend has said, and that it is possible that none of the information is true. Disclosure of such a close Internet friendship would be an indicator to further investigate the child's use of the Internet. While the relationship may be completely harmless, it still should be monitored.

Children and teens are naturally curious, just as adults are. For example, a 12-year-old may want to see nude photos, but does not know the Internet address for these. After entering the Internet, he or she would access a search engine. Then he or she would type in the words, "nude girl" or "nude boy," and touch the appropriate key to tell the engine to search the Internet for sites with nude photographs. Just one search engine could access over tens of thousands of sites, each one containing pictures that can be viewed for free or saved in the computer's memory for later viewing. One could also receive these images via e-mail. Young children most often merely stumble upon adult or pornographic web sites, while teens may be drawn to these sites by their own curiosity or via their participation in online discussions where such sites may be mentioned in conversations dealing with sexual content. The Pew Internet & American Life survey that looked at teenagers' behavior on the Internet found that 15% of teens using the Internet said they lied about their age in order to gain access to a web site (Lenhart, Rainie, & Lewis, 2001). Nineteen percent of males between the ages of 12 and 17 years had lied about their age compared to 11% of females between the same ages. Twenty-five percent of males between 15 and 17 years of age had said they were older to gain access to a Web site (Lenhart, Rainie, & Lewis, 2001).

Search engines and natural curiosity, however, are not the problems. When used appropriately and properly harnessed, search engines and curiosity can help a child with schoolwork, intellectual growth, and hobbies. Supervised usage of the computer and the Internet is needed to ensure appropriate use. Professionals working with children and families need to encourage parental and caregiver supervision of child and teen computer usage as an important aspect of promoting child safety. For example, parents and caregivers should occasionally check the family's computer usage by accessing the cache or history folder in the computer's web browser. These storage areas hold information about the sites that have been visited. The children should be told that this type of periodic supervision will be done, much like checking the family phone bill to see who is being called long distance. Table 12-1 lists instructions for accessing a computer's cache. Parents should also consider keeping the computer in a common room in the household, as opposed to a child's bedroom, to facilitate supervision.

An area of major concern with regard to protecting children on the Internet is the chat room, one of the most popular areas on the Internet, and one that holds potential risk for children. Chat rooms allow users of the Internet to converse in real-time format no matter where they are located. Unlike Instant Messenger services, which also allow for communication in real time, chat rooms provide near total anonymity. Through the Internet, a local telephone call to your service provider allows you to travel virtually anywhere in the world and converse with total strangers by typing messages on the keyboard.

Some of the most frequently used chat rooms exist on the Internet Relay Chat (IRC) or within the databases of Internet service providers, such as America Online (AOL). These chat rooms are listed by name, which usually gives an idea of the topic the room is discussing. To participate, a user selects a screen name by which he or she will be known while chatting. There is no verification that the name chosen reflects who the person really is. Someone could use a name that would indicate he was a 12-year-old girl, when in fact he is a 35-year-old man. After selecting a room, the screen name appears in the room. Most chat formats allow for a brief description or profile of the users. In this area, basic information about the user is stored for viewing by other users. Once a person enters the room, others can check this profile. A pedophile can learn the age or gender of a participating child, and possibly where the child lives and what school the child attends.

A pedophile using a chat room can now begin to profile a potential victim. In the chat room, a predator can observe a child's likes and dislikes or relationship factors, such as if the child has just argued with a parent or friend. The predator may use this acquired knowledge to "befriend" the child. The child can become an easy target and may fall prey to the manipulation of the perpetrator. This manipulative behavior on the part of perpetrators is not new. The electronic age has merely provided a safety net for the offender, who can now remain anonymous as long as he or she desires. More recently, new technology has allowed more private conversations using Instant Messaging Services. This allows real-time, one-on-one private conversations and creates a perception of secrecy and security. The name lists are often referred to as "buddy lists." Children and teens can have safe and valuable conversations about a variety of topics in chat rooms, as can adults. The danger arises when children don't take the anonymity into consideration and don't realize that another person in the chat room could be pretending to be someone else in order to take advantage of the situation. If a mandated reporter observes or suspects this type of activity while supervising a child's or teen's computer usage, immediate action is necessary. Appropriate authorities should be notified, beginning with local law enforcement (Armagh, Battaglia, & Lanning, 2000).

A nationally representative sample of 1501 children and teens between the ages of 10 and 17 years who use the Internet regularly found that 19 percent of these youths were the targets of unwanted solicitation during a one year period of time (Mitchell, Finkelhor, & Wolak, 2001). Those at highest risk are girls, older teens, those having problems, those who used the Internet more frequently, and those who participated in chat room discussions with strangers. Not surprisingly, 25% of the children and teens who were solicited reported high levels of stress following the solicitation. The highest level of distress was seen in younger children (ages 10 to 13 years), in those who were solicited while using a computer away from their home, and in those who received aggressive solicitations defined as the solicitor attempting to make offline contact. Only 10% of the solicitations were reported to the police, ISP, or other officials. Over two-thirds of the parents and over three-quarters

---

Table 12-1. Accessing a Web Browser's Cache

Netscape Navigator and Microsoft Internet Explorer are currently the two most popular web browsers. There are a variety of ways to check what sites the user has visited.

Netscape History

1. Type about:global in the location bar and hit enter; a list of the URLs that the computer has visited will appear on the screen.

2. Hold down the "Control" key and type "H." The history file, or list of URLs visited, will pop up in a new window. The number of days shown in the history file can be changed in the Preferences under Edit.

3. On the toolbar, click "Communicator," then "Tools," then "History." The history file will pop up in a new window.

4. Click the drop-down arrow to the right of the Address Bar for a listing of the URLs most recently typed in. Frequently visited sites are also often saved as "Bookmarks." To find this list, click on the Bookmarks tab on the toolbar.

5. When you first start the browser, it will open to a particular page, which may have been selected by the user as the designated "start page."

Microsoft Internet Explorer History

1. To view recently visited pages, click the History icon on the toolbar (it looks like a sun dial) and then click the appropriate folder.

2. Click the drop-down arrow to the right of the Address Bar for a listing of the URLs most recently typed in.

3. To check cookies, which may contain web site passwords, open the folder C:\windows\temporary Internet files.

---

of the children and teens did not know where they could report the incidents (Mitchell, Finkelhor, & Wolak, 2001). Incidents of inappropriate or illegal activity on the Internet can always be reported to local law enforcement.

The National Center for Missing and Exploited Children (NCMEC) wants to be alerted to the presence of any illegal material online, such as child pornography, threatening messages, or evidence of criminal action. Professionals, parents, and other caregivers can report such activity to NCMEC by calling 1-800-843-5678. ISPs should also be alerted to such observations. ISPs have made progress in policing their sites and are mandated in the United States to report child pornography and crimes against children to the Federal Bureau of Investigation or the United States Customs Service. Federal agencies are working with local law enforcement entities here and abroad to stop the exploitation of children through use of the Internet. Task forces are being formulated and activated all over the United States in an attempt to locate and prosecute perpetrators of child exploitation on the Internet. Some online Internet safety resources for mandated reporters, parents, and children are offered in Appendix II.

◆ Preventive Strategies

The Pew Internet & American Life survey and the Annenberg Public Policy Center survey on computer use by children and children's relationship to parental controls revealed that American parents and youngsters are often at odds regarding supervision of Internet usage and what personal information should be given out over the Internet (Lenhart, Rainie, & Lewis, 2001; Turow & Nir, 2000). As stated previously, children and teens between the ages of 10 and 17 years were more likely than adults to provide personal and family information to commercial web sites, especially when prompted by offers of free gifts. The most effective ways to ensure the safety of children and teens while they use the Internet are to maintain communication between parents or caregivers and children and to provide parental supervision of child computer usage. However, parent-child conversations concerning privacy on the Web and how to avoid divulging information inappropriately are lacking. Children and their parents did not necessarily hold the same attitudes or even recall the same discussions about the topic within the family. It appeared that parent-child conversations about Web privacy issues often consisted of merely "don't give out your name," or "don't talk to strangers" (Turow & Nir, 2000). Such discussions leave children unprepared to deal with strategies such as bartering information for free gifts or extending trust to a person without any factual data as to who that person really is.

For example, in the Pew study:

- 61% of parents said they have rules about Internet use, while only 37% of teens reported being subject to any Internet time-use restrictions.

- 61% of parents reported checking to see what web sites their teens had visited, while 27% of online teens believed they had been checked on.

- 68% of parents said they had sat with their children when they were online, while 48% of children recall such episodes (Lenhart, Rainie, & Lewis, 2001).

The discrepancies in these statistics show that, while parents are attempting to teach their children to use the Internet safely, this communication is not always clear. Parents and mandated reporters who supervise children with access to computers must recognize that no amount of warnings or safety discussions can be as effective as actual supervision of children while they are online. Among investigations carried out by the Maryland Heights Police Department in Missouri, the vast majority of child Internet exploitation or exposure to inappropriate material occurred when children were online unsupervised. The best defense against this is to keep the computer in a common room in the household. A child is less likely to enter a potentially risky personal discussion with a stranger in a chat room or access and view explicit material if a parent or caregiver could look over his or her shoulder at any time.

To minimize the risks faced by children, general safety guidelines should be followed. Below is a sample list of rules from the NCMEC that professionals should encourage parents and caregivers to adopt (Magid, 1998). Children and teens should be counseled to:

- Never reveal your password to anyone online, not even to online service staff members.

- Never reveal identifying information, such as real name (first or last), names of family members, home addresses, details of parents' work, school or team names, telephone numbers, social security numbers, or credit card numbers, in a chat room or in a bulletin board message. Never give this information via e-mail to someone you don't know. Remember: No matter how friendly someone seems on the Internet, that person is a stranger. He or she may even be an adult pretending to be a child.

- Never accept offers of merchandise or give out your street address for deliveries without getting permission from a parent or caregiver.

- Never send a photo of yourself or offer a physical description of yourself or family members over the Internet.

- Never continue a conversation that makes you feel uncomfortable or becomes personal. Hang up on the conversation by going to another area of the Internet. Report what happened to an adult.

- Never answer e-mail, bulletin board system, or Instant Messenger items that are suggestive, obscene, rude, or make you feel uncomfortable in any way. Tell the person in charge if you come across such messages. These messages should be forwarded to the ISP for investigation.

- Never arrange a face-to-face meeting with a person you met online without permission from your parent or guardian. If a meeting is arranged, it is extremely important that a parent or guardian be present and that the meeting be arranged in a public place.

- Be careful when responding to e-mail. Return addresses can be falsified to make the message look innocent. If you cannot verify the sender, do not answer the message.

In an effort to allow children to use the Internet safely, the Federal Trade Commission has established rules for web site operators to ensure that children's privacy is protected while they are online. These rules are part of the Children's Online Privacy Protection Act of 1998, which took effect on April 21, 2000. The rules, along with corresponding parent responsibilities, are outlined in Table 12-2.

BLOCKING OR FILTERING SOFTWARE

Software designed to block access to undesirable sites can be an important aid in preventing Internet safety problems. Some software allows parents to customize the list of "bad sites," but constant updating is required, as new sites are always being created. Updates are frequently available for a certain period of time without extra charge. However, even though software companies review many new web sites, they could never keep up with all the new sites being created each day. Because of this, parents should not depend solely on blocking software to keep their children safe on the Internet (Aftab, 2000; cyberangels.org, 2000).

A strategy some parents try involves Internet filtering products. Filtering software blocks sites by checking for particular keywords that have been deemed inappropriate, as opposed to the blocking software, which just blocks sites on a pre-set list. This helps to prevent newly constructed "bad sites" from getting through the safety net. There is the risk, however, that innocent educational sites containing potentially objectionable keywords will also be blocked (Aftab, 2000; cyberangels.org, 2000). Figure 12-1 offers a quick

Table 12-2. Federal Trade Commission Guidelines from the Children's Online Privacy Protection Act of 1998

Responsibilities of Web Site Operators	Responsibilities of Parents

Privacy Policy
 	
• Web sites directed toward children or that collect information from children under age 13 must post a notice of their information collection practices that includes:
 	
  • types of personal information they collect (e.g., name, home address, e-mail address, hobbies)
 	
  • how they will use the information (e.g., to market to the child, to notify contest winners, to make the information available through a child's participation in a chat room)
 	
  • whether personal information is forwarded to advertisers or other third parties
 	
  • a contact at the site
	Privacy Policy
	
	• Look for a privacy policy on any web site directed to children.
	
	• The policy must be available through a link on the web site's homepage and at each area where personal information is collected. Web sites for general audiences that have a children's section must post the notice on the homepages of the section for children.
	
	• Read the policy closely to learn the kinds of personal information being collected, how it will be used, and whether it will be passed on to third parties. If you find a web site that doesn't post basic protections for children's personal information, ask for details about their information collection practices.

Parental Consent
 	
• In many cases, a site must obtain parental consent before collecting, using, or disclosing personal information about a child.
 	
• Consent is not required when a site is collecting an e-mail address to:
 	
  • respond to a one-time request from the child
 	
  • provide notice to the parent
 	
  • ensure the safety of the child or the site
 	
  • send a newsletter or other information on a regular basis as long as the site notifies a parent and gives them a chance to say no to the arrangement
	Parental Consent
	
	• Decide whether to give consent.
	
	• Giving consent authorizes the web site to collect personal information from your child. You can give consent and still say no to having your child's information passed along to a third party.
	
	• Your consent isn't necessary if the web site is collecting your child's e-mail address simply to respond to a one-time request for information from your child.

Table 12-2. Federal Trade Commission Guidelines from the Children's Online Privacy Protection Act of 1998—*continued*

Responsibilities of Web Site Operators	Responsibilities of Parents
New Uses of Information	**New Uses of Information**

• Web site operators must get new consent when information practices change in a "material" way.
 	
• Web site operators need to notify parents and get consent again if they plan to change the kinds of information they collect, change how they use the information, or offer the information to new and different third parties. For example, new parental consent would be required if the web site decides to:
 	
  • send information from children to marketers of diet pills instead of only marketers of stuffed animals, as covered in the original consent
 	
  • give a child access to a chat room if the parent's original consent was only to send a newsletter
	• Decide whether to approve information collection from your children based on new uses for the information.
	
	• Web site operators will let you know about the need for new consent by sending you a new notice and request. They will do this when they are changing the terms-of-use of the information in a "material" or significant way.

Viewing Personal Information	**Viewing Personal Information**
• Web site operators must allow parents to review personal information collected from their children. • Web site operators must first verify the identity of the requesting parent.	• Ask to see the information your child has submitted. • The site will ask to verify your identity to ensure that your child's information isn't given out improperly.
Revoking Consent	**Revoking Consent**
• Site operators must allow parents to revoke their consent and must delete information collected from their children at the parents' request. • When a parent revokes consent, the web site must stop collecting, using, or disclosing information from that child. The site may end a child's participation in an activity if the information it collected was necessary for participation.	• Understand that you may revoke your consent and have your child's information deleted from the web site at any time. • To stop a web site from collecting additional information from your child, you can revoke your consent, with or without asking the site to delete any personal information it has already collected from your child.

Adapted from Federal Trade Commission, 2000.

summary of six Internet filtering/blocking programs, as well as the parental controls offered by America Online. These ratings were provided in the March 2001 issue of Consumer Reports. They are included here for informational purposes only, and are not intended to endorse any particular product in any way.

Another method of filtering inappropriate sites is site labeling. Site labeling relies on the voluntary labeling of web sites by their owners based on the Internet Content Rating System (ICRA). The major drawback is that many sites have not chosen to label their content and as a result are not blocked even though their content may be objectionable. If a filter is set to block all unlabeled sites, then a large number of legitimate sites are blocked, which makes constructive searching difficult (Consumer Reports, 2001).

More than three-fourths of parents express confidence in their ability to "always know" what their children are doing online (Houston, 1997). Over one-fourth of parents reported using some form of parental-control software, often the controls built into their Web browser or offered through their ISP. Only 4% chose to use software that they bought, installed, and maintained on their own (Houston, 1997). Parents and mandated reporters should be aware, however, that this software should be used only as a supplement and cannot replace the effectiveness of supervision.

◆ CONCLUSION

While the Internet can evoke conflicting feelings in parents—a fear of the risks, yet an appreciation of the benefits—it remains a powerful and pervasive tool in today's society. How parents and children address the risks has been lacking in consistency and clarity. Parents desire to protect their children and set reasonable limits on the data that can be revealed online. Children agree that parents should have control over the information they give out over the WWW, but can be deceived when offered a free gift in exchange for information. Society must set up an equitable system that balances the ethical and legal practices of media and marketers with the safety concerns that have been expressed. Currently, those in the marketplace can freely track, aggregate, and store a much greater variety of information on preteens and teenagers than is allowed to academic investigators, who are obligated by federal and university research guidelines to obtain parental permission to interview persons in these age groups. How to verify whether parental permission has been obtained for the online activity of children and teens presents another hurdle. It also must be determined what consequences might arise with the "electronic carding" of teens or younger children at web sites to identify the ages of site visitors. Some of the issues to be addressed and solutions suggested by the Annenberg Public Policy Center survey are listed in Table 12-3 (Turow & Nir, 2000).

The bottom line for both professionals working with children and parents or caregivers is that supervision of Internet usage by children and teens is essential to their safety. If mandated reporters or parents discover any evidence of illegal activity online or receive reports of such activity from children, they should write down exactly what happened and save any illegal files that come to their attention. They should then inform both the Internet service provider and local law enforcement. The Internet is an extraordinary tool for people of all ages. With the proper guidance and supervision, children and teens should be

What it does. A basic software filter purports to prevent children from reaching inappropriate web sites. Some products add antivirus protection or rudimentary privacy safeguards. America Online includes a "parental controls" filter in its service. Otherwise, filtering software is a product you buy at retail or download.

Choosing the products. Consumer Reports bought nine of the most widely used titles, ranging in price from $39 to $80. Most are written only for Windows computers, not Macintoshes. We also tested AOL's parental controls. Some filters proved to be so simplistic or so complex to set up effectively that we didn't test them fully. And a few dropped off the market while our tests were under way. In the end, we rated six products plus AOL's parental controls. To see whether the filters interfere with legitimate content, we pitted them against a list of 53 web sites that featured serious content on controversial subjects.

Using the ratings. The judgments below tell you how well the tested products blocked inappropriate content (typically preventing both words and images from appearing onscreen) and did not block legitimate content, and how easy the filters were to use. The bottom line: Don't expect miracles.

ONLINE SERVICE

America Online Parental Controls

Part of AOL service, which costs $21.95/month

www.aol.com

Young Teen (ages 13-15)

Protection—Very good

Interference—Poor

Features—Good

Mature Teen (ages 16-17)

Protection—Fair

Interference—Very good

Features—Good

Young Teen is pretty effective, though it will block many legitimate sites. Mature Teen isn't suitable for unattended web filtering.

Young Teen failed to block 14 percent of objectionable sites; Mature Teen, 30 percent. Filtering is hard to defeat because it's handled through AOL's centralized service. For some objectionable sites, both controls blocked images but not text. Young Teen blocked 63 percent of legitimate sites. Neither control can block personal information entered into web sites. FEATURES: Online list of objectionable web sites, automatically updated. Can limit total hours of web access, filter mail. Can also be set for highly restricted Kids Only mode, for ages 12 and under. Available for both Windows and Macintosh.

STAND-ALONE SOFTWARE

All products filter personal information entered into web sites and filter use of chat rooms. Except as noted, these run only on Windows computers, let you limit time spent on the web, and can be configured for multiple users. Products are listed alphabetically.

Cyber Patrol, version 4 $50

Surf Control Inc. *www.cyberpatrol.com*

Protection—Good

Interference—Excellent

Features—Excellent

So-so web blocking; most useful for restricting the time online to certain days and hours or limiting the total number of hours a child can be online.

Failed to block 23 percent of objectionable sites. Feature to protect personal information can be defeated very simply. Can filter mail, sites labeled with content ratings. Blocks selected applications (such as personal-finance or scheduling programs), not just the browser. Online list of objectionable web sites, automatically updated. Only stand-alone software tested that has a Macintosh version. Costs $30/year for site-list updates.

Cybersitter 2000 $40

Solid Oak Software Inc. *www.cybersitter.com*

Protection—Good

Interference—Good

Features—Very good

So-so web blocking; most useful for tracking kids' activity.

Failed to block 22 percent of objectionable sites. Can't be configured for multiple users. Online list of objectionable web sites, automatically updated. Can filter mail, downloads, custom word list. Can select subjects to block from detailed list. Can log activity.

Cyber Snoop $50

Pearl Software Inc. *www.pearlsw.com*

Protection—Poor

Interference—Excellent

Features—Very good

Not suitable for unattended web filtering.

Failed to block 90 percent of objectionable sites. Relies on parents entering lists of objectionable or permissible web sites; changing user requires restarting Windows. Can filter mail, downloads, sites labeled with some content ratings, custom word list. Can log activity.

Internet Guard Dog $39

McAfee Software Division of Network Associates Inc. *www.mcafee.com*

Protection—Fair

Interference—Good

Features—Fair

Not suitable for unattended web filtering; most useful for blocking ads and cookies.

Failed to block 30 percent of objectionable sites. Can't filter newsgroups. Relies on parents entering lists of objectionable or permissible web sites. Can filter sites labeled with content ratings, custom word list. Can block ads, filter cookies, automatically clear web "history" list from browser.

Net Nanny, version 4 $50

Net Nanny Ltd. *www.netnanny.com*

Protection—Poor

Interference—Very good

Features—Very good

Not suitable for unattended web filtering.

Failed to block 52 percent of objectionable sites, in numerous cases blocking words but not images. List of objectionable web sites, automatically updated. Filters custom word list, sites labeled with some content ratings. Can log activity.

Figure 12-1. *Consumer Reports Filtering Products Test Results.*

Norton Internet Security 2001
Family Edition $80

Symantec Corp. *www.symantec.com*

Protection—Good

Interference—Very good

Features—Very good

So-so web filtering; most useful as firewall, antivirus protection, and ad blocker.

Failed to block 20 percent of objectionable sites. Can't limit time of web access; costs $11/year for site-list updates; telephone support costs $30 per problem. Online list of objectionable web sites, automatically updated. Can filter mail, downloads. Can select subjects to block from detailed list. Blocks selected applications that access the Internet, not just the browser. Can block ads, screen viruses ($4/year subscription), act as personal firewall against computer hackers.

The tests behind the Ratings.

Protection is based on the ability to block web sites containing objectionable material, such as sexual content or promotion of crime, bigotry, violence, tobacco, or drugs. Failure to block at least 35 percent of those sites was judged poor. Partial blockage of a site (showing images but no words, or vice versa) was considered less effective than total blockage. **Interference** is based on how often a filter blocked web sites containing potentially controversial but legitimate material, such as sex education, the abortion-rights debate, or gun control. **Features** is based on the number of features related to filtering and child protection. **Price** is the estimated national average.

Figure 12-1—*continued. Consumer Reports Filtering Products Test Results.*

Table 12-3. Policies for Privacy Norms

- Parents and their children should be urged to talk in detail about how to approach requests by Web sites for personal and family information.

- Community groups, libraries, schools, and state and federal agencies should cooperate on campaigns aimed at making information privacy a hot family topic and at bringing community members together to study and learn about it.

- Governmental and nonprofit organizations that care about enriching Americans' Internet experiences should develop strategies that encourage families to surf the WWW together and to hold family discussions about surfing the WWW.

- A Web Freedom of Information Act should be enacted to allow each person access to all data, including click stream data, that a web site connects to his or her individual computer or name. The right of parents to access their children's data should be decided based on public debate of the issue.

- Web sites that target children and teens should be prohibited from tying free gifts, including sweepstakes giveaways, to the provision of personal information.

Adapted with permission from Turow & Nir, 2000.

allowed to safely reap the full benefit afforded them by the vast amount of information and communication available via the Internet.

◆ REFERENCES

Aftab, P. (2000). <u>The parent's guide to protecting your children in cyberspace.</u> New York: McGraw-Hill.

Armagh, D. S., Battaglia, N. L., & Lanning, K. V. (2000). <u>Use of computers in the sexual exploitation of children.</u> Washington, DC: Office of Juvenile Justice and Delinquency Prevention, Department of Justice.

Children's Partnership. (2001). Internet safety guide: Safe surfing for kids. <u>Children's Partnership.</u> Commonwealth of Pennsylvania: The Governor's Community Partnership for Safe Children. Retrieved October 4, 2001 from the World Wide Web: http://www.cp.state.pa.us

Consumer Reports. (2001, March). Digital chaperones for kids: Which Internet filters protect the best? Which get in the way? <u>Consumer Reports,</u> 20-23.

cyberangels.org. (2000). What you always wanted to know about filtering software but were afraid to ask. <u>Cyberangels.</u> Retrieved September 27, 2001 from the World Wide Web: http://www.familyguidebook.com/filtering.html

Federal Trade Commission (2000, February). How to protect kids' privacy online. <u>Kidz Privacy.</u> Retrieved September 27, 2001 from the World Wide Web: http://www.ftc.gov/bcp/conline/pubs/online/kidsprivacy.htm

Fox, S., & Lewis, O. (2001). Fear of online crime: Americans support FBI interception of criminal suspects' e-mail and new laws to protect online privacy. <u>Pew Internet & American Life Project.</u> Retrieved October 4, 2001 from the World Wide Web: http://www.pewinternet.org

Houston, P. (1997, December 1). Survey: Few parents use filtering software. <u>ZDNet News.</u> Retrieved September 27, 2001 from the World Wide Web: http://www.zdnet.com/zdnn/stories/news/0,4586,249786,00.html

Jezycki, M. (1998). How safe is cyberspace: An overview. <u>APSAC Advisor,</u> 11(4), 10-11.

Lenhart, A., Rainie, L., & Lewis, O. (2001). Teenage life online: The rise of the instant-message generation and the Internet's impact on friendships and family relationships. <u>Pew Internet & American Life Project.</u> Retrieved October 4, 2001 from the World Wide Web: http://www.pewinternet.org

Magid, L. J. (1998). Child safety on the Information Highway. <u>National Center for Missing and Exploited Children.</u> Retrieved October 30, 2001 from the World Wide Web: http://www.safekids.com/child_safety.htm

Mitchell, K. J., Finkelhor, D., & Wolak, J. (2001). Risk factors for and impact of online sexual solicitation of youth. <u>Journal of American Medical Association,</u> 285(23), 3011-3014.

Turow, J., & Nir, L. (2000). <u>The Internet and the Family 2000: The view from parents, the view from kids.</u> Philadelphia, PA: The Annenberg Public Policy Center of the University of Pennsylvania.

◆ APPENDIX I: GLOSSARY OF INTERNET AND ONLINE TERMS

Acronyms: Frequently used phrases condensed to their initial letters, often used in instant messaging, chat rooms, and e-mail messages. Some of the most common examples include:

AFAIK – as far as I know

AFK – away from keyboard

BBIAF – be back in a few

BBL – be back later

BRB – be right back

BTW – by the way

IMO – in my opinion

LOL – laughing out loud

RENTS – (abbreviation) parents

ROTFL – rolling on the floor laughing

LTNS – long time no see

OTOH – on the other hand

RTM – read the manual

TTFN – ta ta for now

WB – welcome back

IRL – in real life

BBS (bulletin board system): A computerized meeting and announcement system that allows people to carry on discussion, upload and download files, and make announcements without the people being connected to the computer at the same time.

BPS (bits-per-second): A measurement of how quickly data is moved from one place to another. A 28.8 modem can move 28,800 bits per second.

Browser: Software that is used to look at web sites.

Chat: A system that allows for real-time communication between computer users who are connected to the Internet.

Chat room: A real-time online discussion group.

Click stream: The sequence of clicks or pages requested as a visitor explores a web site.

Cookies: Small file which saves information about web sites on the user's hard drive and directs the hard drive to send information back to the web server. Cookies often include things like records of online purchases.

Cyberspace: Term originated by author William Gibson. The whole range of information resources available through computer networks.

Domain name: The name of an Internet site. Contains at least two components separated by a period. For example, "gwmedical.com" is a domain name.

E-mail (electronic mail): Messages, usually text, sent from one person to another via computer. E-mail can also be sent automatically to a large number of addresses.

Emoticons: A combination of characters that suggests an emotion when read sideways. (Examples: :) smiling face to express humor; :(Frowning face to convey sadness or displeasure; ;) winking smiling face used to convey flirtation or humor.) Often used in instant messaging, chat rooms, and e-mail messages.

FAQ (frequently asked questions): Documents that answer the most common questions on a particular subject.

Flaming: Use of inflammatory or derogatory comments in an online discussion.

FTP (file transfer protocol): A method used to transfer files between Internet-connected computers.

Hit: A single request from a web browser for a single item from a web. Hits are often used as a very rough measure of popularity of a particular document or site, e.g., "Our web site has been getting 300,000 hits per month."

Home page: The main web page for a business, organization, or person—the first screen you see when you enter a web site.

HTML (HyperText Markup Language): The format used to create web pages.

HTTP (HyperText Transfer Protocol): An information retrieval mechanism for HTML documents.

Hyperlink: An object (text or graphic) that you click to get to another web page.

Internet: A vast collection of computer networks allowing any connected computer to communicate with any other.

Intranet: A private network on the Internet reserved for sole usage by a specific organization. Not accessible to the general public.

IRC (Internet Relay Chat): A huge, multi-user live chat facility. There are a number of major IRC servers around the world, which are linked to each other. Anyone can create a channel and all others in the channel see anything that anyone types in that channel. Private channels can be (and are) created for multi-person conference calls. A user can log onto IRC anonymously and chat with other users without any identifying personal information being obvious. IRC chatrooms are one place where pedophiles can contact each other, and it is also a place where children may be at risk of being lured into victimization.

ISP (Internet Service Provider): An organization that provides access to the Internet in some form, usually for a fee.

JPEG (Joint Photographic Expert Group): A visual image file format, often used to share photographic images on the Internet.

Listserv: The most common kind of mail list, listservs are a convenient way for e-mail users to share information with others in a group. Some listservs are "moderated," in which a participant reviews the e-mails for appropriateness prior to them being sent out to all participants.

Login: Noun: The account name used to gain access to a computer system. Not a secret (contrast with Password).

Log in: Verb: The act of entering into a computer system.

Mail List (or mailing list): A (usually automated) system that allows people to send e-mail to one address, whereupon their message is copied and sent to all the other subscribers to the mail list.

MIME (Multiple Internet Mail Extensions): Items that may be included with e-mails, such as audio, visual, and text messages.

Modem: A device that connects to a computer and to a phone line, allowing the computer to talk to other computers through the phone system. Basically, modems do for computers what telephones do for humans. (The contraction comes from Modulate Demodulate.)

MPEG (Moving Picture Experts Group): An animated visual image file format generally used for storing movie files.

Online: To be connected, by way of a modem, to the Internet or other networks, such as America Online. While online services such as America Online, CompuServe, and Prodigy offer access to the Internet, they also provide their own content, chat rooms, newsgroups, and other material, which is accessible only to subscribers of that online service.

Password: A code used to gain access to a locked system. Good passwords contain letters and non-letters and are not simple combinations such as virtue7. A good password might be: Bot$16.

Real time: Synchronous communication in which parties are sharing information visible to both at the same time (compare to e-mail, which is asynchronous).

Search engine: Resource on various web sites (e.g., Google, Excite, Yahoo) which allows users to type in key words or phrases and then searches the WWW for pages on which these key words are found.

Shareware: Software that can be used for free for a trial period after which a small payment is typically expected.

Spam: Messages sent over the Internet to multiple mailings lists and individuals who did not ask for them.

URL (Uniform Resource Locator): Indicates the web address for a specific source of information; a string of characters that is typed into browsers to reach specific web sites.

Web site: A page or set of pages containing text and graphics that can be accessed by anyone with an Internet connection.

World Wide Web (WWW): The universe of hypertext servers (HTTP servers), which are the servers that allow text, graphics, sound files, and others to be mixed together.

Adapted and reprinted with permission from the National Criminal Justice Reference Service (1998) and the Children's Partnership (2001).

◆ APPENDIX II: ONLINE INTERNET SAFETY RESOURCES

America Links Up (www.getnetwise.org/americalinksup/)
A public awareness campaign, sponsored by various non-profit organizations, to teach parents and children how to use the Internet safely.

Chat Danger (www.chatdanger.com)
Explores the issue of safety in anonymous chat rooms.

Child Safety-Net (surfsafely.com/surfsafety)
Online safety resource center. Page of links screened by human editors to assure relevance to online safety.

Children's Internet Protection Act (www.ifea.net/cipa.html)
Public Law 106-554 regarding governmental protection of children on the Internet.

Children's Online Privacy Protection Act of 1998
(www.ftc.gov/ogc/coppa1.htm)
Established by the Federal Trade Commission to protect children's privacy while online.

Cyberangels (www.cyberangels.org)
Comprehensive site on Internet help, including safety and general usage, available in eight languages. This organization is run entirely by volunteers, and the site offers a place to sign up, get information, or ask for help.

CyberTipline (www.missingkids.org/cybertip/index.html)
Online form to report the sexual exploitation of children to the National Center for Missing and Exploited Children.

FBI Publications—A Parent's Guide to Internet Safety
(www.fbi.gov/publications/pguide/pguide.htm)
FBI's official overview for parents, available in English and Spanish.

FBI Safety Tips for Kids on the Internet
(www.fbi.gov/kids/crimepre/internet/internet.htm)
Contains safety tips from the FBI for children. Also links to the FBI Kids and Youth Educational Page, with information on crime prevention, abduction, and gang alerts.

Internet Lifeguard (www.safesurf.com/lifeguard.htm)
Online basics, information on filtering software, a parent-child pledge to sign regarding Internet safety.

Internet School Bus (www.members.home.net/netschoolbus)
Tips for parents to establish family Internet rules, monitor child usage, and talk to kids about safety.

KidShield (www.kidshield.com)
Links to methods of reporting inappropriate material, relevant legislation, and a glossary of Internet terms.

Kidz Privacy (www.ftc.gov/bcp/conline/edcams/kidzprivacy)
Site for kids, parents, and teachers from the Federal Trade Commission, which sponsors a public awareness campaign regarding the Children's Online Privacy Protection Act.

Mothers of America (www.mothersofamerica.com)
Site of organization that started various child safety programs; created by a
family whose child was victimized on the Internet.

National Center for Missing and Exploited Children (www.missingkids.org)
Official site of the NCMEC. Includes resources for the public regarding child
safety, resources for parents of missing children, and a searchable database of
photos of missing children.

NetScrubber (www.netscrubber.com)
This site provides a place to report a web site as inappropriate for children. The
recommendations are sent to the makers of parental control software, ISPs, and
school districts to keep others from coming across inappropriate material
accidentally.

SafeKids.com (www.safekids.com)
Information on child safety and privacy issues; a Family Contract for Online
Safety to print, sign, and post by computer.

SafeSurf (www.safesurf.com/index.htm)
Online safety tips; originator of the Internet's voluntary rating system standard.

Safe Surfing Guide (www.iwf.org.uk/safe/main_safe.htm)
Site designed for those with little previous knowledge of Internet usage.
Includes a glossary of Internet terms for new and inexperienced users.

SafeTeens.com (www.safekids.com/safeteens)
The teen branch of SafeKids.com. Includes safety links and tips for teenagers.

SmartParent.com (www.smartparent.com)
Information on filtering/blocking software, protection tips, links to kid-
friendly sites.

Chapter 13

THE ROLE OF LAW ENFORCEMENT IN THE INVESTIGATION OF CHILD MALTREATMENT

ANGELO P. GIARDINO, M.D., PH.D.
GUS H. KOLILIS, B.S.ED.

◆ THE COMPLEXITIES OF CHILD MALTREATMENT CASES

The role of law enforcement in the investigation of child maltreatment revolves around the criminal aspects of child abuse and neglect (Hammond, Lanning, Promisel, Shepherd, & Walsh, 1997). In most situations, police officers who report and investigate cases of child maltreatment focus a great deal of time and energy on the preservation and collection of evidence for the purpose of criminal prosecution (Pence & Wilson, 1992). Police departments are typically organized in a hierarchical structure with clear lines of authority. Even within this regimentation, however, law enforcement officers are typically permitted to act on their judgment in a given situation. It is the investigative responsibility of the police to prove or disprove allegations. To do so, the police interview parents, caregivers, witnesses, and anyone else who can contribute to the history and circumstances surrounding an incident of alleged child maltreatment. To move beyond a verbal disclosure by the child and denial by the suspect, police officers make every effort to substantiate the report with corroborating evidence (Weston & Wells, 1986). In child maltreatment cases, the police officer determines first if maltreatment has occurred, then attempts to answer the following questions:

- Who is responsible?

- Where did it happen?

- When did it happen?

- How many times did it happen?

- What actions are necessary from a law enforcement standpoint to protect the child?

As well as investigating the alleged abuse, officers must also determine if the victim and other children remain at risk (Pence & Wilson, 1992).

The law enforcement agency plays many roles in the community's response to child maltreatment, including the following:

- **Deterrence:** The criminal justice system delivers the message that child maltreatment is unacceptable behavior and punishable by state and federal laws.

- **Prevention and Advocacy:** Police departments participate in community education efforts to reduce the risk of child maltreatment.

- **Reporting:** Police officers are typically mandated reporters of suspected child abuse and neglect.

- **Immediate Response:** The police are available to rapidly respond to emergency situations 24 hours a day, 7 days a week.

- **Criminal Investigative Role:** Law enforcement agencies have authority to conduct criminal investigations in a collaborative, team approach with child protective services (CPS). Joint investigations, with police working with CPS and other professionals, are ideal.

- **Support to CPS:** Police often accompany CPS case workers as they conduct visits to potentially dangerous locations, provide enforcement of standing court orders, and assist in removing children from the home.

- **Victim Support:** Depending on available victim services, police officers may be called on to help prepare and support the child victim of maltreatment through the entire investigation and prosecution of the case (Pence & Wilson, 1992).

Despite this long list, the investigation of child maltreatment cases is only a small part of the typical law enforcement agency's overall responsibilities. Other than in the largest departments, very few police officers are dedicated to the investigation of crimes against children. Ideally, police officers investigating child maltreatment cases should have specialized training and experience regarding the unique needs of children and families, as well as special issues related to child abuse and neglect (Bockman & Carroll, 1978). Such training should include cognitive and language development of children, non-abusive causes of findings resembling maltreatment, and the typical patterns of disclosure commonly seen in child maltreatment cases (Pence & Wilson, 1992). Additionally, formal training in the value of teamwork with other disciplines should allow for the formation of multidisciplinary teams of police officers, medical personnel, and social workers to provide an efficient and effective approach to these very complex and emotional cases (Bockman & Carroll, 1978; Dinsmore, 1993; Pence & Wilson, 1994).

Child maltreatment investigations can be among the most challenging cases handled by law enforcement agencies (Pena, 1993). Crimes against children are considerably different from crimes involving adult victims. Specifically, the disclosure of the abuse or neglect is seldom deliberate. In most cases children do not report being abused; abuse generally comes to the attention of an adult by way of observed symptoms or injuries. Depending on the child's age and developmental level, the child may not understand what has happened or even the fact that he or she was maltreated. If the abuser is a parent or family member, regardless of maltreatment, the child may still have feelings of love and attachment. Often, child victims are confused, afraid, and intimidated by the perpetrator. Infants and very young children may lack the ability to comprehend or communicate what has occurred to others. Additionally, in many cases, the systems in place to protect children and investigate and prosecute offenders are perceived as being complicated and ineffective. Most reports of adult crimes, on the other hand, are made by victims eager to provide details and information. Adult reporters generally hope that the investigation of the event reported will be successful in identifying the perpetrator and lead to criminal prosecution. The police officers taking these reports usually can initiate effective and appropriate actions with a reasonable expectation of solving the crime. Child maltreatment cases can be more complex and have a number of unique features that revolve around the vulnerability of the child who has been victimized, including:

- Children, because of their inherent dependency on the adults responsible for them and their immature physical, mental, and emotional stages of development, are often unable to adequately "protect" themselves from various forms of abuse, neglect, and exploitation.

- Maltreatment is usually conducted in a private place, such as a home, and in a one-on-one setting, in which few witnesses are present.

- Perpetrators of maltreatment seek to avoid detection and typically keep the abusive activity secretive. Unlike perpetrators of other types of criminal activity, they avoid telling others, who could then inform on them.

- Children may be viewed as less credible or competent than the suspected adult offender and, therefore, a child's disclosures may be dismissed as unbelievable.

- Community members may find it difficult to believe that caregivers would harm children in their care, and may be in denial about the maltreatment of children. Additionally, some adults may not want negative publicity associated with maltreatment to reflect on their community and thus may de-emphasize cases that come to light.

- Interviews of children require special training, understanding, and patience, and are particularly difficult to conduct in cases of alleged sexual abuse.

- Children who are maltreated often do not disclose the abuse, or their disclosure is delayed and/or delivered piecemeal over an extended period of time.

- Children may have conflicting feelings about the perpetrator: while wanting the abuse to stop, they may not want to see the perpetrator or family harmed.

- Maltreatment is often a pattern of abnormal caregiving behavior rather than an isolated incident. It may take place over a long period of time.

- Sexual abuse often leaves no physical or medical evidence. Its recognition frequently rests on the child's disclosure alone.

- Child maltreatment cases often involve joint investigations with CPS agencies that may result in investigative ambiguities and potential conflicts.

- Some maltreatment cases may cross jurisdictional boundaries, such as county lines, making determination of venue difficult for investigators.

- The criminal justice system may not be sensitive to the special needs of children, and children may be frightened and intimidated by the adversarial courtroom and trial process.

Initiating an investigation of suspected child maltreatment begins with a clear allegation. The abuse may be physical, sexual, or emotional, or it may involve some form of neglect.

It is the law enforcement investigator's responsibility to use every legal means to validate the allegation by collecting verifiable evidence and information to prove or disprove that the crime has occurred (Pena, 1993; Weston & Wells, 1986). The majority of information is collected by interviewing the victim(s), witness(es), expert(s), and suspect(s). How these interviews and interrogations are conducted will, in large part, determine the ultimate outcome of the investigation, which will, in turn, determine what interventions are needed to protect the interests of the child. It may also identify other children at risk, as well as crimes not directly associated with the allegation, e.g., weapons, drugs, or child pornography.

♦ INTERAGENCY COLLABORATION

Because of the need for CPS involvement in the investigation of child maltreatment, there will be interaction of law enforcement with other agencies and disciplines. As Pence and Wilson (1992) have made clear, the goal of interagency collaboration is not to create a homogeneous mix of interchangeable disciplines, but rather to create an investigative process whereby police officers and CPS workers each do their mandated work. Through mutual understanding and collaboration, this team produces an investigation in the best interests of the child involved. Lanning and Walsh (1996) make clear that certain police responsibilities cannot be delegated away and that a commitment to teamwork and joint investigation should not blur the line between teamwork and clear-cut law enforcement responsibilities.

The benefits of an effective joint investigation include the following:

- Less "system-inflicted" trauma to children and families.

- Increased agency performance, including enhanced accuracy of investigations and more appropriate interventions.

- Efficient use of limited community resources.

- More capable professionals as they develop collaborative skills and recognize the difficulty inherent in maltreatment-related work. There is also the opportunity to develop a professional network that reduces the sense of isolation and risk of professional burnout (Ells, 1998).

Within the context of a child maltreatment investigation, each discipline and agency has its own roles and responsibilities. Conflict is inevitable as the multidisciplinary team takes shape. Tension frequently revolves around decision-making, interpersonal relationships, competition, territorialism, and perceived lack of cooperation (DePanfilis & Saul, 1992). The success of the team is

---

Table 13-1. Strategies to Resolve Conflict among Team Members

- Don't lose sight of the mission statement and the team purpose it outlines.

- Look forward to opportunity, not backward to blame.

- Be respectful by genuinely considering each person's point of view. Listen to one another. Be sure each position is heard and understood.

- Clarify the opposing point of view. Find something positive in each viewpoint. Don't become defensive.

- State your position clearly, firmly, and without excessive emotion.

- Once you have been heard, do not continue to repeat your position.

- Avoid personalizing your position and stay focused on the issue.

- Offer suggestions rather than criticism of other viewpoints.

- Remember that conflict with a team is natural and work toward a mutually agreeable resolution.

- Base resolutions on consensus, not abdication of responsibility or integrity.

- Keep focused on the team's agreed-upon purpose and refer to your protocol for guidance.

Adapted from Ells, 1998.

---

not measured by the lack of conflict, but rather by the effectiveness with which conflict is resolved (Ellis, 1998; Sands, Stafford, & McClelland, 1990). See Table 13-1 for points to remember when facing such conflict. Of all the agencies involved in multidisciplinary child maltreatment cases, only law enforcement and CPS are likely to have specific mandates regarding child maltreatment investigations. It is essential that beyond collaboration, they coordinate their efforts in order to minimize duplication, conflict, and confusion.

A joint project between the Police Foundation and the American Public Welfare Association identified the types of collaboration seen in joint investigations that have evolved between law enforcement and CPS agencies (Sheppard & Zangrillo, 1996). CPS agencies report that approximately 20% of the CPS investigations of child maltreatment are jointly conducted, whereas law enforcement agencies report that 80% to 95% of police investigations are jointly conducted with CPS (Sheppard & Zangrillo, 1996). This disparity may be explained by the observation that joint investigations occur more frequently in the most severe cases, which are likely to require police involvement. Approximately 42% of cases jointly investigated are substantiated (Sheppard & Zangrillo, 1996). The highest number of joint investigations between CPS and police are seen in cases of sexual abuse (Sheppard & Zangrillo, 1996). Sexual abuse cases were seen as less straightforward when compared to physical abuse and neglect cases mainly because of the relative lack of medical findings in sexual abuse cases, the overarching importance of the child interview in sexual abuse cases, and the difficulty in prosecuting sexual abuse cases that require the child to testify in court (Kinnear, 1995; Sheppard & Zangrillo, 1996).

The models for collaboration between law enforcement and CPS agencies vary in terms of how formalized the protocols are, but most authorities support the development of formal written protocols between the organizations (Bockman & Carroll, 1978; Dinsmore, 1993; Ells, 1998; Pence & Wilson, 1992; Pence & Wilson, 1994; Sheppard & Zangrillo, 1996). The ideal components of formal CPS/law enforcement protocols include the following:

- Statement of purpose.

- Discussion of individual and shared missions as well as agency responsibilities.

- Designation of types of cases that will be jointly investigated.

- Procedures and special investigative techniques.

- Criteria for removing children from the caregiver's home.

- Criteria for the arrest of alleged perpetrators.

- Criteria for police to report suspected maltreatment to CPS.

- Criteria for CPS to inform police of suspected criminal activity around alleged maltreatment.

- Procedures for providing CPS with assistance and support.

- Procedures to follow in conducting joint investigations concerning the timing of steps and defining primary decision-making authority in specific situations.

- Strategy for conducting joint training.

- Operating plans for multidisciplinary team meetings and consultation with other disciplines.

- Coordination procedures for cooperation among various community agencies (Bockman & Carroll, 1978; Dinsmore, 1993; Ells, 1998; Pence & Wilson, 1992; Pence & Wilson, 1994).

The expertise that the police officer brings to the child maltreatment team focuses on the criminal aspects of child abuse and neglect, and specifically includes (1) collecting and preserving evidence, (2) examining crime scenes, (3) taking statements, (4) securing confessions, and (5) exercising the ability to make arrests (Pence & Wilson, 1994). The role and responsibilities of the law enforcement officer are broad, however, and always hinge on the criminal aspects of child maltreatment. According to Pence and Wilson (1994), the law enforcement role includes the following:

- Appropriate response to calls commensurate with the urgency of the situation, stabilization of the crime scene, and taking the initial statements at the scene.

- Collecting and preserving physical evidence at the scene.

- Interviewing witnesses.

- Interviewing child victims (independently or jointly, as decided with the team).

- Facilitating the use of special investigative tools, e.g., monitored telephone conversations.

- Conducting criminal history record checks for alleged perpetrators.

- Interviewing alleged perpetrators.

- Arresting suspects when indicated.

- Presenting evidence in criminal cases.

- Testifying in court.

- Taking the child into protective custody if the child's safety is at risk.

◆ INTERVIEW GUIDELINES
GENERAL INTERVIEW PREPARATIONS

An interview is simply the process of one person obtaining information from another by using a question-and-answer method (Poole & Lamb, 1998). It is important to gather all available case and background information pertinent to the nature of the interview. If necessary, the scene should be revisited and photographs reviewed. Investigators should make certain of the offense and what happened to the victim, never assuming guilt or innocence. Every event should be evaluated and investigated on its own merit.

All persons interviewed must be properly identified in all notes and reports, with the following carefully documented:

- Correct spelling of person's name

- Date of birth and Social Security number

- Home address: apartment number, floor, and location (front or rear)

- Telephone number: both home and work

- Secondary contact person: name, address, telephone numbers—both home and work

The interviewer should attempt to conduct the interview(s) away from other victims, witnesses, or suspected perpetrator(s). Suggested sites include the following:

- A place convenient and familiar to the interviewee.

- A neutral setting; the two most undesirable places for a victim or witness interview are the location of the alleged abuse and the police station. However, the police station is an appropriate place to interview the suspected perpetrator(s).

- With a child interview, a place that is child-friendly and where privacy is assured.

Interviews should take place as soon as possible after the even has occurred so that witness statements are not affected by memory loss or by talking to others. One person should conduct all interviews, if possible. At all times, the interviewer should communicate thoughts clearly and accurately. It is essential that bias not be displayed in nonverbal communications and, above all, that the interviewer remain professional in demeanor.

It is important to determine what information is to be obtained from the person being interviewed and to stay focused on the injury or event being investigated. The interviewer must keep in mind the alleged offense when directing questions. When formulating questions, the following guidelines are helpful:

- Keep questions short, clear, and easily understood.

- Confine questions to one topic at a time.

- Avoid "yes," "no," and leading questions that begin with "did or "does."

- Use comparison-type questions to pinpoint details.

Even though each interview is unique, there are seven general steps to conducting any interview:

1. Develop interview objectives (what needs to be known).

2. Use an introduction and warm-up.

3. Use the opening statement to set the tone of the interview.

4. Ask what happened and then listen.

5. Start over and get specific details (including what occurred before, during, and after the injury or event).

6. Obtain any other information required for the investigation.

7. Bring the interview to a conclusion.

THE VICTIM INTERVIEW

When interviewing a child, the investigator must keep in mind the developmental level and communicative abilities of the child and the circumstances surrounding the interview (Faller, 1993; Poole & Lamb, 1998). It is especially important to be aware of young children's eating and sleeping schedules and to refrain from interviewing them if they are hungry, tired, or otherwise physically uncomfortable. The interviewer should minimize the size difference between himself or herself and the child by getting on the same physical level (e.g., by using a child's table and chairs). It is essential to assure the child that he or she is not in any trouble. Interviewing tools (such as dolls, drawings, paper, crayons, or a dollhouse) may be used but should not detract from the interview. These tools should only be used by an interviewer who has received proper training in their use (Froum & Kendall-Tackett, 1998). Sufficient time should be allotted to conduct the interview.

Information gained before the interview should help in relating to the child on his or her developmental level. The interviewer must keep questions and sentences simple, using words familiar to the child. For example, it is wise to use the child's words for body parts. Interviewers must not assume that a word means the same thing to the child that it means to them. Pronunciation is important, and care must be taken when using pronouns like "he" or "she" and words like "there" and "that," as the child may be unable to follow the meaning. The child should be told that it is okay to answer, "I don't know" or "I don't understand," rather than guess at the answer to a question. It is important to ask questions that encourage the child to give more than a "yes" or "no" answer and to avoid leading questions that start with "did" or "does." Most of all, the interviewer must avoid "why" questions; they imply blame or identify a specific person. The child requires ongoing reassurance that he or she is believed and that he or she is not at fault for what happened.

The interviewer should be aware of the child's nonverbal communication and allow him or her plenty of time to respond to any question asked. Care must be taken in the interviewer's nonverbal communication (i.e., touching, facial expressions, eye contact, body posturing, hand gesturing, body distance) because it can affect the child's responsiveness during the interview. Neither the child's nor the interviewer's body parts should be used to evaluate the child's knowledge of anatomy.

The victim may divulge valuable information concerning the location of evidence or even unrelated contraband. If the interview results in a disclosure, it is extremely important to validate the disclosure with evidence and/or witnesses whenever possible.

If a uniformed officer is to conduct the interview of the child, several issues should be considered concerning the positive or negative impact of wearing the uniform (Pence & Wilson, 1992). First, the uniformed officer may be perceived by the child as an instrument of punishment, especially if the perpetrator has told the child that, if the abuse came to light, the child would be punished. Second, the child's past experience with police may be either positive or punitive. Third, the child may perceive the police uniform as a symbol of protection and an obvious sign of authority, indicating a person who may assist in preventing the perpetrator from harming the child. Fourth, for some children and adolescents, the authority that the uniform symbolizes may be a negative influence on the interview. Finally, small children are often intrigued by uniforms, so it may help establish rapport with the child (Pence & Wilson, 1992).

CONDUCTING THE INTERVIEW

At the beginning of the interview, the interviewer must introduce himself or herself to the child and explain what will happen in the interview. It is essential to take time to establish rapport with the child. Some sample questions that can assist in establishing rapport are as follows:

- What is your name? How old are you?
- Where do you live? Who lives with you? Who visits you?
- What are your mother's and father's names?
- What school do you go to? What grade are you in?
- What is your favorite subject? Your least favorite?
- What is your teacher's name? Who was your teacher last year?
- What makes you happy? Sad? Mad? Scared?
- What do you like best about the people you live with? Least?
- Why are you here today?

The interviewer should try to ask as few direct questions as possible, but attempt to obtain the what, who, how, where, and when of the allegation (Table 13-2). The goal is to obtain information that can be substantiated beyond the verbal disclosure.

CONCLUDING THE INTERVIEW

On completing the interview, the child should be asked if he or she has any questions. These should be answered honestly. It is acceptable to comfort the child, but no promises should be made because promises cannot always be kept.

Table 13-2. Questions That Can Be Asked of the Child Victim

What happened to you?

This question allows the child to describe the event in his or her own words. Help the child expand on the information by asking the following:

- What were you wearing? What was the alleged perpetrator wearing?

- What happened to your clothes? The alleged perpetrator's clothes?

- What did he or she say? What did you say to him or her?

- Who did you tell this to?

Are you hurt or sick now?

Never delay emergency medical care. If the child indicates that he or she is hurt, ask "where?"

What happened next?

This question encourages more detail. When a child begins to disclose, you may prompt him with questions such as the following:

- What else do you remember? What else do I need to know?

- Could you tell me what you mean by _____? I need to understand a little more here.

- Were pictures taken? Of what? By whom? Where are the pictures?

- Were you asked not to tell anyone? Who asked you? What were you asked not to tell?

- Who were you not supposed to tell? This helps to determine the use of threats or bribes.

Who did this to you?

If information is not volunteered, it is important to ask the name and/or relationship of the abuser.

- Were you touched by anyone? Who? Where?

- How do you know him or her?

- Has anyone else done this to you? Who? Where?

How did this happen?

Asking this question will encourage an explanation of the event.

- What were you touched with (an object may have been used)?

It is appropriate to ask the child what he or she expects will happen, then explain what is likely to happen. The child should be told if there will be further contacts or interviews. If additional interviews are needed, it is less traumatic for the child to deal with the same interviewer. It is extremely important that the interviewer not make statements or promises to the child that cannot be kept. Even with the best of intentions, much of what happens to the child is beyond the control of the investigator.

If the child has not disclosed abuse but there are indicators that abuse did take place, it may be necessary to make a referral to a qualified counselor. However, if prosecution is a possibility, counseling, therapy, or other abuse-related treatment (including hypnosis) may be seen as potentially compromising the criminal case. Referrals for such mental health treatment should be discussed with the prosecutor as arrangements for these types of services are being made.

The Witness Interview

Basic Requirements of Witnesses

Some of the more important factors to be considered when conducting an interview with a witness are discussed here. However, before attempting to weigh their effect on the witness' story, it is essential to first determine that the witness meets three essential requirements:

1. The witness was present during the event or a portion of it.

2. The witness was conscious (aware) of what was happening.

3. The witness was attentive to what was happening. (This final element is the most difficult to establish.)

Conducting the Interview

When interviewing the witness, the interviewer must first allow the person to say what happened or what he or she observed in a narrative style. Specific questions can be asked later to gather more detail and to jog the witness' memory.

It is essential to (1) ask the witness for the correct spelling of names and for the addresses and phone numbers of other persons talked about; (2) ask if the victim disclosed the incident to the witness; (3) ask if there is anything that you have failed to ask; (4) ask if there is anything else the witness wants to discuss; and (5) obtain a written statement, if possible.

At the end of the interview, the witness should be told that there are no further questions at this time, but as the investigation continues, he or she may be needed to talk about new information or to clarify what has just been revealed at a later time. The interviewer should encourage the witness to contact authorities with any additional information. Never should the witness be told that by talking now, he or she will not have to appear in court.

Interrogating the Suspected Perpetrator

Procedures or practices should be guided by the investigative agency's rules/procedures, local dictates, and applicable local, state, and federal laws.

A background check on those involved can be invaluable. It is important to gather as much background information as possible before interviewing the suspected perpetrator(s), including:

- Criminal history

- Social history

- Medical history

- Driving record

- Credit history

- Family, friends, hobbies, likes, dislikes, and personal history

- Evidence or previous report of domestic violence in residence

In addition, it is important to read original reports (e.g., police) and check with other professionals (e.g., social worker).

If two interviewers are present, one should conduct the interview, while the other one takes notes and shows support by displaying positive gestures.

CONDUCTING THE INTERVIEW

First, introductions should be made, with care taken to identify why the interview is being conducted. This will set the stage for the interview, so it is important to be candid, honest, and polite. First impressions are lasting impressions. The interviewer should shake the person's hand and take care to communicate on the same level as the person being interviewed. It is unwise to use difficult words to impress or embarrass the other person. The interviewer should be attentive at all times, maintain eye contact, and use reflective listening techniques—mirroring back what is said to indicate an active interest in what the interviewee has to say. It is important to be patient, to make sure sufficient time is scheduled for the interview, and to be empathetic.

If dealing with a person in custody, the interview is initiated by reading the Miranda Rights and having him or her sign and date a waiver. If a person not in custody starts making incriminating statements, he or she should be advised of the Miranda Rights, and sign and date a waiver before the interview continues (Pence & Wilson, 1992). These steps should be guided by the investigative agency's policy and procedures. The Miranda Warning, as prescribed by the Supreme Court, is as follows:

- He or she has the right to remain silent, and need not answer any questions.

- If he or she does answer questions, the answers can be used against him or her.

- He or she has the right to consult with an attorney before or during questioning by the police.

- If he or she cannot afford to hire an attorney, one will be provided without cost (Pence & Wilson, 1994).

During the interview process, it should be the interviewer's goal to build rapport. Openness is encouraged by sharing non-critical information. It is essential to avoid being judgmental; exhibiting personal feelings and emotions, such as anger or disgust, can influence the interview. It is possible to demonstrate interest in the suspected perpetrator as a person through control of actions and reactions. It is useful to allow the suspected perpetrator to talk about himself or herself. As this is done, the interviewer should pay attention to the suspected perpetrator's interests and fantasies, and appeal to his or her emotions. It may be appropriate to show photographs of the victim, but the suspected perpetrator should never be allowed to show disrespect for the victim.

To reduce any feelings of threat, the interviewer can emphasize positive characteristics to bolster the suspected perpetrator's ego. A possible approach is to be open-minded and empathize with the weaknesses and defects of the suspected perpetrator. It may help the suspected perpetrator look at the problem with a lowered level of personal threat if the interviewer states, "I understand how these things can happen; sometimes, we just lose control." The interviewer may suggest that, "There are always two sides to every story. This may be your last chance to tell exactly what happened and why. It's never as bad as you think."

The interviewer must keep in mind that certain information must be obtained: who, what, when, where, why, and how, if possible. It is not advisable to ask the direct question, "Did you do it?" If applicable, the interviewer may ask if drugs or alcohol were used and whether they could be responsible for what happened. It is also appropriate to ask if photographs were taken and/or videotapes made.

Interviewers must look for and recognize the importance of verbal and nonverbal cues. Most of the time, the person being interviewed is looking for help or a release from guilt. He or she may be remorseful, if the correct emotional response can be triggered. It may be necessary to provide a face-saving situation for the suspected perpetrator. When appropriate, the interview should be closed on a cooperative note, remembering that the suspect may have to be interviewed again.

SPECIAL INVESTIGATIVE TECHNIQUES

The use of videotaped or audiotaped recordings during interviews and interrogations is becoming increasingly popular. Recordings may be used as monitoring devices or to document interviews or interrogations. The interviewer should follow investigative agency procedures and check with the prosecutor. If such devices are allowed, it is wise to use the best equipment available and to be proficient in its use (Table 13-3).

Table 13-3. Special Investigative Techniques

- Monitored pretext telephone or personal conversations

  - Two types: Telephone and personal conversation

  - Issues to consider:

    - Authorization, timing, victim maturity/stability, victim preparation, equipment, staffing, perpetrator background

- Polygraphs
- Audiotapes/videotapes of interviews

  - Advantages: accurate record of what was said, actual interview can be reviewed, does not depend on interviewer's notes or memory

  - Disadvantages: can be distracting, small or trivial issues can become major focus that weakens case and obscures more important issues

- Use of anatomically correct dolls

  - Requires specialized training

Adapted from Pence & Wilson, 1992.

The advantages to taping interviews have been described as follows:

- Potentially reduces the number of repeat interviews that the victim must undergo because other investigators and the prosecutor may review the tape, rather than re-interview the child.

- Provides a verbatim account of the statements made, not the interviewer's interpretation or recollection.

- Is useful in potentially breaking down a suspect's defenses and possibly gaining a confession.

- Is useful in convincing the non-offending caregiver of the gravity of the situation and the child's need for protection from the alleged perpetrator.

- Depending on jurisdiction, may be of use in court proceedings. However, this is a contentious area of law and may change, based on appellate court decisions (Pence & Wilson, 1992; Pence & Wilson, 1994).

The disadvantages to taping interviews have been described as follows:

- Videotapes and audiotapes cannot be edited in any way. Everything recorded must remain unaltered if it is to be used as evidence.

- They may have the potential to allow the defense to critique small segments and specific word choices made by the interviewer rather than focus on the overall content of the interview and the child's disclosure.

- They are potentially damaging in court proceedings because the tape records inconsistencies in the child's disclosure as well as denials. Because the disclosure of abusive events, especially events related to sexual abuse, often occurs in a halting, piecemeal fashion peppered with occasional denials by the child, this could be exploited by the defense counsel or defense expert.

- They provide documentation of errors made by the interviewer, such as poorly phrased questions.

- They are often not admissible in court proceedings.

- The taping process and equipment may be distracting to children (Pence & Wilson, 1992; Pence & Wilson, 1994).

◆ CRIME SCENE SEARCH

The law enforcement officer is responsible for searching and collecting physical evidence from the scene of the abuse that could help substantiate the criminal charges (Pence & Wilson, 1992). Following agency guidelines around search procedures, the police investigator should seek the following:

- Instruments of crime used to harm the child (e.g., rod, coat hanger, belt, extension cord, rope).

- Physical traces of the injury (e.g., blood-stained clothing).

- Photographs of the exact location where the abuse occurred (Pence & Wilson, 1992).

Investigators may find crime scene searches particularly helpful in finding evidence that confirms the abusive environment and events. The following are specific places to search:

- Area where the abuse occurred, looking for semen and pubic hair, as well as looking for background evidence discussed in the interview, such as furniture, wallpaper, and lighting fixtures.

- Bathroom where the perpetrator may have washed herself or himself and/or the child.

- Sheets and fabrics from the child's bedroom and locations where abuse may have occurred. If appropriate, fabrics that are not frequently washed, such as the child's bedspread, that might corroborate the child's disclosure should also be submitted to the lab (Pence & Wilson, 1992).

Depending on the circumstances of the case, the suspected perpetrator's residence should be searched for the following:

- "Lures" such as toys, games, and stuffed animals used by the perpetrator to entice the child.

- Child erotica, defined as material related to children that may be arousing to the perpetrator (e.g., sketches, fantasy writings, diaries, and sexual aids).

- Child and adult pornographic material. If child pornography is found, it may require the involvement of other law enforcement agencies, such as postal inspectors and the Federal Bureau of Investigation, because multiple jurisdictions may ultimately become involved (Pence & Wilson, 1992).

- "Souvenirs." Sexual perpetrators are often compelled to keep reminders of the children they molest. These may be in the form of photographs, videos, clothing, or even clippings of hair.

◆ WHEN A CHILD DIES: INVESTIGATING CHILD FATALITIES

The loss of a loved one, particularly a child, is perhaps the greatest loss an individual or family can experience. Many overwhelming feelings follow the death of a child for both the family and the professionals involved with the case. This grief and sadness is a natural and normal reaction to an irreplaceable loss.

Annually, approximately 2000 children are identified as having died from some form of maltreatment (Christoffel, 1992). Most child protection investigators recognize that fatalities related to abuse are the extreme and that for every child homicide, there are literally thousands of infants and children who are injured and disabled, many permanently. The difficulty of investigating serious abuse and fatalities requires investigators to have a thorough knowledge of available professional resources and how and when to access them.

Maltreatment-related child fatalities are closely associated with vulnerability. The safety and well-being of infants and young children are totally dependent on parents and caregivers. Lapses in care and oversight, as well as inappropriate harmful behavior by those in charge of children, dramatically increase the potential fatal risks. Generally speaking, the younger the infant or child, the greater the risk for harm or death (Sedlak & Broadhurst, 1996).

Law enforcement and CPS agencies routinely investigate child deaths that are allegedly related to maltreatment. Whether the death was due to neglect or to injuries, investigators must use every available resource to determine if the fatality resulted from an intentional or unintentional act or omission. In most cases, this requires a close working relationship with medical and other child protection professionals.

A complete history is essential to a correct diagnosis in all cases of child and infant death. The medical personnel who first examine these children and interact with the families or caregivers have the best opportunity to find out what occurred. If the child dies, a major goal of the investigation is to determine if the findings at autopsy are consistent with the past and recent medical history. Social history and witnessed accounts are also essential in determining if the stated causal event is consistent with medical and pathologic findings.

Beyond preliminary investigative information (see Appendix I), infant and child fatalities require special information to document circumstances and evidence at the location of death. The best, most organized method for obtaining comprehensive death scene information is the use of a checklist specific to children (see Appendix II). Death-scene checklists should include as much information concerning the recent and time of death history as possible. While most death-scene checklists are based on a "medical model," the information can be invaluable in a criminal investigation. Checklist information is also an important tool for the pathologist because illness and injury patterns in children are often unique.

Fatal abuse of infants and children can occur in many forms. The most obvious is the battered child who is beaten or bludgeoned to the point of death (Parrish, 1996). Depending on age and the severity of the assault, death can occur immediately or as a result of latent or continuing abuse. It is extremely important to document the child's medical history to establish a pattern of abuse. This may include past treatment as well as injuries that were not treated.

Shaken baby syndrome refers to infants who are shaken violently to the point that there are physiological consequences (Duhaime, Christian, Rorke, & Zimmerman, 1998). Brain movement in the skull can result in immediate death or in long-term or permanent disabilities (e.g., learning, physical, visual, speech, seizures). In most cases, there are no visible signs of injury. If it is suspected that an infant or young child is the victim of violent shaking, specialized medical examination is imperative. To assist in identifying the person responsible, a time line of the child's life and those with access to him or her is extremely important. It will assist the doctor or pathologist in evaluating the explanation of how the injury occurred.

The cause of sudden infant death syndrome (SIDS) is not known, but it is generally believed to be the result of multiple risk factors, as opposed to a single cause (Farley & Reece, 1996; Committee on Child Abuse and Neglect, 2001). For the investigator, it is important to separate SIDS deaths from other causes that in themselves cannot be readily identified (Dix, 2001). Most SIDS-type deaths mimic infant suffocation. Generally, the pathologist cannot differentiate between accidental suffocation (e.g., rollovers, wedging, bedding entanglement) and deliberate suffocation.

While there are many similarities, the circumstances of every child fatality are in some way unique. The investigator of suspected maltreatment-related child death must form trusting partnerships with other child protection professionals in order to identify more accurately not just the *cause* of death, but, equally important, the *manner*. The circumstances surrounding the death help determine if the event was natural, accidental, intentional, or unintentional. In some states, multidisciplinary Child Fatality Review Programs concurrently review child deaths and contribute to more accurate determinations of cause and manner of death (Kolilis, 1998). The investigative checklist used in the state of Missouri for child deaths is in Appendix II at the end of this chapter.

◆ PREPARING A REPORT

All of the information obtained is assembled into a logical sequence of events, accurately reflecting the results of the entire investigation. Observations, statements, evidence, sketches, photographs, and medical and technical findings should clearly portray all the known facts of the case. If new or additional information becomes available, it is best to prepare a supplemental report and distribute it to all participating agencies.

All investigative results (interviewing, disposition of evidence, names of responders and what they did) are recorded according to the policy and procedures of the investigative agency. It may be necessary to take handwritten notes, record electronically, videotape, or use a combination of all these methods. Whatever the means, it is important to record and document every step of the investigation.

While the primary role of law enforcement in the investigation of child maltreatment is to investigate alleged crimes, the ultimate responsibility is to identify and protect children at risk. Beyond the case being investigated, law enforcement officers should be alert to any situation that puts a child in harm's way. The assessment and immediate actions taken by law enforcement may save a child's life and improve the opportunity to preserve the family.

◆ CONCLUSION

The criminal justice system and law enforcement agencies cannot successfully deal with child maltreatment alone. The resolution of a given case requires collaboration with other agencies and disciplines. A number of factors set child abuse and neglect cases apart from other "adult" criminal activity that police routinely confront. These factors may be summarized as follows:

- The investigation of child maltreatment first involves the need to make a determination that a crime has actually occurred, based on state law, as well as where and when it happened.

- The investigator in child maltreatment must have the ability to interact with children and must be an effective communicator with children at different developmental levels.

- In cases of child maltreatment, joint investigations are the rule rather than the exception. Effective teamwork between CPS staff and other child protection professionals is essential when investigating allegations of child maltreatment.

- Judgments made by investigators about the evidence in child maltreatment cases depend significantly on information provided by other disciplines, such as physicians, psychologists, coroners, and social workers. Investigators must know what resources are available and how to access them.

- Multiple jurisdictions and courts may be involved in child maltreatment cases, including juvenile/family court, criminal court, and civil court (Pence & Wilson, 1992).

In addition to all of these unique aspects, the fact that child maltreatment deals with children being harmed places a significant emotional burden on the investigators and other professionals involved.

◆ REFERENCES

Bockman, H. R., & Carroll, C.A. (1978). The law enforcement's role in evaluation. In B. D. Schmitt (Ed.), The child protection team handbook (pp.149-152). New York: Garland Publishing, Inc.

Committee on Child Abuse and Neglect. (2001). Distinguishing sudden infant death syndrome from child abuse fatalities (RE0036). Pediatrics, 107(2), 437-441.

Christoffel, K. K. (1992). Child abuse fatalities. In S. Ludwig and A. E. Kornberg (Eds.), Child abuse: A medical reference (2nd ed.) (pp. 49-59). New York: Churchill Livingstone.

DePanfilis, D., & Salus, M. K. (1992). A coordinated response to child abuse and neglect: A basic manual. Washington, DC: U.S. Department of Health and Human Services, National Center on Child Abuse and Neglect.

Dinsmore, J. (1993). Joint investigations of child abuse: Report of a symposium. Washington, DC: U.S. Department of Health and Human Services, National Center on Child Abuse and Neglect.

Dix, J. (2001). Death investigators manual. Columbia, MO: Academic Information Systems.

Duhaime, A. C., Christian, C. W., Rorke, L. B., & Zimmerman, R.A. (1998). Nonaccidental head injury in infants—The "shaken-baby syndrome." New England Journal of Medicine, 338(25), 1822-1829.

Ells, M. (1998). Forming a multidisciplinary team to investigate child abuse. Portable guide to investigating child abuse. Washington, DC: U.S. Department of Justice.

Faller, K. C. (1993). Child sexual abuse: Intervention and treatment issues. Washington, DC: U.S. Department of Health and Human Services, National Center on Child Abuse and Neglect.

Farley, R. H., & Reece, R. M. (1996). Recognizing when a child's injury or illness is caused by abuse. Portable guide to investigating child abuse. Washington, DC: U.S. Department of Justice.

Froum, A. G., & Kendall-Tackett, K. A. (1998). Law enforcement officers' approaches to evaluations of child sexual abuse. Child Abuse and Neglect, 22(9), 939-942.

Hammond, C. B., Lanning, K. V., Promisel, W., Shepherd, J. R., & Walsh, B. (1997). Law enforcement response to child abuse. Portable guide to investigating child abuse. Washington, DC: U.S. Department of Justice.

Kinnear, K. L. (1995). Childhood sexual abuse. Santa Barbara, CA: ABC-CLIO, Inc.

Kolilis, D. M. (1998). Child fatality review teams. In J. A. Monteleone and A. E. Brodeur (Eds.), Child maltreatment: A clinical guide and reference (2nd ed.) (pp.509-515). St. Louis, MO: GW Medical Publishing, Inc.

Lanning, K. V., & Walsh, B. (1996). Criminal investigation of suspected child abuse. In J. Briere, L. Berliner, J.A. Bulkey, C. Jenny, and T. Reid (Eds.), The APSAC handbook on child maltreatment (pp.246-270). Thousand Oaks, CA: SAGE Publications.

Parrish, R. (1996). Battered child syndrome: Investigating physical abuse and homicide. Portable guide to investigating child abuse. Washington, DC: U.S. Department of Justice.

Pena, M. S. (1993). Practical criminal investigation (pp.257-259). Incline Village, NV: Copperhouse Publishing.

Pence, D., & Wilson, C. (1992). The role of law enforcement in the response to child abuse and neglect. Washington, DC: U.S. Department of Health and Human Services, National Center on Child Abuse and Neglect.

Pence, D., & Wilson, C. (1994). Team investigation of child sexual abuse: The uneasy alliance. Thousand Oaks, CA: SAGE Publications.

Poole, D. A., & Lamb, M. E. (1998). Investigative interviews of children: A guide for helping professionals. Washington, DC: American Psychological Association.

Sands, R. G., Stafford, J., & McClelland, M. (1990). "I beg to differ": Conflict in the interdisciplinary team. Social Work in Health Care, 14(3), 55-72.

Sedlak, A. J., & Broadhurst, D. D. (1996). The third national incidence study of child abuse and neglect (NIS-3 final report). Washington, DC: U.S. Department of Health and Human Services; U.S. Government Printing Office (Contract # 105-94-1840).

Sheppard, D. I., & Zangrillo, P. A. (1996). Coordinating investigations of child abuse. Public Welfare, 54(1), 21-31.

Weston, P. B., & Wells, K. M. (1986). Criminal investigation (pp. 253-259). Upper Saddle River, NJ: Prentice-Hall, Inc.

◆ Appendix I: Multidisciplinary Preliminary Investigative Checklist for Serious Children's Events

Checklists are an excellent investigative aid to facilitate a more timely and comprehensive assessment of the case. They act as reminders to obtain specific information and provide a means to organize and measure the status of the investigation. Checklists can be adapted to meet most agency requirements. This checklist outlines generic information essential to the investigation of suspected child maltreatment. Field investigators are encouraged to evaluate the list and make modifications appropriate to specific case needs and objectives. This checklist is only a reminder and guide. Every effort should be made to verify and expand on information as it becomes known. It is essential to a credible investigation to differentiate between investigative leads and verified facts. Individual agency policies and procedures have precedence over these investigative suggestions.

PRELIMINARY INVESTIGATIVE CHECKLIST
WHAT IS THE NATURE OF THE ALLEGATION(S)?
- Who?

- What?

- When?

- Where? (What is the exact location and venue where the alleged event took place?)

- How?

- How many times?

HOW WAS ALLEGATION OR REPORT RECEIVED?
- By whom?

- Has a child abuse and neglect hotline report been made?

- Incident number?

- Date?

- Reporter? (NOTE: In most states, the name of the child abuse and neglect reporters, by law, are confidential.)

- County of incident?

VICTIM(S)—FULL PEDIGREE?
- Date of birth?

- Name?

- Gender?

- Race?

- Social Security number?

- Child protective services client number?

- Home address, phone number, county?

- Residence of child(ren) at the time of this report (e.g., foster care)?

- Is the victim at risk?

- Protective custody taken?

- Has the victim been injured? If so, is the victim in need of medical treatment?

- Are there sibling(s) in the home?

- Are the sibling(s) at risk?

MEDICAL EXAMINATION/TREATMENT—WAS IT NEEDED?
- Apparent nature of the illness/injury/event?

- When did it occur?

- Where did it occur?

- How was it conveyed?
- By whom?
- Name/location of medical facility?
- Were photographs taken of an injury? By whom? When? Present location?
- Is there a diagnosis/prognosis?
- By whom?

Parent(s)—Full Pedigree?

- Father and mother's name?
- Date of birth?
- Gender?
- Race?
- Social Security number?
- Child protective services client number?
- Home address, phone number, county?
- Employer? Work phone number?

Name of Guardian/Caretaker(s)—Full Pedigree (If Other Than Parent)?

- Date of birth?
- Gender?
- Race?
- Social Security number?
- Child protective services client number?
- Home address, phone number, county?
- Employer? Their work phone number?
- Relationship to the victim?

If Sexual Abuse Is Alleged, Has a Sexual Assault Forensic Examination Been Completed on the Victim?

- When?
- Where?
- By whom?
- Findings?
- Colposcope or other image documentation used?

Has the Victim Been Interviewed?

- By whom?
- When?
- Where?
- Recorded by audio or video?

- If appropriate, is a "Cool call" considered? (Is it appropriate for the victim to make a monitored and recorded phone call to the suspect? Is the child developmentally and emotionally able to make such a call?)

- Was information obtained that would justify seeking a search warrant? (If the suspected perpetrator is no longer on the premises, a "permission" search may be possible.)

SUSPECTED PERPETRATOR(S)—FULL PEDIGREE?

- Name(s)?
- Date of birth?
- Gender?
- Race?
- Social Security number?
- Child protective services client number?
- Home address, phone number, county?
- Employer? Work phone number?
- Relationship to victim?

RECORD CHECKS COMPLETED?

- Local?
- State?
- FBI?
- Other applicable state(s)?
- Social history?
- Child abuse and neglect hotline prior reports?
- Medical and health records?

IS THERE PHYSICAL EVIDENCE?

- Description?
- Seized by and chain of custody?
- Evidence photographed?
- Is laboratory examination required?
- Present location?

ARE THERE WITNESSES?

- Name(s)?
- Date of birth?
- Gender?
- Race?
- Social Security number?

- Child protective services client number?

- Home address, phone number, county?

- Employer? Work phone number?

- Relationship to victim?

Have Documented Statements Been Taken From Witnesses and Others?

- From whom?

- By whom?

- Where were they taken?

- How were they documented?

Child Protective Services/Juvenile Court Actions Taken to Date?

- Investigation in progress?

- Sibling risk assessment?

- Protective measures taken?

- Criminal justice actions taken?

- Charges pending?

- Charges filed (what and by whom)?

- Arrest(s) made (by whom and for what)?

What Agencies and Investigators Are Involved in the Investigation?

- Who are the agency contacts?

- What are their responsibilities?

◆ APPENDIX II: DEATH-SCENE INVESTIGATION CHECKLIST FOR CHILD FATALITIES

Adapted from the Missouri State Technical Assistance Team, 2001.

MISSOURI DEPARTMENT OF SOCIAL SERVICES
DIVISION OF FAMILY SERVICES
MISSOURI CHILD FATALITY REVIEW PROGRAM

615 HOWERTON COURT
JEFFERSON CITY, MO 65109
(314) 751-5980
(800) 487-1626

DEATH-SCENE INVESTIGATIVE CHECKLIST FOR CHILD FATALITIES

(CORONER/MEDICAL EXAMINER SHOULD PREPARE AND SUBMIT TO CERTIFIED CHILD DEATH PATHOLOGIST PRIOR TO AUTOPSY.)

INSTRUCTIONS:
Complete each numbered item by providing the appropriate response and by marking the completed or not completed box in the left-hand margin. Make every attempt to obtain as much information as possible. For assistance, call (800) 487-1626.

COMPLETED / NOT COMPLETED

1. ☐ ☐

NAME OF DECEDENT ___ / (MI) ___ / (LAST)

RACE ☐ — W = WHITE / B = BLACK / O = OTHER / U = UNKNOWN

SEX ☐ M ☐ F

DATE OF BIRTH (MM/DD/YY): ___ DATE OF DEATH (MM/DD/YY): ___

TIME OF DEATH: ___ ☐ AM ☐ PM

SCENE/EVENT ADDRESS (STREET, CITY, ZIP):

COUNTY OF SCENE/EVENT:

DECEDENT DISCOVERED BY (NAME):

DATE DISCOVERED (MM/DD/YY): TIME: ___ ☐ AM ☐ PM

RELATIONSHIP TO DECEDENT:

DATE SCENE INVESTIGATION CONDUCTED (MM/DD/YY): TIME: ___ ☐ AM ☐ PM

DEATH SCENE PHOTOGRAPHS OF DECEDENT OR SILHOUETTE TAKEN BY (NAME & TITLE):

DATE PHOTOS TAKEN (MM/DD/YY)? TIME ___ ☐ AM ☐ PM

PRESENT LOCATION OF FILM/NEGATIVES/PRINTS:

WHO PRONOUNCED DECEDENT DEAD (NAME & TITLE)?

WHERE PRONOUNCED (HOME, MEDICAL FACILITY, ETC.) ADDRESS:

DFS HISTORY CHECKED BY (NAME & TITLE)? DATE (MM/DD/YY): TIME ___ ☐ AM ☐ PM

CFRP CRITERIA PREVIEWED? ☐ NO ☐ YES ☐ UNKNOWN

CERTIFIED CHILD-DEATH PATHOLOGIST CONSULTED (NAME)?

AUTOPSY REQUESTED? ☐ NO ☐ YES ☐ UNKNOWN

BODY DELIVERED TO PATHOLOGIST BY (NAME & TITLE):

DATE DELIVERED (MM/DD/YY) TIME ___ ☐ AM ☐ PM

INVESTIGATOR(S) (NAME & TITLE):

INVESTIGATING AGENCY/DEPARTMENT

REPORT NUMBER

ASSESSMENT OF HISTORY AND CIRCUMSTANCES

2. ☐ ☐

MEDICAL ASSISTANCE SUMMONED? ☐ NO ☐ YES ☐ UNKNOWN

IF YES, WHO WAS SUMMONED?

WHO PLACED THE CALL (NAME & RELATIONSHIP)?

DATE (MM/DD/YY): TIME: ___ ☐ AM ☐ PM

3. ☐ ☐

CONVEYED TO MEDICAL FACILITY? ☐ NO ☐ YES ☐ UNKNOWN

NAME AND ADDRESS OF MEDICAL FACILITY?

4. ☐ ☐

WAS DECEDENT PHOTOGRAPHED AT MEDICAL FACILITY? ☐ NO ☐ YES ☐ UNKNOWN

PHOTOS TAKEN BY (NAME & TITLE):

TIME: ___ ☐ AM ☐ PM DATE (MM/DD/YY):

PRESENT LOCATION OF FILM/NEGATIVES/PRINTS:

5. ☐ ☐

RESUSCITATION BY EMS? ☐ NO ☐ YES ☐ UNKNOWN

ANYONE ELSE (NAME & RELATIONSHIP)?

IF NOT EMS, WAS PERSON CPR CERTIFIED? ☐ NO ☐ YES ☐ UNKNOWN

WHERE WAS RESUSCITATION INITIATED (HOME, NEIGHBOR'S HOME, HOSPITAL, ETC.)? FOR HOW LONG?

6. ☐ ☐

DESCRIBE IN DETAIL, LOCATION WHERE DECEDENT WAS FOUND (BED, FLOOR, HOUSE, YARD, VEHICLE, TRASH CONTAINER, ETC.):

MO 886-3228N (6-00)

PAGE 1

7. ☐ ☐	DESCRIBE ANYTHING UNUSUAL FOUND ON OR AROUND THE BODY, ESPECIALLY ANYTHING THAT MAY HAVE INFLUENCED THE DEATH (MEDICINE, BABY BOTTLE, CLEANING AGENT, BED CLOTHING, ETC.).

SEIZED? ☐ NO ☐ YES ☐ UNKNOWN	IF YES, BY WHOM (NAME & TITLE)?	PRESENT LOCATION OF EVIDENCE:

8. ☐ ☐	WAS DECEDENT MOVED FROM ORIGINAL POSITION? ☐ NO ☐ YES ☐ UNKNOWN	MOVED BY WHOM (NAME AND RELATIONSHIP)?

WHY MOVED?

9. ☐ ☐	RIGOR MORTIS (RIGIDITY) ☐ NO ☐ YES ☐ UNKNOWN	WHERE OBSERVED ON DECEDENT?	DATE OBSERVED (MM/DD/YY):	TIME OBSERVED: _____ ☐ AM ☐ PM

(DO NOT ATTEMPT TO MOVE OR STRAIGHTEN FIXED EXTREMITIES)

10. ☐ ☐	LIVOR MORTIS (SETTLING OF BLOOD)? ☐ NO ☐ YES ☐ UNKNOWN	WHERE OBSERVED ON DECEDENT?

TIME OBSERVED: _____ ☐ AM ☐ PM	CONSISTENT WITH POSITION WHEN FOUND? ☐ NO ☐ YES ☐ UNKNOWN

11. ☐ ☐	APPROXIMATE ENVIRONMENTAL TEMPERATURE AT LOCATION OF DEATH (IN FAHRENHEIT DEGREES)? °	TIME OBSERVED: ☐ AM ☐ PM	DATE OBSERVED (MM/DD/YY):

IF OUTSIDE, GENERAL WEATHER CONDITIONS: ☐ RAINING ☐ SNOWING ☐ SUNNY ☐ OTHER: (DESCRIBE)_____

12. ☐ ☐	TO THE TOUCH, APPARENT BODY TEMPERATURE OF DECEDENT AT LOCATION OF DEATH? ☐ WARM ☐ SWEATY ☐ COLD	DATE OBSERVED (MM/DD/YY):	TIME OBSERVED: _____ ☐ AM ☐ PM

13. ☐ ☐	DATE DECEDENT LAST SEEN ALIVE (MM/DD/YY)?	TIME: _____ ☐ AM ☐ PM	BY WHOM (NAME & RELATIONSHIP)?

WHAT WAS THE CONDITION OF THE DECEDENT WHEN LAST SEEN ALIVE?

14. ☐ ☐	WAS DEATH WITNESSED? ☐ NO ☐ YES ☐ UNKNOWN	IF YES, BY WHOM (NAME & RELATIONSHIP)? DESCRIBE DETAILS IN NARRATIVE SECTION.

15. ☐ ☐	WHAT WAS THE DECEDENT'S ACTIVITY PRIOR TO DEATH (e.g., SLEEPING, PLAYING, ETC.)?

16. ☐ ☐	APPEARANCE OF DECEDENT WHEN OBSERVED: ☐ CLEAN ☐ DIRTY ☐ OTHER:

DESCRIBE:

17. ☐ ☐	CLOTHING WORN? ☐ CLEAN ☐ DIRTY ☐ TORN OR DAMAGED	APPROPRIATE? ☐ NO ☐ YES

DESCRIBE:

18. ☐ ☐	CLOTHING SEIZED AND PACKAGED? ☐ NO ☐ YES ☐ UNKNOWN	IF YES, BY WHOM (NAME & TITLE)?

PRESENT LOCATION OF EVIDENCE:

19. ☐ ☐	BODY POSITION WHEN DISCOVERED: ☐ ON STOMACH ☐ ON BACK ☐ SEATED UPRIGHT ☐ LEFT SIDE ☐ RIGHT SIDE	IF APPLICABLE, BODY WAS: ☐ VERTICALLY PINNED ☐ HORIZONTALLY PINNED ☐ OTHER WEDGING ☐ N/A

PINNED OR WEDGED BY WHAT?

20. ☐ ☐	USUAL SLEEPING POSITION? ☐ ON STOMACH ☐ ON BACK ☐ SEATED UPRIGHT ☐ LEFT SIDE ☐ RIGHT SIDE

21. ☐ ☐	POSITION OF FACE (NOSE/MOUTH) WHEN DISCOVERED: ☐ FACE DIRECTLY UP ☐ FACE TO RIGHT ☐ FACE DIRECTLY DOWN ☐ FACE TO LEFT	WERE PHOTOS TAKEN? ☐ NO ☐ YES ☐ UNKNOWN

IF PHOTOS TAKEN, WHO TOOK THEM (NAME & TITLE)?	DATE (MM/DD/YY):	TIME: ☐ AM ☐ PM	PRESENT LOCATION OF FILM/NEGATIVES/PRINTS:

22. ☐ ☐	WAS DECEDENT'S FACE IN CONTACT WITH WET SUBSTANCE? ☐ NO ☐ YES ☐ UNKNOWN	SUBSTANCE APPEARED TO BE: ☐ MUCUS ☐ VOMIT ☐ BLOODY FROTH ☐ FOOD ☐ SALIVA ☐ DRIED SECRETION ☐ FORMULA ☐ FROTH ☐ BLOOD TINGED SECRETION OTHER: _____

23. ☐ ☐	**SUBSTANCE OBSERVED IN NOSE?** ☐ NO ☐ YES ☐ UNKNOWN	

SUBSTANCE APPEARED TO BE:
☐ MUCUS ☐ VOMIT ☐ BLOODY FROTH OTHER:
☐ FOOD ☐ SALIVA ☐ DRIED SECRETION
☐ FORMULA ☐ FROTH ☐ BLOOD TINGED SECRETION

24. ☐ ☐ **SUBSTANCE OBSERVED IN MOUTH?**
☐ NO ☐ YES ☐ UNKNOWN

SUBSTANCE APPEARED TO BE:
☐ MUCUS ☐ VOMIT ☐ BLOODY FROTH OTHER:
☐ FOOD ☐ SALIVA ☐ DRIED SECRETION
☐ FORMULA ☐ FROTH ☐ BLOOD TINGED SECRETION

25. ☐ ☐ **ANYTHING OBSTRUCTING FACE, NOSE OR MOUTH?**
☐ NO ☐ YES ☐ IF YES, DESCRIBE

26. ☐ ☐ **SECRETIONS FOUND ON:**
☐ PILLOW ☐ BLANKET ☐ SHEET ☐ MATTRESS ☐ CLOTHING ☐ OTHER:

APPEARED TO BE:
☐ MUCUS ☐ VOMIT ☐ BLOODY FROTH OTHER:
☐ FOOD ☐ SALIVA ☐ DRIED SECRETION
☐ FORMULA ☐ FROTH ☐ BLOOD TINGED SECRETION

27. ☐ ☐ **HEMORRHAGE OF EYES?** ☐ NO ☐ YES ☐ UNKNOWN | **HEMORRHAGE OF EARS?** ☐ NO ☐ YES ☐ UNKNOWN
DESCRIBE:

28. ☐ ☐ **IS THERE A VISIBLE CREASE ON FACE, NECK OR HEAD FROM PILLOWS, CLOTHING, BEDDING, OR OTHER OBJECT?**
☐ NO ☐ YES ☐ UNKNOWN
EXPLAIN:

29. ☐ ☐ **SKETCH POSITION OF DECEDENT AS FOUND, AND IDENTIFY IF IN BED OR OTHER IDENTIFIABLE LOCATION. (INDICATE DIRECTION OF DECEDENT'S HEAD; CIRCLE DIRECTION INDICATOR.)**

30. ☐ ☐ **IF APPROPRIATE, DESCRIBE BED/CRIB/BASSINET/COUCH/FLOOR/WATER MATTRESS/BEAN BAG OR OTHER SLEEPING ARRANGEMENT INCLUDING ALL SHEETS, PILLOWS, PLASTIC COVERS, BLANKETS, DEFECTS OF MISCELLANEOUS OBJECTS IN OR NEAR BEDDING WHERE DECEDENT WAS FOUND. NOTE: IF A CRIB, DESCRIBE ANY DEFECTS, DAMAGE AND/OR INAPPROPRIATE MATTRESS SIZE.**

31. ☐ ☐ **WAS ANYTHING SEIZED? DESCRIBE:** _____ | **BY WHOM (NAME & TITLE)?** | **PRESENT LOCATION OF ITEM(S):**
☐ NO ☐ YES ☐ UNKNOWN

32. ☐ ☐ **IF SLEEPING, WAS THE DECEDENT SLEEPING ALONE?**
☐ NO ☐ YES ☐ UNKNOWN
IF NO, WHO WAS DECEDENT SLEEPING WITH? (NAME(S), RELATIONSHIP(S), AND AGE(S) NEEDED.)

33. ☐ ☐	ANY POSSIBILITY OF OVERLAYING? ☐ NO ☐ YES ☐ UNKNOWN IF YES, REPORTED RECENT ALCOHOL CONSUMPTION OR DRUG/MEDICINE USAGE BY PERSON SLEEPING WITH CHILD? ☐ NO ☐ YES ☐ UNKNOWN
34. ☐ ☐	IN GENERAL, DO LIVING CONDITIONS APPEAR OVERCROWDED? ☐ NO ☐ YES ☐ UNKNOWN EXPLAIN:
35. ☐ ☐	IF ANY INJURY IS NOTED, HOW IS IT ALLEGED TO HAVE OCCURRED?
36. ☐ ☐	FULLY DESCRIBE ANY INDICATIONS OF TRAUMA OR INJURY INCLUDING BRUISES, SCRAPES, CUTS, RASHES, BURN MARKS, SWELLING, ETC. INCLUDE COLORS, SHAPES, SIZES AND LOCATIONS ON BODY. (IF NOT AT SCENE, INDICATE LOCATION WHERE BODY VIEWED?)

37. ☐ ☐	IF INJURY WAS INFLICTED, APPARENT OBJECT OR WEAPON USED?	WHO INFLICTED INJURY (NAME & RELATIONSHIP)?
	WAS OBJECT SEIZED? ☐ NO ☐ YES ☐ UNKNOWN	SEIZED BY WHOM (NAME & TITLE)?
	PRESENT LOCATION OF OBJECT/WEAPON:	

38. ☐ ☐	IF INJURY RESULTED FROM A FALL, DESCRIBE WHAT DECEDENT FELL FROM, THE DISTANCE OF THE FALL AND SURFACE DECEDENT FELL ON (CARPET, CONCRETE, GROUND, ETC.). USE NARRATIVE SECTION, IF NECESSARY.
39. ☐ ☐	IF INJURY RESULTED FROM A BURN, DESCRIBE APPARENT CAUSE (HOT WATER, CIGARETTE, CHEMICAL, ETC.):
40. ☐ ☐	HAS DECEDENT HAD OTHER SERIOUS INJURIES DURING THE LAST YEAR? ☐ NO ☐ YES ☐ UNKNOWN EXPLAIN:
41. ☐ ☐	HAS DECEDENT HAD A RECENT ILLNESS? ☐ NO ☐ YES ☐ UNKNOWN EXPLAIN:

42. ☐ ☐	Has decedent been exposed to any contagious disease recently? ☐ NO ☐ YES ☐ UNKNOWN If yes, explain: _____ Symptoms Noted: ☐ Appetite change ☐ Wheezes ☐ Fussy ☐ Sniffles ☐ Cough ☐ Diarrhea ☐ Cold ☐ Irritability ☐ Runny nose ☐ Congestion ☐ Other: _____ ☐ None noted ☐ Fever ☐ How high? _____

43. ☐ ☐	WAS DECEDENT TAKEN FOR TREATMENT FOR PREVIOUS SYMPTOMS? ☐ NO ☐ YES ☐ UNKNOWN WHERE WAS TREATMENT RECEIVED (NAME OF FACILITY)? WHO PROVIDED TREATMENT (NAME & TITLE)? IF YES, WHAT DIAGNOSIS WAS RENDERED?

44. ☐ ☐	HAS DECEDENT BEEN ON MEDICATION? IF YES, NAME OF MEDICATION: ☐ NO ☐ YES ☐ UNKNOWN HAS DECEDENT RECEIVED RECENT IMMUNIZATION? IF YES, WHAT TYPE? ☐ NO ☐ YES ☐ UNKNOWN IF YES, NAME OF MEDICAL PRACTITIONER/CLINIC:

45. ☐ ☐	ANY KNOWN ALLERGIES OR PREVIOUS REACTIONS TO SHOTS OR MEDICATIONS? ☐ NO ☐ YES ☐ UNKNOWN IF YES, EXPLAIN:

46. ☐ ☐	WHEN HAD DECEDENT LAST EATEN? DATE (MM/DD/YY): TIME: WHAT WAS EATEN OR INGESTED? QUANTITY EATEN? ANY FEEDING/EATING DIFFICULTIES (PAST OR RECENT)? Describe:

47. ☐ ☐	ANY KNOWN FOOD INTOLERANCE? ☐ NO ☐ YES ☐ UNKNOWN IF YES, WHAT FOODS?

48. ☐ ☐	IF INFANT, WAS DECEDENT BREAST FED? FORMULA FED? IF YES: ☐ NO ☐ YES ☐ UNKNOWN ☐ NO ☐ YES ☐ UNKNOWN FORMULA BRAND: ____

49. ☐ ☐	HAD DECEDENT RECEIVED ANY OF THE FOLLOWING WITHIN THE LAST 48 HOURS? ☐ COW'S MILK ☐ GOAT'S MILK ☐ HONEY ☐ WATERED DOWN FORMULA ☐ UNKNOWN OTHER: _____

50. ☐ ☐	HAS DECEDENT BEEN UNDER ROUTINE CARE OF A MEDICAL PRACTITIONER? ☐ NO ☐ YES ☐ UNKNOWN IF YES, PRACTITIONER'S NAME/CLINIC: DESCRIBE CHILD'S GENERAL TEMPERAMENT (e.g., COLICKY, FUSSY, HYPERACTIVE, QUIET, ETC.):

51. ☐ ☐	NAME, AGE, AND ANY KNOWN SERIOUS MEDICAL CONDITIONS OF NATURAL PARENTS: MOTHER (INCLUDE MAIDEN NAME): FATHER:

MO 886-3228N (6-00) PAGE 5

52. ☐ ☐	WHO DOES DECEDENT LIVE WITH IF DIFFERENT FROM PARENT(S) (NAME, ADDRESS & RELATIONSHIP)?
53. ☐ ☐	NAME, AGE, DOB AND ANY KNOWN SERIOUS HEALTH CONDITIONS OF SIBLINGS?
54. ☐ ☐	WHO ARE THE DECEDENT'S REGULAR PLAYMATES (NAMES & ADDRESSES)?
55. ☐ ☐	IF PARENT(S) EMPLOYED, WHO ROUTINELY PROVIDED CHILD CARE FOR THE DECEDENT (NAME/ADDRESS/RELATIONSHIP)? WAS SIBLING RESPONSIBLE FOR CARING FOR THE DECEDENT AT TIME OF DEATH? IF YES, WHICH SIBLING(S)? ☐ NO ☐ YES ☐ UNKNOWN
56. ☐ ☐	KNOWN MATERNAL PRE-NATAL HEALTH PROBLEMS (DIABETES, HYPERTENSION, ETC)? ☐ NO ☐ YES ☐ UNKNOWN IF YES, DESCRIBE: WAS MOTHER TAKING PRESCRIPTION MEDICATION FOR ABOVE MEDICAL CONDITION DURING PREGNANCY? ☐ NO ☐ YES ☐ UNKNOWN IF YES, WHAT TYPE MEDICATION?
57. ☐ ☐	PRE-NATAL MATERNAL CIGARETTE, ALCOHOL OR DRUG USAGE? ☐ NO ☐ YES ☐ UNKNOWN IF YES: ☐ HEROIN ☐ MARIJUANA ☐ METHAMPHETAMINE ☐ ALCOHOL ☐ CIGARETTES ☐ COCAINE OTHER: _____
58. ☐ ☐	KNOWN COMPLICATIONS OF PREGNANCY OR DELIVERY? ☐ NO ☐ YES ☐ UNKNOWN IF YES, EXPLAIN: LOCATION OF BIRTH AND NAME OF ATTENDING MEDICAL PRACTITIONER:
59. ☐ ☐	BIRTH DEFECTS OR OTHER ABNORMALITIES OF DECEDENT AT BIRTH; DESCRIBE:
60. ☐ ☐	ANY FAMILY HISTORY OF SIDS OR OTHER INFANT DEATH? ☐ NO ☐ YES ☐ UNKNOWN IF YES, DESCRIBE DETAILS INCLUDING DATE OF DEATH & LOCATION OF OCCURRENCE: FAMILY MEMBER OR OTHER CARE GIVER WITH KNOWN HISTORY OF AIDS? ☐ NO ☐ YES ☐ UNKNOWN IF YES, PROVIDE NAME AND RELATIONSHIP:

MO 886-3228N (6-00)

NARRATIVE

61. ☐ ☐ PROVIDE ADDITIONAL COMMENTS (TO INCLUDE NAME(S) AND PEDIGREE(S) OF ALL PERSONS AND RESPONDERS AT SCENE), CONTINUED ANSWERS TO QUESTIONS (INCLUDE QUESTION NUMBER BEING RESPONDED TO) OR ANY OTHER INFORMATION PERTINENT TO THE DEATH SCENE INVESTIGATION. USE ADDITIONAL PAGES AS NEEDED.

SIGNATURE OF INVESTIGATOR:	PHONE NUMBER	DATE (MM/DD/YY):
▶		

MO 886-3228N (6-00)

Chapter 14

LEGAL ISSUES

DAVID KATNER, J.D.
HENRY J. PLUM, J.D.*

The identification and investigation of alleged child abuse and neglect for purposes of medical treatment, social service intervention, or criminal prosecution are likely to involve some aspect of the legal system. First, various state statutory provisions give definitions of "child abuse" and "child neglect," although they may differ both from state to state and within a given state, depending on the objective in making the identification. The three general objectives are: reporting to child protection agencies, establishing a standard for juvenile court intervention, or defining behavior deemed unlawful and meriting punishment through the criminal justice system. Second, state laws and regulations, as well as other legal rules, prescribe how child abuse and neglect cases are handled. They address both the method of reporting the incident to the appropriate state agency and how that agency is to respond to the report. Third, the legal system not only controls what may transpire in a juvenile, criminal, or divorce court setting, but also dictates some of what should occur in medical facilities.

*Original chapter authors: Jesse A. Goldner, M.A., J.D.; Cassandra K. Dolgin, B.A., J.D.; and Sandra H. Manske, R.N., M.A., J.D.

♦ AN HISTORICAL PERSPECTIVE

The United States initially adopted the legal view that children were the property of their parents from English common law. Under common law, children under age 7 years were considered incapable of possessing criminal intent, but children older than that age were subject to arrest, trial, and (in theory) punishment similar to that for adult offenders. Although the law did recognize the parental obligation to maintain, educate, and protect one's own child, the widely accepted maxims "a man's home is his castle" and "spare the rod and spoil the child" reflected the reality that parental duties were relatively free from legal restrictions. Consequently, only cases of severe child abuse, involving cruel and merciless punishment or permanent physical injury, resulted in intervention and criminal prosecution.

During the Industrial Revolution, there was a greater willingness to recognize the need for child protection. Legislation limited child labor and provided for other forms of child protection. In the early nineteenth century, state statutes were adopted that authorized the removal of children from neglectful environments. Although the first reported criminal cases involving child abuse in the United States date back to the 1600s, the first documented civil cases involving child protection did not appear until 1874 (Trost, 1998). Not until 1874, with the founding of the Society for the Prevention of Cruelty to Children, an outgrowth of the Society for the Prevention of Cruelty to Animals, was there a significant push for legislative reform in child maltreatment.

State juvenile court systems, modeled after the Illinois Juvenile Court Act of 1899, emerged in the early 1900s. The development of these courts represented a direct exercise of the state's parens patriae authority, which justifies state intervention, over parental objection, in order to protect children. The exercise of such state power over a child is generally controlled by three principles:

1. It is presumed that children lack the mental competence and maturity possessed by adults.

2. Before intervening, the state must show that the child's parents or guardians are unfit, unable, or unwilling to care for the child.

3. The state may exercise the parens patriae power solely to further the best interests of the child.

The development of juvenile courts corresponded with the movement toward professionalism in social work and increased social services directed at child protection. However, with the decision and influence of the In re Gault case (387 U.S. 1, 1967), the three principles have given way to a more due process model in dealing with children coming into the legal system. Today the juvenile court exercises jurisdiction over minors brought within the system due to alleged abuse, neglect, abandonment, incorrigibility, and delinquency. However, recent legislative changes have resulted in an increase in removing juveniles from the juvenile justice system and sending them into adult criminal courts for prosecution as though they were adults. We have come full circle with respect to the treatment of juvenile offenders; that is, we have returned to treating many juveniles as adults, at least with respect to criminal misconduct or delinquent behavior.

These courts, as opposed to those which are part of the criminal justice system, afford the judge broad discretion in addressing the problems encountered by invoking state coercion to achieve the social welfare system's goal of rehabilitation and treatment of abusive and neglectful parents and other caretakers. The court's determination that a child needs supervision or assistance may result in court-ordered family services, placement of the child in foster care or a state youth facility, or, in extraordinary circumstances, termination of parental rights.

Differentiating between physical abuse and symptoms or injuries resulting from disease processes or accidents often proved to be a difficult task. The work of two physicians provided guidance. Radiologist Dr. John Caffey, in the early and mid-twentieth century, related previously unexplained x-ray findings to trauma that may have resulted from parental action (Caffey, 1946). In the 1950s and early 1960s, Dr. C. Henry Kempe and his colleagues at the University of Colorado Medical School defined the "battered child syndrome" as an observable clinical condition that could be diagnosed according to medical principles (Kempe, Silverman, Steele, Droegemueller, & Silver, 1962). Together, these discoveries had legal as well as medical significance.

Medical identification of certain nonaccidental physical injuries contributed to increased criminal prosecutions and to legislative efforts to require reporting of suspected cases of child abuse. In 1963, the Children's Bureau of the United States Department of Health, Education and Welfare (now Health and Human Services) developed a model child abuse reporting statute. By 1967 each state had enacted such a law. The aim of these first reporting statutes was simply to identify suspected child abuse, and only physicians were designated as mandated reporters. As knowledge regarding child abuse increased, however, states refined these laws, expanding their purpose beyond mere identification to investigation and intervention, and broadening the group of mandated reporters.

Recently, the rehabilitative approach to dealing with child abuse and neglect cases, which has been favored in the treatment of physical and sexual abuse, has been subject to extensive attack. Some critics have cited frustrations with the courts' ability to effectively intervene in many cases where such intervention seems necessary. Other critics point to the inability of professionals working in the area of mental health and child protection to change deviant behavior, particularly in a cost-effective way.

Consequently, attention is shifting in two other directions: First, over the last decade, in an effort to increase the success of reliance on the judicial system to aid in the handling of these cases, many jurisdictions have passed statutes or issued judicial rulings designed to make testimony by a child easier and less traumatic in some or all of the proceedings involving child abuse. These generally involve efforts to minimize the need for the child to be in the presence of the alleged abuser, while at the same time protecting the rights of defendants and others involved in these cases. Options include the use of closed circuit cameras, videotaped testimony and courtroom screens, and the increased admissibility of hearsay evidence. Some limitations on the use of such techniques are reviewed later. Second, increased efforts are being made to focus on prevention as perhaps the most cost-effective way of dealing with child abuse and neglect in the long run.

Generally, it is the state that responds to child maltreatment, but during the past quarter century federal legislation has greatly influenced the states' legal response to child maltreatment. Beginning in 1974, the National Center on Child Abuse and Neglect was established by Congressional mandate (Child Abuse Prevention and Treatment Act, 1974). The law imposed various requirements on the states as a condition for receiving federal funds for "developing, strengthening, and carrying out child abuse and neglect prevention and treatment programs." Presently, eligibility for funding under the legislation requires the establishment of the following: state reporting laws, statutory immunity provisions for those who report suspected cases of abuse and neglect under state law, a state agency responsible for carrying out investigatory and treatment procedures, a state-wide central child abuse registry, provisions for confidentiality of registry records, and the appointment of a guardian ad litem for the child in cases involving judicial proceedings.

In 1980, additional federal legislation was passed (Adoption Assistance and Child Welfare Act, 1980) that requires states to make reasonable efforts to avoid removing maltreated children from parental custody and mandates court or administrative review of state-supervised foster care placement at least every 6 months. This review determines the continuing necessity for and appropriateness of the placement, the compliance with an established case plan, and the extent of progress made toward alleviating or mitigating the cause of the placement. The review must also include a projected date for the child's return home or, when return to the biological parents' home is unlikely, recommend placement for adoption or legal guardianship. The need for permanence was re-emphasized with the passage of additional legislation (Adoption and Safe Families Act, 1997). This expanded the principles of permanency planning initiated in the earlier legislation by requiring that, when a child is placed out of the parental home for a total of 15 months, the agency is mandated to initiate steps to make a permanent placement. In addition, the enactment of federal statutes concerning Native Americans requires state agencies to make "active efforts" to provide services "designed to prevent the breakup of the Indian family" (Indian Child Welfare Act, 1977).

Finally, federal legislation has enhanced intervention in child sexual abuse cases. Recent statutory measures impose criminal sanctions on any person who uses, or assists another in using, a minor to engage in sexually explicit behavior for the purpose of producing physical depictions of this behavior with the intent to distribute the material in interstate commerce (Federal Protection of Children Against Sexual Exploitation Act, 1977).

◆ REPORTING STATUTES AND CHILD PROTECTIVE SERVICES

The identification of abuse and neglect, the assessment of family social service needs, and the implementation of treatment programs and other intervention strategies for abused children and their families are carried out predominantly by state and county child protective service (CPS) agencies. Authorization for such action is typically found in state laws that establish and provide funding for these agencies and define the criteria for and mode of intervention. The primary purposes of CPS agencies are "(1) to protect and insure the safety of children who have been or are at risk of maltreatment, and (2) to provide services to alter the conditions which create risk of maltreatment in the future."

A report to the state's child abuse and neglect hotline, made either by a professional involved with the child or by a neighbor or other non-mandated reporter, generally results in a referral to a CPS agency. Often such a referral results from a report to the local police. Occasionally the report is initiated by one parent with respect to the other in the context of a child custody dispute.

Child abuse and neglect reporting laws dictate how referrals are made to the CPS agency and also how the agency is to respond. Additionally, the statutes mandate other duties and rights of healthcare personnel and other reporters. These laws govern the central registries that maintain information regarding cases that have previously been investigated by the CPS agency. Finally, the laws often define the relationship between the CPS agency, the juvenile court, and various law enforcement agencies.

REPORTING STATUTES

Each state, as well as the District of Columbia, Puerto Rico, and the United States Virgin Islands, Guam, American Samoa, and the Virgin Islands, has enacted its own child abuse and neglect reporting legislation. As a result, there is a lack of uniformity in statutory language and in the effect of the various laws. In particular, the statutes vary as to the precise definition of child abuse and the standards and procedures used for reporting suspected cases. All of the statutes, however, share a common purpose and tend to follow a similar format based on the federally mandated requirements.

The purpose of every child abuse and neglect reporting statute is to protect the child from additional injury. Accordingly, statutes are written to encourage and facilitate reporting suspected abuse or neglect. They are designed to promote early identification of the child in peril so that adequate investigation, intervention, and treatment of the child, as well as of the family, when appropriate, can begin.

Every state reporting statute contains essentially the same elements, including the following:

1. What must be reported (reportable conditions/definition of child abuse)

2. Who must or may report

3. When a report must be made (including the degree of certainty a reporter must have)

4. Reporting procedures

5. The existence and operation of a central registry

6. Rules regarding protective custody

7. Immunity for good faith reporters

8. The abrogation of certain privileged communication rights which might otherwise apply

9. Sanctions for failure to report

10. Confidentiality requirements concerning the use and accessibility of such reports.

In addition, many child abuse reporting statutes provide for the taking of photographs or x-rays of the child when physical abuse is suspected, even in the absence of parental consent.

WHAT MUST BE REPORTED

Every state reporting statute requires that mandated reporters report suspected child abuse and neglect. Each state, however, defines child abuse and neglect differently; therefore, reportable conditions vary among the states. In general, reportable conditions include nonaccidental physical injury, neglect, sexual abuse, and emotional abuse.

WHO MUST REPORT

Each state reporting statute designates who is required to report suspected child abuse and neglect. Typically, these individuals include physicians, healthcare professionals, educators, social work professionals, and law enforcement personnel. Many states, however, have an even broader base of mandated reporters, including such professionals as coroners, dentists, probation officers, child care workers, and other persons responsible for the care of children, as well as lawyers (Beyea, 1999). The legislative trend has been to create a more expansive list of mandated reporters; over 20 states require "any person" to report. In addition, the majority of state reporting statutes also provide for permissive reporting by nonmandated reporters. In 1996, child protective agencies in the 50 states and the District of Columbia investigated more than two million reports alleging the abuse of more than three million children. According to the National Child Abuse and Neglect Data System (NCANDS) 1996 data collection, there was an 18% increase in the number of cases of child abuse between 1990 and 1996 (Beyea, 1999).

WHEN A REPORT MUST BE MADE

Child abuse reporting statutes dictate when a report must be made. Most statutes require reporters to make an immediate oral report by telephone, followed shortly thereafter by a written report to the appropriate state agency. This procedure facilitates an immediate investigatory response by the CPS agency, ensuring that the child is protected. It also establishes a permanent record of the alleged incident.

The degree of suspicion a reporter must reach before making a report is set out in the reporting statute and likewise varies from state to state. The original child abuse reporting statutes provided for a report to be made when there was "reason to believe" that a child had been abused. Many states have expanded the requirement and now use language such as "cause to believe" or "reasonable cause to suspect" that a "child has been or may be subjected to abuse or neglect or observes a child being subjected to conditions or circumstances which would reasonably result in abuse or neglect." Practically, "cause to believe" and "reasonable cause to suspect" mean essentially the same thing for reporting purposes. As noted later, however, there may be a distinction in cases where civil liability for failure to report is at issue.

REPORTING PROCEDURES

Each state statute designates at least one agency to receive reports of suspected child abuse and neglect. Traditionally, four different agencies have served as potential recipients for child abuse reports: social service agencies, police departments, health departments, and juvenile courts.

Most states have specified the department of social services, or a division within that department, as the appropriate agency to ultimately receive these reports. Some states designate only the department of social services, while other states designate two or more agencies, such as the police and the department of social services, to receive reports. These states generally require that all reports ultimately flow into the department of social services. A few states, however, permit reporting to two or more agencies without requiring the coordination of information by any agency.

In many states the reporting statute specifies what information is to be included in the report. In other states the receiving agency determines, on a case-by-case basis, what information is required. Required information typically includes name, age, address, present location of the child, type and extent of the injuries, name and address of the parent(s) or caretaker(s) if known, and any other information that the reporter believes might be relevant. Most states require a mandated reporter to divulge his or her name and position.

Reporting statutes generally prescribe the time within which the CPS agency must initiate its investigation. In most instances this is within 24 hours of the receipt of a report.

CENTRAL REGISTRIES

Reports received by a state's child abuse hotline are recorded in a central registry. Central registry records usually contain additional case information such as prior reports of child abuse and neglect and CPS case outcomes, treatment plans, and final dispositions at the CPS level. Nearly every state has established a central registry of child protection cases.

State law generally deems central registry records confidential and regulates their disclosure because they contain highly private data about individuals and families. Three general statutory approaches govern record accessibility: (1) Only individuals within a CPS agency may have access; (2) the CPS agency may issue regulations authorizing access by certain persons outside of the agency; or (3) state law may enumerate precisely which persons may have access. This third approach is most prevalent today. Those typically having access are law enforcement personnel investigating a report of child maltreatment, the treating physician, the CPS agency, the court, and persons conducting bona fide research. In addition, the child's attorney or guardian ad litem generally is permitted to review registry records in instances when the CPS agency or law enforcement personnel refer the case to juvenile court and court involvement ensues. Registry information often is available for purposes of screening applicants for licenses to establish child care facilities, agencies, or services, or applicants for employment or volunteer work with such operations or with schools. Almost all states provide that prohibited disclosure is punishable as a misdemeanor.

PROTECTIVE CUSTODY

Nearly every state authorizes certain categories of individuals to take a child into protective custody if the individual concludes that the child would be seriously endangered if he or she remained with or was released to the parent or other caretaker. The child abuse reporting statutes designate who may take the child into custody, when, and under what circumstances. Depending on the particular statute, such individuals may include one or more of the following: police officers, physicians, juvenile court or probation officers, and CPS professionals.

Some states require a court order, at least over the telephone if not in writing, before taking the child into custody against the parent's wishes. Other states directly authorize protective custody, provided that written notice or another document is filed with the juvenile court within 24 to 48 hours after the action is taken. In either case, a custody hearing will typically be held at the juvenile court within a short period of time thereafter to review the initial decision to hold the child. Some states provide for protective custody when an authorized individual deems that there "is an imminent danger to the child's life or health." Other states allow protective custody when returning the child to his parent "would endanger his health or welfare." In addition to this review, the agency or prosecuting attorney seeking a protective or removal order must also file a petition with the juvenile court asserting facts that allege the child to be "dependent, neglected, or a child in need of protection or services." The particular "status" or category is defined within each state's juvenile or children's code.

IMMUNITY FOR GOOD FAITH REPORTERS

Individuals may be reluctant to report suspected child abuse. Potential reporters may fear that the suspected perpetrator will bring a lawsuit against them if the abuse is unconfirmed. To encourage reporting and alleviate this fear, every state's reporting statute extends some type of immunity from civil and criminal liability to persons making reports. Although such immunity provisions may not completely insulate the reporter from a lawsuit (that is, they cannot prevent the filing of an action against a reporter), they can make the successful litigation of such suits nearly impossible.

Some jurisdictions grant absolute immunity to mandated reporters. This means that the mandated reporter is protected even if the report was false and the reporter knew it to be false. Most jurisdictions, however, provide immunity only to an individual making a good faith report. In these states, a reporter is liable only when the plaintiff can prove that the reporter made a false report and that the reporter knew that the report was false, or otherwise acted in bad faith or with a malicious purpose.

ABROGATION OF PRIVILEGED COMMUNICATIONS

Certain professionals owe their patients or clients a duty of confidentiality. This duty is incurred by virtue of the ethical obligations which the individual undertakes on becoming a professional and adopting the standards of that profession. Any breach of this obligation would ordinarily lead to a malpractice suit against the professional in which money might be awarded to the patient or client as compensation for damages sustained as a result of the breach of confidentiality. If the disclosure is mandated by a state statute, as in the instance of child abuse, however, no liability will result. Moreover, as discussed later, in such instances, the failure to make the disclosure, even in the face of an otherwise existing obligation of confidentiality, may, in fact, result in civil or criminal liability.

In addition to this obligation of confidentiality, certain professional communications are protected by a judicially or legislatively created testimonial privilege. Generally, a privilege operates to exclude information obtained in the course of a particular relationship from being presented as evidence at judicial proceedings.

The most common types of privileged communications are those between doctor-patient, husband-wife, attorney-client, social worker-client, and clergy-penitent. States differ, however, as to which communications are protected by testimonial privilege. Most states abrogate all types of privileged communications in a child abuse case, except attorney-client. Many states also refuse to intrude on the clergy-penitent relationship. Legislative changes that include attorneys as mandated reporters may challenge these exceptions. Additionally, the United States Supreme Court has recognized a psychotherapist-patient evidentiary privilege in cases litigated in federal courts. This privilege was established in *Jaffee v. Redmond*, 518 U.S. 1, 116 S.Ct. 1923 (1996).

Mandatory reporters must report suspected abuse or neglect, regardless of whether the abuse or neglect became apparent as a result of a confidential communication with the patient or client. Also, the professional must testify in juvenile court child protection cases when subpoenaed. In many jurisdictions, this requirement to testify may also exist in criminal cases and in child custody cases in which allegations of child abuse are involved. Failure to testify when a judge orders that the testimony be given is likely to result in holding the witness in contempt and jailing the witness. In some states, however, if a claim of privilege is appropriately made, the testimony may be limited to information required to be reported under the reporting statute rather than to more extensive information of which the witness may have become aware.

CRIMINAL SANCTIONS FOR FAILURE TO REPORT

Most states have provisions in their reporting statutes that make it a crime for a mandated reporter to knowingly fail to report suspected child abuse. Almost all of these statutes classify the offense as a misdemeanor and specify a maximum fine and/or jail sentence. Although criminal prosecutions for failure to report are rare, courts have ruled that physicians, including psychiatrists, may be subject to criminal penalty under the child abuse statute for failure to report suspected child abuse. The inclusion of a penalty provision serves a useful function for some reluctant professionals. They may find it more palatable to report suspected child abuse if they can explain to the child's family or caretaker that it is a crime for them not to make the report.

SOCIAL SERVICE AND LAW ENFORCEMENT RESPONSE

A report of suspected child abuse or neglect to a state-wide telephone hotline or to a local office in accordance with the state's child abuse reporting statute usually initiates the CPS process. At this early stage of the process, child abuse and neglect are often broadly defined. Individual local CPS offices and workers exercise wide discretion in how the agency will respond to individual reports of child maltreatment.

VALIDATION OF REPORTS

As noted in the preceding discussion of reporting procedures, each state has enacted legislation prescribing criteria for case follow-up, which generally requires an investigation within a limited period of time. The primary aim of the investigation is to determine the validity of the report. If the case is "substantiated," "founded," or "indicated," a decision must be made regarding how to proceed.

If the child is not in the protective custody of a physician, the police, or the juvenile court at the time of the investigation, the CPS investigator must determine if the child is safe or if there is imminent risk of harm to the child that would warrant the child's immediate removal from the home. If such action is needed, the police or the juvenile court may be contacted to facilitate this removal.

If the available evidence is insufficient to merit a finding of abuse or neglect, or if the investigation could not be completed, the case may be deemed "unsubstantiated" or "unfounded." The case may then be closed and all references to the report and case deleted from the central registry within a designated period of time, if no additional reports are made.

Central registries involve state collection of potentially inflammatory personal information. This gives rise to constitutional concerns regarding the rights to privacy and due process. Accordingly, many states have enacted procedures, by statute or state regulation, for the expungement of registry records. Expungement of records is based on the child's attainment of a certain age, or passage of a designated period of time since services were terminated, or on a finding by the CPS agency that the report was unsubstantiated. In some states, individuals may formally challenge information contained in the registry through administrative or court procedures for the expungement or modification of records.

INVESTIGATIVE PURPOSES AND PROCEDURES

Reporting statutes often detail the purpose of the investigation. Generally the goal is to evaluate the nature, extent, and cause of the abuse or neglect and to identify the person responsible. Efforts are also made to ascertain the names and conditions of other children in the home, the nature of the home environment, and the relationship of the subject child to the parents or other caretakers.

The investigative caseworker typically begins the process by contacting the individual who made the hotline report to confirm the information originally provided and to obtain additional information. The investigation consists of a series of interviews. Often the child is the next person interviewed. Preferably, this takes place in a neutral setting. The parents are also interviewed, often during a home visit. Thereafter, other persons named in the report who may have relevant information are questioned. These persons typically include teachers, physicians, neighbors, and other relatives.

The CPS purpose when responding to a report of child maltreatment is distinct from the objectives of the criminal justice system. Yet, as noted, law enforcement personnel may be contacted by the CPS worker during the investigative stage, or they may already be otherwise involved. This is true in cases involving serious abuse, where there is a reason to believe that the parents are or may likely be resistant to CPS intervention, or if the CPS caseworker is concerned for his or her own safety.

State law provides the authority for CPS home visits, either expressly or implicitly. If individuals refuse to cooperate, a warrant or court order may be needed to gain access to a home. In addition, many states' statutes, regulations, or case laws authorize CPS or law enforcement investigators to conduct examinations of the child without parental permission or to refer the child for evaluation by medical personnel.

CONSTITUTIONAL CONCERNS

Constitutional considerations are raised in the CPS investigative stage because the Constitution protects individuals against state action. CPS caseworkers act under "color of state law": that is, they carry out their investigative tasks pursuant to legislative authority. Protection under both federal and state constitutions may be implied in such areas as home visits, child and parent interviews, and examinations of the child.

Search warrants are generally not required to conduct such visits or examinations. The burden of obtaining a warrant would seriously impair the state's effort to protect the child, particularly in emergency situations. However, there may be constitutional limits on the nature and circumstances under which investigative visits take place. Usually the parent or guardian consents to the caseworker's or police officer's entry into the residence. Absent consent, or if the search exceeds the scope of the consent, any evidence that is found may be deemed inadmissible in any subsequent criminal proceeding. Similarly, statements made to investigators by a parent or other perpetrator may be inadmissible if a court finds that, at the time of the questioning, the individual was in custody or otherwise deprived of his freedom in some significant way. Nevertheless, it is important to note that juvenile court hearings are civil in nature rather than criminal, and the rules regarding the admissibility of evidence may be different.

Treatment and Referral Options

Following a determination of the validity of the allegation of abuse or neglect, a report is made to the agency's central registry. If the hotline referral is substantiated, a CPS caseworker, who may or may not have been involved in the initial investigation of the report, is usually assigned to the case. The caseworker develops a treatment plan and presents it to the family. CPS agencies offer various mental health and social services and seek voluntary acceptance of these recommended services. If the parent or guardian does not cooperate with the CPS agency, or if such voluntary treatment will not adequately protect the child, the investigative or treatment caseworker will request that a county juvenile prosecutor or agency attorney file an abuse or neglect petition with the juvenile or family court. Such an action will seek court intervention with the child and his or her family. Intervention may include temporary removal of the child from the home, court-ordered treatment, or, in some circumstances, termination of parental rights.

When the police have not been involved in the investigation, referral to a local law enforcement agency upon completion of the CPS investigation may be mandated under state law when the abuse is "substantiated" or meets the statutory requirements for criminal child or sexual abuse. In the absence of legislative direction, CPS regulations may require referral to prosecuting authorities or the police.

Civil Liability and Child Maltreatment

Health care professionals and others engaged in protective services may be exposed to civil liability during the identification and investigation of alleged child abuse.

Failure to Report by Mandatory Reporter

Violation of a statutory duty, such as the duty imposed on a mandated reporter to report suspected child abuse or neglect, is negligence per se (negligence in itself). Under this theory, an injured child and his family could successfully sue a doctor or another mandated reporter for willingly or negligently failing to detect and report known or suspected child abuse. The suit could result in a judgment awarding monetary damages to compensate the patient for all injuries that occurred as a result of abuse or neglect after the time when a report should have been made.

OTHER BASES OF LIABILITY OF REPORTERS AND POTENTIAL DEFENSES

In rare instances, civil actions may also be brought against healthcare professionals or others based on their conduct in connection with a child abuse or neglect case. Typically these lawsuits allege that the physician, social worker, or police officer and their respective agencies negligently acted under the reporting statute, thereby causing harm to the parent or the child. A parent or child may bring an action seeking monetary damages for a wrongful report of child abuse, defamation and slander, negligent diagnosis or treatment, breach of confidentiality, overly intrusive investigation, wrongful removal of a child from his or her home, wrongful institution or prosecution of an alleged offender, and wrongful examination of the child for signs of abuse. Willful conduct may also be alleged, including battery, false imprisonment, and/or malicious prosecution.

These claims are usually based on state tort (private or civil wrong or injury) law, which, through statute or common law (judicial precedent), recognizes that individuals in certain situations owe duties to one another. Violation of these duties can form the basis of an action for monetary damages. Similarly, an alleged violation of constitutional rights, either federal or state, may form the basis of a claim for damages.

As previously noted, all jurisdictions provide absolute or limited immunity for the reporting of suspected child abuse. The same immunity provisions typically apply to other authorized actions taken by any individual in connection with the making of the report. Such actions include, for example, the taking of photographs and x-rays, the removal or retaining of the child, the disclosure of otherwise confidential or privileged information to CPS investigators, and the participation in any judicial proceedings that result from the reporting. Immunity provisions may preclude liability, but they cannot prevent the initiation of a civil action.

Initially, the court assumes that the plaintiff's allegations in the petition or complaint regarding the defendant's actions are true, without hearing any testimony. The court then determines if the immunity granted by the child abuse reporting statute was applicable. In jurisdictions that have adopted a rule of "absolute" immunity for statutorily prescribed activities of the defendants, the judge will dismiss the proceeding. If, however, the jurisdiction has adopted a rule of "qualified" immunity (that is, immunity only for actions undertaken in "good faith"), the court will allow the case to go to trial. The jury or the judge acting as the finder of fact will then hear testimony on behalf of each party from various witnesses regarding the allegations of the petition. If the alleged actions are proved to be true, but the trier of fact concludes that they were taken in good faith, the proceeding will be dismissed. Liability attaches only if the facts adduced at the trial prove both that the defendants engaged in the alleged behavior and that the defendants did not act in good faith.

ADDITIONAL CAUSES OF ACTION BASED ON FAILURES TO PROTECT THE CHILD AND RELATED DEFENSES

In situations involving state-employed child protection workers resulting in the death or additional serious injury to the child, the child and an innocent parent or guardian may bring an action alleging that the public employees should have taken various steps to protect the child. The lawsuits may allege a failure to accept reports for investigation, a failure to adequately investigate reports, a failure to remove the child from the home, a failure to protect the child following return to the home or to foster care or to a child care facility, or a failure to provide services leading to the return of the child. These actions are also typically brought under state tort law.

Similar suits for damages have been brought charging violations of the federal Constitution. The typical allegation is that the officials' failure to act deprived them of their liberty in violation of the Due Process Clause of the Fourteenth Amendment to the United States Constitution. Specifically, the plaintiffs assert that substantive due process requires state agents to protect children referred as abused to child protection agencies. Nevertheless, in 1989, the United States Supreme Court limited the type of suit that could be brought in some of these cases (*DeShaney v. Winnebago County Department of Social Services*, 1989). The Court concluded that a state's failure to protect a child not in the actual custody of the state against violence generally will not constitute a violation of the Due Process Clause because the clause imposes no duty on the states to provide members of the general public with adequate protective services. While the clause forbids the state from depriving individuals of life, liberty, and property without due process of law, it only limits the state's power to act and does not impose an affirmative obligation to ensure any minimal level of safety and security. Thus the constitutional issue is not whether the CPS agency or another public actor was aware of the danger to the child, but rather whether it limited or prevented the child from acting on his or her own behalf. Liability still could be found, however, under state rather than federal law in instances of negligent conduct or of a child within the custody of a state agency.

In addition to any immunity provided under the reporting statute, civil liability may also be precluded by the "public duty" doctrine or rule. This rule generally applies only to health care professionals or other child care workers who are state employees. The rule provides that a public official is generally not liable to individuals for his or her negligence in discharging public duties. The rationale behind the rule is that the duty is owed to the public at large, rather than to any one individual.

Liability will attach, however, where the duty is specifically owed an individual under state tort law. A special relationship between an individual and a public official or agency may be sufficient to give rise to liability for negligence in carrying out that duty. State reporting laws may be viewed as creating such a duty. Consequently, the public duty doctrine generally will not protect a physician or other health care professional employed by a public agency who undertakes to treat a child but then fails to report child abuse or otherwise fails to comply with the specific requirements of the reporting statute.

Finally, in addition to legislating a statutory immunity for actions taken by reporters under the child abuse reporting laws, a number of states have enacted general immunity statutes that protect public employees from liability for injuries caused while acting within the scope of their employment. The underlying rationale is that the fear of being sued will infringe on the individual's discharge of his or her duty. In addition, even in the absence of a statutory provision, as a matter of common law, immunity may be affirmatively pled and judicially invoked by public employees.

As with the immunity provisions under the reporting statutes, "absolute immunity" applies to "public officials whose special functions or constitutional status requires complete protection from suit" and extends to judges, legislators, and prosecutors acting within their official capacity. Only "qualified" or "good faith immunity," on the other hand, is available to officials performing discretionary functions. But even such limited immunity may be sufficient to terminate a lawsuit based on insubstantial claims involving bare allegations of malice by government employees.

◆ THE LITIGATION OF CHILD ABUSE AND NEGLECT CASES

Court involvement in child abuse or neglect cases may occur in the form of a civil proceeding under specific child abuse or neglect statutes in a juvenile or family court, or in a criminal proceeding for homicide, assault or battery, or criminal child abuse or neglect. The issue may also be litigated in a child custody case related to a dissolution of marriage proceeding. Usually, the state's goal of protecting the child in peril is met in a civil proceeding that takes place in a juvenile court or a family court.

This section reviews how child abuse cases generally proceed in juvenile, criminal, and divorce courts. It concludes with a discussion of the evidentiary rules that may arise in any trial dealing with child abuse.

THE ROLE OF THE JUVENILE COURT AND ITS PROCEDURES

The role of the juvenile court or family court in child abuse cases is to (1) protect the child from further injury; (2) provide a fair and impartial hearing on the allegations in the petition; (3) consider recommendations of the child protection agency and other social service agencies; (4) implement a treatment and reunification plan for the child and/or the parent(s) when appropriate; and (5) protect the constitutional rights of both the child and the parents. The function of the court is not to punish but, rather, to work closely with the social service agencies to effect a treatment plan designed to protect the child. Generally, the court attempts to improve the family situation so that the family is preserved unless the child has suffered serious harm and would continue to be endangered if allowed to remain within that family.

Statutory provisions give these courts their specific powers. Typically, juvenile courts are authorized to adjudicate proceedings involving claims of abuse and neglect, dependency, and delinquency, as well as requests for the termination of parental rights. There has been a long-standing debate, however, on whether the focus of juvenile court jurisdictional statutes, from a policy perspective, should be directed to intervention when the parents or caretakers have shown potentially harmful behavior or only when the child shows harmful effects of such behavior.

Some states have structured their juvenile justice system around family courts. Family courts generally have a broader jurisdiction than juvenile courts, including divorce and child custody, intrafamily assaults, and juvenile traffic offenses. Juvenile courts and family courts are courts of limited jurisdiction, and thus they are involved only in cases the state's statutes specifically authorize the court to hear. Moreover, these courts can issue orders only as specifically authorized by statute. Separate sets of state and local court rules may also govern the conduct of juvenile and family court procedures.

Child abuse and neglect proceedings usually involve bifurcated hearings. For the court to take any action with respect to the child, it first must determine that the child has, in fact, been abused or neglected and thus qualifies to be a "ward" or "dependent" of the court for care and protection. This is often referred to as the "adjudication" stage or phase of the proceeding. In many cases, if all parties are in agreement, there may be a stipulation that the child or children are adjudicated as dependent or children in need of care, and it is not necessary to conduct a trial. However, if a parent, a child, or the state does not wish to enter into such a stipulation, the case will proceed to trial, or an adjudication hearing. This adjudication hearing is usually conducted before a judge. However, several jurisdictions allow for a jury to make this determination. If the court concludes that abuse or neglect has taken place, the child is considered to be under the jurisdiction of the juvenile court as dependent or a child in need of care, and the second phase, or dispositional hearing, is held. The dispositional hearing is designed to determine the appropriate intervention and to initiate a treatment plan.

The court may then order one or more of a variety of dispositions for the child. Additionally, the court may order dispositions for one or both of the parents. Generally, if the parent fails to comply with the juvenile court's order, the court cannot punish the parent with fines or imprisonment, but is restricted to conditioning the child's return to the home on the parent's obeying the court's order. In very limited instances, in which the remedy of changing custody is not available or appropriate, the court may be authorized to hold the parent in contempt and jail the parent until the parent complies with the court's order.

Although most juvenile court proceedings are confidential and closed to the public and the press, many states have opened up delinquency adjudications to the public and the media, especially in cases involving more serious felony charges. In most instances, only those individuals directly involved are allowed access.

PARTICIPANTS IN THE JUVENILE COURT PROCESS

Participants in a juvenile court child abuse proceeding may include the judge, the petitioner, the child, the parent or parents, an agency or county prosecuting attorney for the petitioner, an attorney for the parent(s), a guardian ad litem, and sometimes an attorney for the child.

Judge

Child abuse cases in juvenile court are heard by a judge who may be elected or assigned to the juvenile court on a permanent or a rotating basis, or by an attorney who is appointed to hear cases in juvenile court. These attorneys are called commissioners, masters, or referees.

The judge's initial responsibility in juvenile court child abuse cases is to protect the child's well-being, and in seeking to attain that goal, to see to it that proper procedures are observed. In addition, the judge is the trier of fact. Generally, there are no juries. The judge rules on the admissibility of evidence and then decides, based on the evidence that has been admitted, whether the child should be adjudicated and placed under the jurisdiction of the juvenile court. In the dispositional hearing, the rules of evidence are often relaxed and the judge reviews the various recommendations and determines the appropriate disposition for the child.

Petitioner

State statutes often restrict who may bring actions in juvenile court. Generally, a suit may be filed by probation officers, juvenile officers, officials of the state or local social service agency, or local county or prosecuting attorneys. In some states "any interested person" can initiate a proceeding. The decision to initiate juvenile court proceedings is based on a variety of factors, including the following: (1) the nature of injury involved; (2) the attitude of the family toward voluntary cooperation with social service agencies; and (3) prior history of abuse or neglect within the family.

Child

The child is the subject of the juvenile court proceeding. The case is often named or "styled" "In the Interest of John Doe, a Child." The child may be called as a witness at the hearing by any of the parties and may be subject to cross-examination by other parties. This would obviously not occur in cases involving preverbal infants or toddlers. Nonetheless, most state evidence codes presume that any witness called to testify in court is competent until proven otherwise.

Parents

Each parent of the child is entitled to notice of the hearing and, in most jurisdictions, is considered a party in the case. The parent, too, can be called as a witness and would then be subject to cross-examination. A parent can claim his or her constitutional right under the Fifth Amendment to refuse to respond to any question that might tend to be incriminating. However, since such proceedings are civil in nature, refusal to answer questions generally allows the court to draw a negative inference against the parent. Additionally, the right to refuse to answer may be limited if the state grants immunity to the parent, whereby testimony given by the parent cannot then be used against him or her. In addition, the United States Supreme Court has held that, even without such a grant of immunity, a parent can be required to produce a child in his or her custody for a court hearing, at least in those instances where a parent has custody of a child pursuant to a court order resulting from child protection proceedings. Such action can be mandated even though it might tend to incriminate the parent and aid the state in criminally prosecuting the parent.

Attorney for the Petitioner

In most juvenile courts there will be a county, city, or corporation attorney who is employed full-time to represent the party instituting the court action. In some jurisdictions, CPS agencies have their own attorneys whose functions include bringing such juvenile court actions. In some locales the government contracts with private attorneys for representation. The petitioner's attorney drafts and files the petition and other necessary pleadings or motions. At the adjudicatory hearing, the attorney for the petitioner attempts to establish, through the presentation of evidence, that the allegations in the petition are true. Then, at the dispositional hearing, the attorney attempts to convince the court to follow the recommendations of the petitioner regarding the child's future.

Attorney for the Parent(s)

Because it is often the parent who is suspected of inflicting the harm or neglecting the child, the parent will typically want to be represented by an attorney in the juvenile court proceeding. In every state the parent has a right to be represented. In most jurisdictions the state will appoint an attorney if the parent is indigent, although this is not required by the United States Constitution. The right of a parent to appointed counsel may be granted by state statute. The United States Supreme Court has held that the Constitution does not require the appointment of counsel for parents in every parental termination proceeding (*Lassiter v. Department of Social Services*, 1981). The Court ruled that in the absence of an applicable state statute or rule regarding the appointment of an attorney for indigent parents, the decision to do so must be made by the trial judge on a case-by-case basis.

The attorney for the parent, of course, is required to protect the interests of the parent. In the adjudicatory hearing, the parent's attorney usually tries to persuade the court that no abuse or neglect occurred, that any injury sustained was accidental, or that the perpetrator was someone other than the parent and the parent cannot be faulted for the perpetrator's conduct.

If the child is determined to be within the jurisdiction of the juvenile court, the parent's attorney in a dispositional hearing will typically seek to have the child remain in the custody of his or her client or otherwise minimize the extent of official intervention in the family. The attorney must also protect the other interests of his client. The attorney must caution the client not to make statements which could be used against himself or herself in a later criminal prosecution. If there is a conflict of interest between the parents, it may be necessary for each parent to have his or her own attorney.

Representation for the Child

Many states have enacted statutes providing representation for the child in child protection proceedings. State laws vary, however, as to whether the child is to be represented by a guardian ad litem (guardian for this particular law suit), an attorney, or both. In some jurisdictions, a guardian ad litem must be an attorney. Although the role and responsibility of the two differ, both the guardian ad item and the attorney may present evidence and question witnesses at the adjudicatory hearing. Moreover, both may offer recommendations regarding the child's placement and treatment at the dispositional hearing.

The guardian ad litem represents the child's best interest in the child abuse or neglect proceeding. He or she must use independent judgment to determine the best interest of the child. The guardian ad litem is not the child's legal guardian and has no duties after the proceeding. An attorney must be an advocate for his or her client, in this case the child, and when the child is mature enough to express an opinion, counsel must generally advocate what the child determines to be in his or her own best interest.

JUVENILE COURT PROCEDURES
Petition

A juvenile court case involving abuse or neglect usually begins with the filing of a petition or complaint that alleges one or more specific instances of child abuse, neglect, or dependency. The petitioner is usually a juvenile probation officer or a representative of the state's department of social services charged with the investigation of allegations brought to the court by social service personnel, police, or other individuals. With the assistance of the attorney, the petitioner decides whether or not to file the action.

Custody Hearing

The juvenile court will typically conduct a custody or detention hearing within a short time after a petition is filed. This allows the judge to review the initial decision to hold the child and to authorize continued placement outside the home. The hearing occurs only if the child has not been returned to his or her home pending further proceedings but, rather, remains in a hospital, other temporary shelter, or with relatives without the parents' consent. The temporary placement may have been authorized or arranged by the juvenile court, a probation officer, or a CPS worker. Before ordering the continuation of the protective custody, the judge generally must ascertain, pending a full hearing, that there is a substantial risk of immediate harm to the child and that there is no viable alternative for reducing that risk.

Adjudicatory Hearing

In an adjudicatory hearing, the state presents the evidence of abuse or neglect to the court. The only issue to be resolved is whether the child has been abused, neglected, or abandoned, or otherwise comes within the jurisdiction of the court either as dependent or a child in need of care. In many instances the parent will admit the allegations or at least a sufficient part of them for the court to conclude that it is authorized to take jurisdiction or to adjudicate the child to be a ward of the court. In other situations, however, it is necessary for the attorney representing the petitioner to call witnesses to substantiate the facts alleged in the petition. Typical witnesses are doctors, police, teachers, child protection workers, relatives, or parents. Often, a subpoena is issued to compel the witnesses' attendance at the proceedings.

The burden of proving child abuse or neglect in a juvenile court is on the party or petitioner asserting the abuse or neglect, typically the state. The petitioner does not have to prove that a specific individual committed a certain abusive act, but only that the child's environment is injurious to his or her welfare or that those legally responsible for the child's care did not carry out their legal responsibility.

The standard of proof refers to the level of certainty by which the trier of fact must be convinced that the allegations in the petition are true. In a juvenile court child abuse case the standard is not that of "beyond a reasonable doubt," as in a criminal matter. State laws differ, however, as to whether the petitioner must prove child abuse or neglect by the standard of a "preponderance of the evidence" or by "clear and convincing evidence." "Clear and convincing" is higher than preponderance but lower than "beyond a reasonable doubt." Proof by a "preponderance of the evidence" means that the petitioner must convince the judge that it is more likely than not that certain facts are true, that is, by a 51% degree of certainty. A "clear and convincing evidence" standard requires proving that it is highly probable that the existence of those facts is true. The United States Supreme Court has concluded, however, that a burden of proof of at least "clear and convincing evidence" is constitutionally necessary when the petitioner seeks to terminate parental rights. Some states, however, do require the highest standard of proof of "beyond a reasonable doubt" for termination of parental rights. This same standard applies in Termination of Parental Rights proceedings when the child qualifies as an "Indian Child" under the Indian Child Welfare Act.

In most jurisdictions, the judge has the authority to exclude individuals from the courtroom upon a finding that it is in the best interests of the child to do so. A judge may, for example, exclude a parent when the child is testifying to acts of abuse or neglect. Similarly, the judge may exclude a child, who might otherwise be entitled to be present, during medical or other testimony.

Rules of evidence do apply in juvenile court proceedings, but, depending on the particular state, their application may be less strict and court procedures less formal than in criminal cases. They are often relaxed in the context of dispositional hearings and dispositional review hearings; otherwise they are generally followed as in any court proceeding. Direct evidence—that is, evidence by an eyewitness to the incident—is not necessary to prove child abuse or neglect; circumstantial evidence can be sufficient. The inference of abuse or neglect can be drawn from a combination of evidence such as the nature and extent of the injuries, the lack of explanation for the injuries consistent with medical knowledge, the age of the child, and the fact that the parent was the custodian of the child at the time of the alleged abuse. The introduction of medical diagnoses such as "battered child syndrome," "shaken baby syndrome," or "Munchausen syndrome by proxy," among others, are frequently received into evidence to support the legal conclusion of child abuse. If the state fails to establish child abuse or neglect by the requisite standard of proof, the case is dismissed and no further action is taken. If, however, the child is adjudicated and the court takes jurisdiction over the child, the case proceeds to disposition.

Dispositional Hearing

The appropriate placement for the child and the appropriate treatment, if any, for the child and the parent are determined at the dispositional hearing. The hearing may take place immediately after the adjudication or may be scheduled for a later date, pending the collection of additional information that might aid the judge in deciding the terms for the court order. Evidence submitted at the hearing usually focuses on the recommendations made to the judge by a court social worker, and in some situations by the guardian ad litem, regarding placement and treatment. Generally, state statutes give juvenile courts the authority to order a broad range of dispositions, but the specific powers granted to the court differ from state to state. Additionally, some states add a phrase such as "and such other orders as the court deems necessary." Common dispositional powers include the following:

1. Returning the child to the home with or without supervision

2. Giving physical custody to a relative

3. Transferring legal custody to an agency

4. Placing the child in foster care

5. Ordering reunification services

6. In severe cases, terminating the rights of the parent to the child

Once a child has been adjudicated a ward of the juvenile court, the court retains "jurisdiction," or control over the child, until the child either reaches the age of majority (as defined by state law, usually 18 years) or until the jurisdictional status is otherwise terminated by the court. Most juvenile courts hold periodic reviews to measure the progress of the case and to determine the need to modify previous orders. Review hearings are usually scheduled every 6 or 12 months. As a result of the legal requirements under the Adoption and

Safe Families Act of 1997 (ASFA), placement of a child in foster care may not continue indefinitely. After a period of 15 months in foster care, except under limited circumstances, the agency must institute a plan for the child to return home or proceed to a termination of parental rights.

The most drastic measure a state may take to protect an abused or neglected child is the termination of parental rights. In essence the court orders that the parent(s) no longer has any rights or duties with respect to the child. Termination of parental rights may be either voluntary or involuntary. State statutes define the grounds and the specific circumstances under which parental rights may be terminated. Involuntary termination is usually a disposition of last resort.

The most common grounds for termination of parental rights are abandonment, child abuse, or neglect. Statutes specify what conditions constitute abandonment for termination purposes. In some states termination of parental rights is not an authorized disposition in the initial child abuse or neglect proceeding. Rather, it can only be ordered in situations where there is chronic failure to support the child or a consistent pattern of specific unacceptable parental behavior with respect to the child. Ordinarily, the parent must be given sufficient time and opportunity to become a more adequate parent before termination. In some states a parent's severe chronic mental illness, rendering him or her unable to adequately care for the child, may also be grounds for termination of parental rights.

CHILD ABUSE AND NEGLECT IN CRIMINAL COURT

The prosecution of individuals accused of crimes perpetrated against children, while not necessarily commonplace, has increased in recent decades, particularly in the area of child sexual abuse. This increase is, in part, due to advances made in identifying battered and sexually abused children and to the relaxation of evidentiary rules relating to victim competency, in-court testimony, and certain out-of-court statements.

Although the juvenile court's involvement in these cases is based on the legal doctrine known as "parens patriae," the criminal justice system's (CJS) involvement is exercised under the state's police power, which authorizes official action to prevent identified harms to society. The use of this power serves to dissuade private retribution on the part of victims by placing the responsibility for prosecuting alleged violations of the criminal law solely with the government. CJS activities include law enforcement investigations, criminal prosecutions, and sentencing proceedings. The substantive criminal law defines what conduct is criminal and provides the punishment to be imposed on an adjudication or finding of guilt.

SUBSTANTIVE CRIMINAL LAW

State legislatures are responsible for declaring what conduct within their own jurisdictions is deemed criminal and subject to punishment. Similarly, the United States Congress provides for the punishment of activity determined to be harmful to society that occurs within certain territories under federal supervision.

In most jurisdictions, "child abuse" or "child neglect" is viewed as violating the prohibition of one or more of the following statutory crimes: murder, homicide, manslaughter, felonious restraint, false imprisonment, assault, battery, rape, statutory rape, deviant sexual assault, sexual assault, incest, indecent exposure, child endangerment, reckless endangerment, or corruption of minors. A majority of jurisdictions do, however, have specific crimes of child abuse and child neglect. Depending on the alleged conduct and resulting harm to the victim, a criminal prosecution may be sought for one or more of these offenses. Conviction of more than one substantive crime arising from the same series of actions may be authorized, if the proof of each particular crime overlaps.

Crimes are further differentiated as felonies and misdemeanors. The boundary between which offenses constitute felonies and which constitute misdemeanors varies from state to state. In some jurisdictions, the distinction between the two is based on whether ordered incarceration will take place in a local jail or in a state penitentiary, but more frequently the difference is in the prescribed minimum penalty in the event of a conviction. In general, a felony offense is typically punishable by 1 year or more of imprisonment. Sanctions imposed for a misdemeanor conviction usually involve incarceration for less than a year and/or a fine of $500 or less. The distinction between misdemeanors and felonies is not only relevant to the potential punishment, but also to the resulting procedural consequences. Greater constitutional protection is offered to defendants in felony prosecutions, such as the right to a trial by a 12-person rather than a six-person jury. Defendants are entitled to appointed counsel for all felonies and in misdemeanors where the convicted defendant's punishment involves confinement.

PROCEDURE IN CRIMINAL CASES

The precise procedure in criminal cases varies somewhat from state to state, but the sequence is basically the same. Most frequently, the initial stage in the CJS process is the police investigation. In cases of alleged child abuse, police involvement may (1) precede reporting to the CPS agency; (2) coincide with or accompany the CPS investigation; or (3) follow the CPS agency's substantiation of a reported allegation of maltreatment and referral to juvenile court and/or the law enforcement agency. Regardless of the time and manner in which law enforcement officers are notified of a suspected case, the police investigation is directed at goals separate from those of child protection investigations. The law enforcement agency's primary function is to determine whether a crime has occurred and, if so, whether there is sufficient evidence indicating the guilt of a particular person to justify arresting and charging the individual. CPS agencies are concerned with the identification of abuse for prevention and intervention purposes.

Investigation

Police officers use a variety of investigative techniques, including pre-arrest questioning of possible suspects, interviewing witnesses or others with pertinent information, and collecting physical evidence (see Chapter 13).

Care must be taken, however, to ensure that a healthcare professional does not breach the obligation of confidentiality in an effort to cooperate with law enforcement personnel. Access to an individual's medical records or information should not be given to law enforcement personnel without a valid release of information, specific statutory authority, or a court order.

Healthcare professionals may wish to obtain a release of information authorizing the disclosure of information to police and prosecutors. Only half of the state statutes explicitly authorize and require the reporting of child abuse cases to the police. Such statutes may permit disclosure to certain law enforcement agencies or personnel of either specific facts or general medical or other reliable information known to healthcare personnel. In the absence of such specific authority, on occasion, police sometimes attempt to gain access to this information by threatening the healthcare professional with criminal charges based on other statutes. Such threats ought to be resisted.

A few states still have misprision of felony statutes, which create an affirmative obligation to report a felony on the part of anyone with knowledge of its occurrence. Although some jurisdictions have statutes prohibiting the obstruction of justice or the hindering of prosecution, these, as well as misprision of felony laws, generally require an affirmative interference with an officer's lawful discharge of duties in order for the statute to apply. Thus, it would be permissible for the healthcare professional to refuse to disclose to the police otherwise confidential or privileged information.

On occasion, healthcare personnel may be presented with a subpoena duces tecum commanding the production of medical records. Subpoenas are generally issued in the name of a court clerk at the request of an attorney, but at this stage there has been no judicial determination that the record should, in fact, be disclosed without consent. In the absence of a release of information from an authorized individual such as a parent, a judge should be asked to rule on the question of whether the medical record should be released to avoid the possibility of liability for breach of confidentiality. In the same way, portions of an agency child abuse record that contain confidential information protected by statute may also be subject to an in camera or in chambers inspection to determine the admissibility of this information at trial (*Pennsylvania v. Ritchie,* 1987).

As the police proceed with their investigation, possible suspects may be questioned. If an individual has been taken into custody or otherwise deprived of his freedom of action in any significant way, the suspect must be given his "Miranda warnings" before questioning by law enforcement officials. These warnings contain specific cautionary language informing the individual that he has a right to remain silent, that anything he says may be used against him in a court of law, that he has a right to an attorney, and that if he cannot afford an attorney, one will be appointed for him. If the warnings are not given, or if any statement or confession made was not voluntary, then the information may be excluded from evidence in any subsequent related criminal trial.

Arrest and Booking

Before making an arrest, that is, formally taking an individual into custody, law enforcement officers must have probable cause to believe that the arrestee is committing or has committed a felony, or that the arrestee committed a misdemeanor in the officer's presence. If, however, the crime is a misdemeanor not committed in the officer's presence, the police officer must obtain an arrest warrant from a magistrate or other judicial officer.

Once the police have probable cause to justify an arrest, they usually take the suspect into custody and process or "book" him or her. Fingerprints are made and "mug shots" or booking photos are taken. How long the suspect can be held without judicial review is determined by state law. If an arrest warrant is not issued by a court before the termination of the prescribed time period, the police must release the suspect. In many jurisdictions, an individual arrested has the right to have a bond commissioner or judge decide if he or she is to be released on personal recognizance, or if a bail amount is to be set pending prosecutorial review of the case and the possible issuance of formal charges.

Prosecutorial Discretion

The investigating police officer presents the case to the prosecutor's office. The prosecutor possesses broad discretion regarding whether or not to file formal charges. This latitude finds support historically in American law. A number of factors generally influence the decision to file charges, including the strength of the available evidence, the harm caused by the offense, the victim's attitude toward pressing the case, the arrestee's prior criminal record, and the adequacy of alternative remedies apart from prosecution.

Prosecutors sometimes are particularly reluctant to prosecute child abuse cases. Sometimes there is the belief that a criminal prosecution of a parent may impede treatment and reunification of the family. More importantly, the victim or the primary or sole witness is frequently a young child, and concerns arise regarding both the child's credibility and the absence of other admissible evidence. Extensive cross-examination of a child witness may lead to confusion. Fears also exist that the child may be highly suggestible to influence by the perpetrator or other family members, causing an alteration of the content of the child's testimony at trial from the description of events provided earlier to the police and prosecutors. Sex abuse cases generate concerns that the jury will view the child as being prone to fantasy or being curious about sexuality and therefore apt to be confused. The extent to which these notions are valid is debatable. Many prosecutors, however, believe that the jury's possible concerns make it difficult to establish the elements of a criminal offense to the satisfaction of a jury "beyond a reasonable doubt." With the use of DNA evidence, prosecutors have had greater success in prosecuting sexual abuse cases. Because of the frequent need for testimony from the victim, the majority of prosecutions in child sexual abuse involve victims older than age 7 years. However, the criminal prosecution of physical abuse typically involves those cases in which the acts of the perpetrator are egregious, regardless of the victim's age.

Over the past decade, many prosecution offices have organized special units or assigned a limited number of prosecutors to pursue these cases. In such instances, expertise with these cases is developed and successful prosecutions may be more likely to occur.

If the prosecutor elects to bring criminal charges, a complaint is filed, and if an arrest warrant has not previously been obtained, the court generally will issue one upon the filing of the complaint. Further screening out of cases may occur as a result of a preliminary hearing of grand jury action, as described later in this chapter.

Initial Appearance

The arrestee, now referred to as the defendant, is presented before the court and advised of the formal charges contained within the complaint. This proceeding must occur within a specified period of time after arrest, as prescribed by law. At this hearing, bail and other possible conditions of release will be set or reviewed if initial determinations on these issues were made earlier. In felony cases, a date will be set for a preliminary hearing on the charges, as described later in this chapter, unless such a hearing is waived by the defendant or a grand jury issues an indictment in the interim. Defendants charged with misdemeanors are generally not entitled to preliminary hearings or grand jury indictments, and the case will be brought based solely on the prosecutor's charge.

Right to Counsel

At the initial appearance, the court will generally inquire whether the defendant has retained counsel or wishes to do so. If the defendant is indigent, the court will appoint an attorney to represent the defendant. The attorney will either be a public defender or an attorney in private practice who has agreed to represent indigents. In either instance, the attorney will be paid by the state.

Bail

Bail is usually viewed as a means of securing the defendant's presence at subsequent proceedings, and it also has come to be viewed as a way of helping to ensure the safety of the community. State and federal statutes may specify factors for the court to consider in determining whether bail should be set and in what amount. Typically, these factors include the seriousness of the offense, the strength of the case, the defendant's prior criminal record, and the defendant's background. The court may impose additional conditions of release. Appropriate conditions in child abuse cases may include a prohibition on contact with the victim, other members of the victim's family, or other witnesses.

Sometimes, particularly in homicide cases, the court will refuse to set bail or other conditions of release and instead will order that the defendant be held in jail pending the trial. Such preventive detention may be warranted upon a finding of future dangerousness or when there is a serious likelihood that the defendant will flee or otherwise attempt to obstruct justice. This measure may be appropriate in child abuse cases when there are concerns that the perpetrator will return to the child's home and either engage in further abuse or attempt to influence the child to recant accusatory statements.

Preliminary Hearing

The preliminary hearing or grand jury is the next stage in the process. In many jurisdictions, individuals accused of crimes have a right to an adversarial preliminary hearing before a magistrate or judge. There the court determines, based on the evidence presented, whether probable cause exists to believe that a crime was committed and that the defendant was the perpetrator. Both the prosecution and the defense have the right to present evidence by subpoenaing witnesses and questioning them, as well as by the submission of documentary evidence such as medical and other reports.

The government carries the burden of proof. The defendant rarely presents affirmative evidence on his own behalf at this stage, although prosecution witnesses may be rigorously cross-examined. Probable cause will be found in practically all cases because the magistrate or judge generally does not have to weigh the credibility of the various witnesses unless the testimony is implausible or incredible. The only question is whether or not a jury, if it believed even some of the evidence presented, could find that a crime was committed and the defendant did it. If the judge concludes that a jury could so find, then the case is "bound over" for trial. The prosecutor will then issue a charge, usually called an information, based on what took place at the preliminary hearing. If no probable cause is found, the case must be dismissed and the defendant released.

The preliminary hearing gives the defendant an opportunity to review the likely testimony to be presented against him. This may play a significant role in inducing him to enter a guilty plea. The defendant, of course, is entitled to attend the proceedings, although as described below, in some cases involving child abuse, limits may be placed on this right.

Grand Jury

In federal felony prosecutions, the Fifth Amendment to the United States Constitution requires that the case proceed only upon issuance of a grand jury indictment. A number of state constitutions contain comparable provisions. In some of those jurisdictions the preliminary hearing may be bypassed by the presentation of the case to a grand jury.

Grand jury review, whether or not subsequent to a preliminary hearing, also serves to provide a means of determining whether there is probable cause to proceed with prosecution against the defendant. But, unlike a preliminary hearing held before a judicial officer, the grand jury consists of a selected group of private citizens who review cases over a legislatively determined period of time.

The grand jury screening process differs fundamentally from the preliminary hearing in the manner in which it is conducted. The grand jury meets in closed session and only hears testimony from witnesses whom it or the prosecutor subpoenas. Members of the grand jury and the prosecutor may question the witnesses, but the defendant and his counsel are not permitted to attend the proceeding. The grand jury mechanism may be preferable in cases involving child maltreatment because if the child is to be a witness, the grand jury procedure protects the child victim from the trauma of an additional confrontation with a perpetrator and an additional cross-examination by defense counsel. In some jurisdictions it may not even be necessary for the child victim to appear before the grand jury because a parent or law enforcement officer may be permitted to testify to what the child has stated, or a videotape of the child's statement may be used in lieu of live testimony.

When a majority of the grand jurors find sufficient evidence to justify prosecution, an indictment is signed by the members of the grand jury and designated a "true bill." The indictment, which sets forth a description of the offense, is then filed with the trial court. Return of a "no true bill" requires dismissal of the charges against the defendant.

Arraignment

After the filing of either the prosecutor's information or the grand jury indictment with the court, the defendant is formally arraigned. The defendant appears before the court and is informed of the charges now pending against him or her. The defendant then enters a plea of not guilty or guilty. The question of the propriety of bail and other release procedures may again be explored.

Pre-trial Motions

Between entering a plea and the commencement of trial, the criminal defendant typically makes one or more pre-trial motions, challenging such technical matters as the institution of the prosecution; the sufficiency of the indictment; the admissibility of expected physical evidence, statements, or confessions; the court's jurisdiction; and the physical location of the trial. In addition, the defendant will seek to "discover" certain materials from the prosecution and otherwise obtain information from witnesses who may testify against him. The extent to which this occurs depends on applicable law.

Plea Bargaining, Guilty Pleas, and Dismissals
Before the arraignment, plea bargaining between the prosecutor and defendant frequently occurs. Agreements derived from plea negotiations may take various forms. Such agreements can involve a plea of guilty to a less serious offense, a plea of guilty to the charged offense with a promise by the prosecutor to recommend a reduced sentence, or a plea of guilty to one or more charges in exchange for dismissal of other charges or a promise not to file additional charges. Justification for plea bargaining is found in the notion that it provides a quick disposition of cases necessitated by a system of justice that is already heavily overburdened. Plea bargaining is an important tool for the prosecutor when the child witness is reluctant to testify or the physical evidence of the crime is less than compelling.

The vast majority of criminal cases are disposed of by a guilty plea or by the dismissal of charges. In one study that examined a set of criminal filings in three counties across the country during the mid-1980s, 68% of the defendants entered guilty pleas to some or all of the charges and another 20% were dismissed before trial. These figures are consistent with national trends for all felony cases; in 1989, 86% of federal cases resulted in a plea bargain, as did 91% of state felons in the 75 most populous U.S. counties in 1988 (Maguirs & Flanagan, 1990).

Diversion
Diversion programs have emerged as a possible alternative to adjudication within the CJS. Diversion involves halting or suspending formal criminal proceedings against a defendant without a formal conviction and requiring his or her participation in a therapeutic program. Diversion programs are a response to the difficulties in successfully prosecuting child maltreatment cases, particularly those involving sexual abuse.

Diversion generally is used only for misdemeanors or less serious or first felony complaints and typically when the victim and the accused are family members. It may begin before the arrest or at any other stage before trial. Individuals selected for diversion are generally viewed as likely to participate in treatment and likely to benefit from it. Typically they are offered counseling directed at the abusive behavior, as well as career development, education, and supportive treatment services. If the participant responds favorably for a specified period of time, the court, the prosecutor, or both will dismiss the case. If the defendant fails to meet the program's obligations, prosecution is resumed on the original criminal charge.

Jurisdictions vary in their use, if any, of diversion programs. Some states, by statute, specifically authorize diversion for particular crimes if certain criteria are met, while other jurisdictions provide for some degree of prosecutorial discretion or specific court involvement. Similar schemes may be used as part of a condition of probation after a guilty plea or conviction at trial.

Constitutional and Related Issues at Trial
The trial of any criminal case raises a broad array of constitutional and related issues, practically all of which are designed to protect the defendant and to ensure a fair and impartial trial.

Presumption of Innocence and Burden of Proof

The defendant is entitled to a presumption of innocence. This means that the prosecution has the burden of producing evidence of guilt and must persuade the trier of fact (the jury or the judge alone in a "bench trial") of the truth of each of the elements or legally significant facts of the offense with which the defendant is charged. Moreover, each of the elements must be proven by a high degree of evidence—"beyond a reasonable doubt." Although it is difficult to define this standard, it is usually said that there must be "an abiding conviction, to a moral certainty, of the truth of the charge."

Privileges

The Fifth Amendment to the United States Constitution protects the defendant against compelled self-incrimination. This protection includes the right of the defendant not to take the witness stand and be forced to testify against himself.

In addition, statements admitting responsibility for abuse which are made to spouses, physicians, and other healthcare professionals may be excluded as a result of a claim of privilege. The privilege may apply in criminal cases with respect to at least some of the information provided to healthcare professionals, even in the face of an abrogation of the privilege for civil child protection proceedings under a state's reporting statute.

Searches, Seizures, and Confessions

As briefly noted in the discussion of social service and police response to reports of child abuse and neglect, an investigation of alleged child maltreatment may implicate various constitutional issues that affect the admissibility of evidence at trial. These concerns are commonly based on activities such as the examination of the child, a search of a perpetrator's home, and statements obtained from the child's parent(s), guardian(s), or other possible perpetrators. The constitutional issues come into play not only in the context of potential civil liability of healthcare and child protection professionals, but also in criminal cases involving charges brought against perpetrators of child abuse and neglect.

Generally, constitutional provisions protect against intrusions by state authorities. Such authorities may include the police, child care workers, and even medical personnel employed by or acting on the direction of law enforcement or other state agencies. If such constitutional violations do occur, evidence obtained as a result of the violation may not be admitted in criminal prosecutions. Thus physical evidence that implicates a defendant may be excluded if it was seized in violation of the defendant's rights to be free from unreasonable searches and seizures under the Fourth Amendment to the United States Constitution. Similarly, confessions made in the absence of required Miranda warnings or as a result of police coercion may not be admissible at a criminal trial.

Confrontation Clause

The Confrontation Clause of the Sixth Amendment to the United States Constitution is an area of constitutional law that has recently attracted attention from the United States Supreme Court. The Clause often has impact on the trial of criminal cases involving allegations of child abuse. The Clause provides, in part, that "[i]n all criminal prosecutions, the accused shall enjoy the right . . . to be confronted with the witnesses against him." The Clause confers on a criminal defendant a right to confront witnesses at trial, both face-to-face and through cross-examination, and is designed to increase the defendant's ability to challenge the charges against him and to ensure an adversarial proceeding at trial. Confrontation Clause rights are also buttressed by rights under the Fourteenth Amendment's Due Process Clause, which prohibits a state from depriving an individual of liberty without due process of law.

The tension between the right to confrontation and attempts by both legislatures and individual judges to protect child victims from the potential trauma of confronting the abuser at trial or in pre-trial proceedings is evident. Unlike the situation that may occur in both juvenile court and divorce-related hearings, where the court may be authorized in some circumstances to allow a child to testify "on camera" or in chambers and outside the presence of the alleged perpetrator, such testimony in a criminal case may violate the defendant's right to a public trial under the Sixth Amendment to the Constitution. It may also violate his right to confront witnesses and be present at trial under the Confrontation Clause. Finally, the First Amendment rights of the press and related rights of public access to trials may likewise be implicated.

A number of states have passed legislation providing for closed circuit and videotaped testimony in an effort to balance the competing interests of the child victims and the rights of criminal defendants. In addition, as discussed in the evidentiary section later, the Confrontation Clause may play a role in connection with the creation of various exceptions to the hearsay rule.

A violation of the Confrontation Clause may occur when the defendant is denied face-to-face confrontation with the witness. Although the defendant's right to be present extends to every stage of the trial, some exceptions do exist. The United States Supreme Court (*Kentucky v. Stincer*, 1985) failed to find a violation of the Confrontation Clause when the defendant (but not his lawyer) was denied access to a pre-trial hearing to determine the competency of two children who were victims of an alleged sex offense. The Court noted, however, that the questions asked did not relate to the crime itself and therefore the lack of the defendant's participation did not bear a substantial relationship to the defendant's opportunity to defend himself at trial. Moreover, the same questions were asked at trial where the defendant was present and there was full and complete cross-examination.

The problem surrounding face-to-face confrontation is more likely when a child victim gives live testimony at trial, out of the presence of a defendant. In another case (*Coy v. Iowa*, 1988), the United States Supreme Court reversed the conviction when a state law permitted a trial judge to order the placement of a large screen between the defendant and two 13-year-old girls who testified that he had sexually assaulted them. The Court noted that the screen improperly prevented the witnesses from seeing the defendant and only allowed him to dimly perceive them. Justice O'Connor, who agreed with the reversal but filed a separate opinion, pointed out that the statute presumed that trauma would occur any time a young victim testified. She suggested that had there been an individualized finding by the trial judge that the child witnesses needed special protection, a different result might have ensued.

Soon thereafter, the United States Supreme Court upheld a conviction under somewhat similar circumstances. In a 1990 case (*Maryland v. Craig*, 1990), a state statute provided for a one-way television procedure if the trial judge decided that face-to-face testimony "will result in the child suffering serious emotional distress such that the child cannot reasonably communicate." The statute provided that once this finding was made, the witness, prosecutor, and defense counsel would withdraw to a separate room, while the judge, jury, and defendant remained in the courtroom. The defendant could watch direct and cross-examination of the child over a video hookup and remain in electronic communication with his counsel.

The Court concluded that the central concerns regarding the Confrontation Clause were addressed under such a procedure. The Court acknowledged the "growing body of academic literature documenting the psychological trauma suffered by child abuse victims who must testify in court." It concluded that as long as the trial judge decided, on a case by case basis, that such trauma would result if the child was faced with the defendant, and procedures such as those provided were followed to ensure the defendant's rights were respected, there was no constitutional violation.

Trials

Defendants charged with felonies or misdemeanors punishable by more than 6 months in jail are entitled to jury trials. Juries generally comprise 12 persons, but in some jurisdictions, in certain cases, a jury of six is permissible. A defendant can waive his right to a jury trial and be tried by a judge alone. A jury verdict either of guilt or acquittal, at least in felony trials, must be unanimous. If the jury cannot come to a unanimous agreement, a mistrial results, and the prosecution is terminated without a decision on the merits of the case. The state may not retry the defendant after an acquittal, but a subsequent prosecution may follow a mistrial.

Sentencing

Following a guilty verdict, a sentencing hearing is scheduled. Before the hearing, a pre-sentence report is completed, usually by the state's probation and parole department, to guide the judge in the sentencing decision. The report includes information about the defendant based on interviews with a variety of individuals who have had contact with the defendant. The report may include the results of psychological testing or interviewing.

Both state and federal law define the range of permissible sanctions that may be imposed for the offense committed, including whether probation is available. In some jurisdictions, in some circumstances, the jury will recommend a punishment, which the judge can follow or choose to ignore in favor of a less severe penalty.

In some situations, the defendant may receive a prison sentence, but the sentence may be suspended with the defendant being placed on probation (with or without some limited period of incarceration) under the supervision of the probation department. A typical condition of probation in child abuse cases is a requirement for treatment of the defendant. The defendant's failure to attend or to participate in the treatment program can be viewed as a violation of probation, and the court might then reinstate the prison term originally decreed. Other conditions of probation may include an order to stay away from the victim and required payment to the victim for his or her treatment costs.

Appeals and Post-Conviction Action

Following a criminal conviction, direct appellate review is limited to a statutorily defined period of time and allows challenges to any alleged errors committed by the judge that occurred at trial. These include the judge's rulings on various motions which the defendant's attorney made before or at trial, on objections made to the admissibility of evidence, and on instructions the judge gave to the jury regarding the applicable law in the case. If the defendant's appeal is unsuccessful, he may make a "collateral attack" on the conviction. A collateral attack is usually based on constitutional challenges, such as a claim of ineffective assistance of counsel at trial or on appeal. The state, however, may not appeal from an acquittal.

CHILD CUSTODY DISPUTES AND ALLEGATIONS OF ABUSE
ARENAS OF LITIGATION

Sometimes allegations of child abuse arise in child custody disputes. They often include claims of sexual abuse. The parents may have been residing together as a family unit at the time, or the alleged behavior may have occurred subsequent to the breakup but pending judicial resolution of custody and visitation rights. Alternatively, the alleged incident might have taken place after a temporary or final custody decree, while the child was in the custody of a custodial parent, or during the course of visitation by the child with the noncustodial parent.

If no dissolution of marriage action has been filed, but there is a dispute concerning child custody, its resolution is likely to take place in the context of a juvenile court child protection proceeding as described previously. In addition, most states have enacted legislation that provides for "civil orders of protection" for victims of domestic violence. Many of these statutes provide for judicial determination of custody rights with respect to the children of the parties involved in the context of such litigation.

Finally, the issue of child abuse may appear in any one of a number of stages of a court action related to the dissolution of a marriage of the child's parents. For example, together with or shortly after the filing of a petition for divorce, a motion may be filed requesting the court to issue an order providing for temporary custody and visitation pending the final hearing on the petition for a decree of divorce. At the final hearing, in which the court must determine provisions for joint or sole custody and visitation rights, the issue of child abuse may also be contested. Subsequent to the court issuing a final custody order, one or both of the parents may file motions to modify that order, alleging a change in the circumstances of the child or custodial parent. There, too, the question of child abuse may be litigated. State law or state or local court rules will determine whether it will be a juvenile or family court or a court of general civil jurisdiction that will rule on the custody issue in each of these contexts.

Litigation of child custody disputes in each of these situations differs from that in the juvenile court/child protection context or the criminal context. The court here is engaging in a private dispute settlement function where it must choose between two or more individuals, each of whom claims an associational interest with the child. In the other situations described previously, the court is enforcing standards of behavior believed necessary to protect the child or the greater society at large and, perhaps, to punish a wrongdoer.

PROCEDURAL AND EVIDENTIARY RULES

The state's power to adjudicate private custody disputes, like its power in child protection cases, derives from the common law concept of the state as parens patriae. Each state, through legislation and judicial precedent, has prescribed both procedural and evidentiary rules that regulate how the issue is to be litigated, as well as substantive rules that guide the court in determining what its orders regarding custody should be.

Depending on the particular state, rules exist that permit or require the appointment of a guardian ad litem in child custody disputes. Similarly, under more or less restrictive circumstances, the trial judge may order that an investigation and report regarding custodial arrangements for the child be made by employees of public or private social service agencies or by other competent individuals. The child may be referred to professionals for diagnosis by the court or by the individual conducting the custody investigation. The investigator may consult with and obtain information from medical, psychiatric, or other experts who have previously dealt with the child. The judge may conduct in chambers interviews with the child to ascertain custodial preferences or seek the advice of professional personnel in an effort to elicit such information most effectively. Some jurisdictions require the consent of all parties, in some circumstances, for the application of one or more of these unique procedural devices in a given child custody case. The manner in which a given state approaches these issues affects the court's ability to ascertain whether or not abuse or neglect has taken place. This, in turn, will control the extent to which the abuse or neglect then plays a role in the court's ultimate determination of contested custody questions.

Evidentiary rules control the extent to which professional privileges such as that between physician and patient, psychologist and client, and husband and wife limit the amount of information available to a court in making a child custody determination. Although most state reporting statutes seem to abrogate these privileges in child custody situations involving known or suspected child abuse or neglect, the precise language of the statutory provision that abrogates the privilege in a given state and possible judicial interpretations of that language could still affect whether or not related evidence is deemed admissible.

SUBSTANTIVE STANDARDS

A majority of states currently provide that custody decisions turn on "the best interests of the child," or comparable language, as the substantive standard for making custody determinations. Likewise, visitation rights may be subject to a similar analysis. "The best interests of the child," however, can be an ambiguous standard. This standard essentially requires that a prediction be made in relation to the child's needs and each parent's ability to meet them.

The analysis of the phrase, when specified by the legislature, may provide guidelines that take into account a lengthy list of factors. These include matters such as the following:

1. The wishes of the child's parents as to custody

2. The wishes of the child

3. The interaction and interrelationship of the child with his parents, siblings, and any other person who may significantly affect the child's best interest

4. The child's adjustment to his home, school, and community

5. The mental and physical health of all individuals involved, including any history of abuse of any individuals involved

6. The needs of the child for a continuing relationship with both parents, and the ability and willingness of parents to actively perform their functions as mother and father to meet the child's needs

7. The intention of either parent to relocate his or her residence outside the state

8. Which parent is more likely to allow the child frequent and meaningful contact with the other parent

9. Other considerations of environment, physical and emotional needs, intellectual stimulation, financial resources, moral development, and family makeup

When custody is contested, the judge must choose among various alternative arrangements, allocating between the two parents the rights and obligations relating to the child that were formerly shared by them. Although most jurisdictions now authorize awards of "joint custody" under which the parents continue to share rights and responsibilities with respect to the child after divorce, such an award is not required. In cases where child maltreatment is alleged, the court necessarily seeks to determine the truth of the accusations. When the allegations are substantiated, the judge should, of course, choose a custody arrangement that will maximize the child's safety.

REVIEW AND MODIFICATION

Custody decisions are generally viewed as matters best left to the sound discretion of the trial court because of the fact-sensitive nature of the determinations, combined with the general lack of firm guidelines controlling "the best interests of the child" analysis. The wide latitude traditionally afforded to a trial court allows for a necessarily individualized case-by-case decision. It does, however, limit the scope of review of an appellate court to that of reversal only for an "abuse of discretion." Thus, on appeal, a higher court generally will not re-evaluate the facts to determine whether, in its own view, a finding of child abuse perpetrated by the accused should have been made.

Legislation providing for modification of a child custody or visitation order commonly requires a showing of a "substantial or material change of circumstances" and that a modification will be in "the best interests of the child." Allegations of abuse, formerly raised when custody was initially decided, will generally not constitute a change of circumstances, without new evidence of abuse.

EVIDENTIARY ISSUES

The law of evidence is the system of rules and standards that regulates the admission of proof at the trial of any lawsuit. In response to efforts to introduce various types of evidence, in the nature of both testimony and physical exhibits (sometimes called "real" evidence), objections may be made by opposing counsel. The trial judge must then rule on these objections and determine what actual evidence the finder of fact (which may be the jury, as in criminal cases, or the judge himself or herself, in juvenile court child protection cases or divorce cases) will be allowed to consider. The judge will rely on established rules that are part of the law of evidence in making these determinations.

General rules of evidence may affect virtually any question that is asked of a witness during the trial. Particularly unique and difficult evidentiary issues do arise, however, in cases involving child abuse and neglect, and these warrant specific attention here. These issues include the possible use of circumstantial evidence, the competency of child witnesses, the use of hearsay testimony, limits regarding the scope of admissible expert testimony, and the use of various types of demonstrative evidence such as photographs and anatomically correct dolls.

Generally, the applicable rules of evidence in criminal child abuse prosecutions, civil juvenile court child protection proceedings, and child custody cases are the same. The rules may be somewhat "relaxed" in noncriminal proceedings in juvenile court or in divorce cases because a judge rather than a jury in the majority of jurisdictions is the fact finder and, at least theoretically, has been trained to ignore inadmissible evidence in making his or her determination.

DIRECT AND CIRCUMSTANTIAL EVIDENCE

Child abuse often does not yield a great deal of evidence which, under U.S. rules of evidence, would be admissible in any of the trials or hearings related to child abuse. Most cases of child abuse occur in the child's home, and often the only people present are the child and the perpetrator. Even when others are present at the time of the incident, in many instances it is a member of the immediate family, such as a spouse who may be unwilling to testify or to testify truthfully, or a young child who is too immature to take the witness stand. Frequently the victim is too young or too immature to testify. Even if the child is mature enough to testify, he or she may be reluctant to do so or will change or recant his or her story. The alleged adult perpetrator typically contends that the child's injuries were accidental. Therefore, direct evidence is usually sparse or nonexistent. Direct evidence is evidence which, if believed, resolves the matter in issue.

Most of the available evidence in child abuse cases is circumstantial. Circumstantial evidence is evidence not based on actual personal knowledge or observation of facts or events in controversy. Rather, it is based on facts from which deductions may be drawn, showing indirectly that certain events did take place or that certain other facts sought to be proved are true. Circumstantial evidence, even if believed, does not resolve the matter in issue. Additional reasoning must be applied to reach the proposition to which it is directed.

For example, a witness' testimony that he saw X beat a child with a belt is direct evidence of whether X did, indeed, beat the child. Testimony that the child had belt marks on his back and legs, that the child was in X's custody, and that no one else had access to the child during the time when the marks were acquired would be strong circumstantial evidence that X beat the child. A case of child abuse may be proven entirely by circumstantial evidence, but there still must be sufficient evidence to convince the trier of fact.

In juvenile court proceedings, some courts have applied the doctrine of res ipsa loquitur to support an inference of child abuse. Res ipsa loquitur means "the thing speaks for itself." For example, child abuse may be inferred from the mere fact that the child sustained a particular injury, given the character of the injury and the surrounding circumstances.

COMPETENCY

An individual must be competent to testify as a witness at any trial or hearing. Competence to testify involves four factors: (1) the mental capacity, at the time of the occurrence in question, to observe or receive accurate impressions of the event; (2) memory sufficient to retain an independent recollection of the observations; (3) the capacity to communicate that memory in words and to understand questions about the event; and (4) a present understanding of the difference between truth and false testimony and an appreciation of the obligation to speak the truth.

Historically, courts and legislatures created presumptions, depending on age, regarding the competency of children to testify. More recently, however, the trend has been to presume that all witnesses are competent to testify and to resolve doubts as to the credibility of the witness in favor of allowing the testimony and having the trier of fact decide what weight to give that testimony. A party can still challenge a witness, however, and the trial judge may prohibit the testimony if the judge finds that the witness did not meet one of the criteria listed. Because judges would otherwise have the discretion to exclude testimony on the basis of competence, a number of jurisdictions have recently passed legislation that makes admissible all testimony by a child regarding evidence of child sexual abuse.

HEARSAY

In general, a witness can only testify to those facts about which he or she has personal knowledge. The witness may not testify to what others have said in an out-of-court or extrajudicial statement to prove the truth of the matter stated. Such second-hand information is called hearsay. Hearsay evidence is usually inadmissible in a judicial proceeding. Hearsay is excluded to prevent the introduction of statements made by out-of-court declarants whose statements were not made under oath and whose credibility cannot be evaluated by the jury.

There are, however, certain recognized exceptions to the hearsay rule. Each of these exceptions has been recognized in some or all jurisdictions. The exceptions typically have been created when the situation and the circumstances surrounding the declarant's statement increase the reliability of the out-of-court statement and thereby make the statement more trustworthy. For such statements to be admissible, however, they must meet the jurisdiction's requirements for that particular hearsay exception and, in criminal cases, not violate the Confrontation Clause of the Sixth Amendment to the United States Constitution. A number of the recognized exceptions to the hearsay rule are important in child abuse and neglect cases, as acknowledged by the U.S. Supreme Court in *White v. Illinois* (1992).

Excited Utterances and Statements of Physical and Mental Conditions

One recognized hearsay exception is that for excited utterances. This exception allows for the admission of nonreflective statements regarding a startling event made while the declarant is still in a state of excitement. For example, a statement made by a child to a neighbor or the police that her mother beat her with a belt may be admissible if the court finds that the statement was made while the child was still excited and that the statement was impulsive and spontaneous rather than a product of reflective thought.

A related exception, recognized in most jurisdictions, is for statements made to anyone regarding then existing physical conditions, including pain or other physical sensations. These are admissible to prove the truth of the statement.

That is, they are admissible to prove that the physical condition or pain existed at the time the statement was made. Thus a statement made by a child to her mother, while pointing to a genital area, that "it hurts" could be admissible under this exception.

Similarly, most jurisdictions admit statements of the declarant's then existing state of mind or emotion. Thus, for example, in child custody litigation incident to a divorce, a child's statement to another individual regarding affection for or dislike of a parent will be admissible. Similarly, statements indicating fear of an abusive parent may also be admitted.

Statements for Medical Diagnosis

In most jurisdictions there is a separate recognized exception authorizing the admission of statements made for purposes of medical diagnosis and treatment. Statements admissible under this exception may pertain to present or to past conditions, if they are made to a physician or the physician's agent, such as a nurse, technician, or receptionist. Such statements are admissible on the assumption that one generally does not fabricate statements to healthcare providers because the success of the patient's treatment depends on the accuracy of the information provided. Thus an affirmative response by a child to a question asked by a physician of whether anyone "touched you there" would be admissible as evidence to prove that the molestation had taken place.

Some courts will also admit statements that refer to the cause of the condition for which the declarant is seeking treatment if the statements are reasonably pertinent to the diagnosis and are made in connection with the treatment. In the child abuse situation, a number of courts have reasoned that because the treatment of child abuse includes removing the child from the abusive setting, the doctor should attempt to ascertain the identity of the abuser. Therefore a child's statement to a physician to the effect that "Daddy hurt me" would be admitted.

Present Sense Impressions

A few jurisdictions recognize an exception for "present sense impressions." These are statements describing or explaining an event or condition that were made while the declarant was perceiving the event or condition or immediately thereafter. For example, if a child was rescued while the abuse was taking place and immediately began to describe to the rescuer what had occurred, his or her statement may be admitted.

Admissions by Parties

Another recognized exception to the hearsay rule is when the out-of-court statement is that of a party to the litigation and is relevant to the party's defense. For example, a parent-perpetrator may tell a neighbor, "I beat my child because he wet his pants." In a criminal case against the parent, the neighbor could testify to this statement. Its admission in a juvenile court proceeding may depend on whether the parent is considered a party under the state's juvenile court rules.

Business and Medical Records

Finally, an additional exception to the hearsay rule allows the introduction of business records. This generally includes medical records. When business records are used to prove the truth of their contents, this constitutes hearsay. Such records, however, often will be admitted under a recognized exception to the hearsay rule for records kept by a business in the regular course of its operation. The theory is that if the "business" itself will rely on the accuracy of such records in carrying out its operations, a court should do likewise. For the record to be admitted, there must be "foundational testimony" to the effect that the entry to the records was made accurately and promptly, it was made in the course of usual business activity, and the person recording the information had first-hand knowledge of the matter.

In most instances, medical records may be admissible as substantive evidence of the child's diagnosis, condition, medical history, and laboratory and X-ray findings under the business records exception to the hearsay rule. Medical records may also be used to refresh the physician's memory regarding the specific case when the physician is testifying at trial or when giving evidence in a deposition. This use is appropriate whether or not the record is otherwise admissible as a business record.

Many courts are reluctant, however, to admit prognostic statements or statements about the cause of a condition that are contained in the medical record unless the doctor who wrote the statement is available for cross-examination or the statement was based on objective data rather than on data requiring speculation. For example, it would probably not be necessary to have a radiologist testify in court that the child has a spiral fracture of the femur. In this situation the record would be admissible to show that the child had the spiral fracture. Conversely, a doctor's statement that the spiral fracture of the femur was caused by child abuse rather than by an accidental fall would probably not be admitted into evidence unless the doctor was available for cross-examination.

Residual Exception

Some jurisdictions have recognized a so-called "residual" exception to the hearsay rule. This permits the receipt of "reliable" hearsay evidence, which does not fit into an established exception, under limited situations, as long as the statement has "equivalent circumstantial guarantees of trustworthiness" to the recognized exceptions. Courts have sometimes relied on this exception in litigation involving children.

Sexual Abuse Hearsay Exception

A number of jurisdictions, through legislation or by judicial decision, have created a new hearsay exception that authorizes the admission of out-of-court statements by children about sexual abuse. Often the sexual abuse hearsay exception's applicability is limited to criminal or juvenile court proceedings or both. This exception is similar to the residual exception, but only applies to children's statements about sexual abuse. The time, content, and circumstances of the statement must provide sufficient guarantees of trustworthiness. In addition, the child must either testify at the hearing or must be unavailable. When unavailable, there must be additional corroborative evidence of the act that is the subject of the child's statement. These statutes allow a parent, doctor, or other individual to whom a child has made a statement regarding sexual abuse to testify to the child's description of what occurred, irrespective of whether or not the statement otherwise meets the requirements of another hearsay exception.

Videotaping Statutes

Some state legislatures have passed statutes permitting a child's testimony to be preserved on videotape for presentation to a jury, thus enabling the child to avoid repeated appearances in court. The statutes exempt from the ban on hearsay an audiovisually recorded statement of a child victim or witness that describes an act of sexual abuse or physical violence if certain requirements are met. The court must find that (1) the minor will suffer emotional or psychological stress if required to testify in open court; (2) the time, content, and circumstances of the statement provide sufficient guarantees of trustworthiness; and (3) certain other procedural requirements were met. Generally, the presence of the judge, the accused, or counsel is not required at the taping, and any person can conduct the interview. The admission of the statement, however, does not preclude the court from allowing a party to call the minor as a witness, if justice requires. On the defendant's request, the court must provide for further questioning of the minor.

In addition, these statutes authorize presenting the evidence of the statement of the child as the equivalent of testimony in the case, either by audiovisually recorded deposition or by closed circuit television. Such statutes specify who is to be present at the recording and authorize the exclusion of a party on a finding that his presence may cause severe emotional or psychological distress to the child. The use of such a recording is permitted, provided the defendant can observe and hear the testimony and can consult with his lawyer.

Confrontation Clause Issues

Although the rules regarding hearsay and its exceptions are generally applicable in juvenile, criminal, and divorce cases, particular note should be made of the interplay between these hearsay rules and a criminal defendant's rights under the Confrontation Clause of the Sixth Amendment to the United States Constitution. As noted in the discussion of criminal trials as well as in the discussion of hearsay, state legislatures and trial courts have endeavored to reduce the trauma a child might sustain from testifying in a criminal trial. Such protective measures may, however, violate the Confrontation Clause.

The Confrontation Clause and the hearsay rules are not one and the same, but they do advance a number of similar values. As a matter of constitutional law, the right to confrontation (1) ensures that the witness will give his statements under oath, thus impressing him with the seriousness of the matter and guarding against a lie by the possibility of a penalty for perjury; (2) forces the witness to submit to cross-examination, which aids in the discovery of truth; and (3) permits the jury to observe the demeanor of the witness in making his statement, allowing it to assess his credibility.

When the state seeks to admit hearsay evidence in a criminal case, the proper inquiry under the Confrontation Clause is said to be twofold. First, if the declarant was available as a witness at trial, it must be asked whether the defendant was permitted an adequate opportunity for cross-examination. Second, and more important for present purposes, if the declarant was not present as a witness at trial, it must be asked whether the absence of the witness was necessary and whether there was sufficient "indicia of reliability" surrounding the out-of-court statement. When the declarant is a child victim, the prosecutor must produce evidence of a good faith effort to obtain the presence of the witness or establish that the witness is "not capable of testifying" as defined by state law. This may involve a showing that the witness is incompetent or that the child should be excused from testifying because the experience will cause additional trauma.

In a 1990 United States Supreme Court decision (*Idaho v. Wright*, 1990), a female defendant and her companion were convicted of lewd conduct against the companion's 2 ½-year-old daughter. The conviction was successfully challenged by the female defendant on the grounds that the trial court should not have admitted the pediatrician's testimony that the victim suggested to him that her father had abused her. The critical statements were made in response to the doctor asking whether her daddy touched her with his "pee-pee." The girl responded that "daddy does this with me. . . ." The trial judge determined that the daughter was incompetent to testify and refused to allow her testimony, but he concluded that her statements to the pediatrician were reliable and admitted them under the state's "residual exception" to the hearsay rule.

On appeal, the Supreme Court held that incriminating statements such as these, although otherwise admissible under an exception to the hearsay rule, may be prohibited under the Confrontation Clause. To be admitted, the prosecution must produce the declarant for cross-examination or establish the declarant's unavailability, as well as demonstrate that the statement bears adequate indicia of reliability.

The Court assumed that given the incompetency finding, the child had in fact been "unavailable" for testimony. The question then became one of the reliability or trustworthiness of the statements. The Court refused to adopt any hard and fast rules for professional interviews, such as a requirement that the statements be videotaped or that leading questions could not be used. It ruled that, in determining reliability, factors relating to whether the child was likely to be telling the truth when the statements were made were to be considered and that these included the declarant's mental state, spontaneity, and consistent repetition; motive or lack of motive to make up a story; and the use of terminology unexpected of a child of that age.

In this particular case, the Court pointed out that the doctor had conducted the interview in a suggestive manner. Given the presumptive unreliability of the statements, the Court concluded that there was no special reason for supposing that the statements were particularly trustworthy.

EXPERT TESTIMONY

Generally, a witness is only permitted to testify to factual matters and may not offer an opinion or conclusion regarding the meaning of those facts. An expert witness, however, is allowed to give opinions in areas related to his or her expertise when the judge determines that such testimony is beyond the common knowledge of the trier of fact and will aid the trier of fact in deciding the issues in the case. An expert witness is someone with specialized knowledge obtained through training and/or experience. To qualify as an expert, the witness will be required to state facts about his or her education and experience. The opposing attorney or the judge may ask additional questions regarding the expertise of the witness. The trial judge is given great discretion in deciding whether the witness qualifies as an expert on the particular matter in issue.

Generally, physicians and perhaps other licensed or certified healthcare professionals have sufficient training and experience to express a medical opinion to help the judge or jury understand the medical aspects of the case. Therefore, in most situations, an individual with a medical degree will qualify as an expert witness. There is no requirement for subspecialization. The weight the fact finder, be it a judge or a jury, gives the physician's testimony, may, however, be affected by such factors as board certification in the particular area involved, experience, publications, and the clarity of the witness' presentation on the pertinent condition.

Battered Child and Failure-to-Thrive Syndromes

When physical abuse is alleged, expert medical testimony is often essential to establish that the injury was not accidental. In child abuse cases, a physician usually qualifies as an expert who can give his or her opinion as to the nature of the child's injuries. Medical testimony that the child's injuries are consistent with "battered child syndrome" is often allowed on the grounds that it is an accepted medical diagnosis. The United States Supreme Court acknowledged the admissibility of this diagnosis to determine that certain injuries were caused intentionally and were not accidental (*Estelle v. McGuire,* 1991). For example, patterned abrasions (belt, cord, stick) and certain fractures in young children (posterior rib fractures in different stages of healing) are powerful evidence of nonaccidental injury and child abuse. In *Estelle v. McGuire* (1991), the United States Supreme Court upheld the defendant's second-degree murder conviction for the death of his daughter and admitted "battered child syndrome" evidence to prove that the death was the result of an intentional act and not simply an accident.

"Failure-to-thrive" syndrome is another diagnosis generally recognized by the medical community and the courts. The syndrome describes a condition in which a young child's height and weight are consistently below the third percentile on the standard growth chart. Although similar growth patterns may be indicative of certain organic disease processes, they also may be due to parental neglect or deprivation, such as inadequate feeding and poor nutrition. Courts generally have accepted an expert's conclusion that the problem results from neglect when, subsequent to the child's hospitalization and receipt of proper nutrition, the child has gained substantial weight in a relatively short period of time.

Other Abuse-Related Syndromes

Psychologists, social workers, and other mental health professionals may be called as expert witnesses in child abuse cases to testify to matters within their competence. Such areas include testimony regarding the emotional status of the child, conditions of the child's home, and parenting techniques. "Child abuse family profile," "child sexual abuse accommodation syndrome," and the "battering parent syndrome" are terms used to denote specific behavior patterns and characteristics common to children and families where child abuse has occurred. In a very few jurisdictions testimony regarding the presence of these characteristics and syndromes common in abused children or in families in which abuse occurs may be offered into evidence by an expert to indicate the probability that the child has been abused. Other syndrome evidence that has been admitted in child abuse cases includes Munchausen syndrome by proxy— a term coined in 1977 by British pediatrician Roy Meadow—or "pediatric condition falsification" in which a caretaker falsifies or induces illness in a child for the purposes of gaining medical attention (Goldman & Yorker, 1999; Firstman & Talen, 1998).

"Shaken baby syndrome" is a term dating back to pediatric radiologist John Caffey's 1972 description of a constellation of clinical findings in cases with common injuries including retinal hemorrhage, subdural and/or subarachnoid hemorrhage, and minimal or absent signs of external cranial trauma. Estimates suggest that shaken baby syndrome accounts for 10% to 12% of all deaths attributed to abuse or neglect (Hatina, 1998). Courts in many jurisdictions are reluctant, however, to admit expert testimony regarding these syndromes because such syndromes are based on psychological factors that are speculative as compared to physical factors that are either concrete or qualitative. Because the introduction of these syndromes generally requires the prior presentation of evidence proving the abuse, these syndromes are usually introduced as rebuttal evidence.

Demonstrative Evidence

Demonstrative evidence consists of things rather than assertions of witnesses about things. Demonstrative evidence, such as photographs, medical illustrations or diagrams of the child's injuries, and x-rays, frequently helps in assisting the trier of fact in child abuse cases to understand a particular issue.

Photographs, Drawings, and X-rays

Generally, demonstrative evidence will be admitted if a proper foundation is laid. That is, it must be shown that the demonstrative object is a fair and accurate representation of the thing it purports to represent or illustrate. For example, if a physician testifies about a child's bruises and cuts observed in the hospital and then is shown a picture of the child taken at approximately the same time the physician examined the child, the physician will be allowed to testify that the photo is a "true and accurate representation" of what he or she saw. Consequently, the photograph can then be admitted into evidence and shown to the trier of fact. Similarly, drawings that indicate the location of injuries may be admitted when the proper foundation is laid.

In a criminal prosecution for child abuse, admission of photographs of the child's injuries is left to the discretion of the judge because such photographs may inflame and prejudice a jury. The judge must balance the probative value of the pictures against their prejudicial effect in ruling on admissibility.

Generally, the child's x-rays will be admitted into evidence if accompanied by testimony explaining their relevance. X-rays may reveal certain types of fractures, which, when found in a young child, are indicative of child abuse rather than accidental injury. For example, posterior rib fractures in different stages of healing in a young child are highly suggestive of physical abuse. Conversely, an x-ray may indicate an accident rather than child abuse. A fractured clavicle accompanied by bruises on the arms is indicative of an accidental fall.

Additional diagnostic tools that may be admitted into evidence include computed tomography (CT) scans and magnetic resonance imaging (MRI), which are often used in tandem to comprehensively evaluate patients.

Often, evidence collected by Child Death Review Teams will be admitted in these proceedings. Started in 1978 by Dr. Michael Durfee, a child psychologist in Los Angeles, California, local or statewide multi-agency review teams comprising various professionals, including medical examiners, law enforcement agencies, prosecuting attorneys, child protective services, pediatricians, and health professionals, examine the factors surrounding the untimely deaths of children and infants in at least 45 states at this time. (Durfee, Gellert, & Tilton-Durfee,1992).

Anatomically Detailed Dolls

The use of anatomically detailed (AD) dolls is designed to reduce the trauma to child witnesses in sexual abuse cases (Goodman, Quas, Bulkley, & Shapiro, 1999). The dolls may ease the child's experience of testifying and assist the child who has difficulty relating events using appropriate sexual or physiological terms to the trier of fact. Some states have enacted legislation expressly permitting the use of such dolls during children's testimony. In addition, expert witnesses are sometimes permitted to describe or comment on a child victim's interactions with the dolls. Because the use of such dolls has sometimes been viewed as controversial, some jurisdictions bar their use in the courtroom.

◆ REFERENCES

Adoption Assistance and Child Welfare Act (AACWA). (1980). PL 96-272.

Adoption and Safe Families Act (ASFA). (1997). PL 105-89.

Beyea, A. (1999). Competing liabilities: Responding to evidence of child abuse that surfaces during the attorney-client relationship. <u>Me L Rev, 51,</u> 269, 274-275.

Caffey, J. (1946). Multiple fractures in the long bones of infants suffering from chronic subdural hematoma. <u>American Journal of Roentgenology, 56,</u> 163-173.

Child Abuse Prevention and Treatment Act (CAPTA). (1974). PL 93-247.

Coy v. Iowa, 487 U.S. 1012, 108 S.Ct. 2798, (1988).

DeShaney v. Winnebago County Department of Social Services, 489 U.S. 189 109 S.Ct. 998 (1989).

Durfee, M. J., Gellert, G. A., & Tilton-Durfee, D. (1992). Origins and clinical relevance of child death review teams. <u>JAMA, 267</u>(23), 3172-3175.

Estelle v. McGuire, 502 U.S. 62, 112 S.Ct. 475 (1991).

Firstman, R., & Talen, J. (1998). <u>The death of innocents.</u> New York: Bantam Books.

Goldman, L. H., & Yorker, B. C. (1999). Mommie dearest? Prosecuting cases of Munchausen syndrome by proxy. <u>Crim Just, 13,</u> 26.

Goodman, G. S., Quas, J. A., Bulkley, J., & Shapiro, C. (1999). Innovations for child witnesses: A national survey. <u>Psychol Pub Pol'y & L, 5,</u> 255, 260.

Hatina, J. D. (1998). Shaken baby syndrome: Who are the true experts? <u>Clev St L Rev, 46,</u> 557, 560.

Idaho v. Wright, U.S., 110 S.Ct. 3139 (1990).

In re Gault, 387 U.S. 1, 87 S.Ct. 1248 (1967).

Indian Child Welfare Act (ICWA). (1978). U.S. Code Title 25, Indians Chapter 21.

Jaffe v. Redmond, 518 U.S. 1, 116 S.Ct. 1923 (1996).

Kempe, C. H., Silverman, F. N., Steele, B. F., Droegemueller, W., & Silver, H. K. (1962). The battered-child syndrome. <u>JAMA, 181,</u> 17.

Kentucky v. Stincer, 474 U.S. 15 (1985).

Lassiter v. Department of Social Services, 452 U.S. 18 (1981).

Maguirs, K., & Flanagan, T. J. (Eds.). (1990). <u>Sourcebook of criminal justice statistics-1990</u> (pp. 502, 526). Washington, DC: U.S. Department of Justice.

Maryland v. Craig, 497 U.S. 836; 110 S.Ct. 998 (1990).

Pennsylvania v. Ritchie, 480 U.S. 39, 107 S.Ct. 989 (1987).

Protection of Children Against Sexual Exploitation Act (PCASEA). (1977). 18 USC 2252.

Trost, C. T. (1998). Chilling child abuse reporting: Rethinking the CAPTA amendments. <u>Vanderbilt Law Rev, 51,</u> 189.

White v. Illinois, 502 U.S. 346, 112 S.Ct. 736 (1992).

Chapter 15

After the Call: Children and the Child Welfare System
Community and In-Home Services or Out-of-Home Placement

Heather Forkey, M.D.
Karen Hudson, M.S.W., L.S.W.
Patricia H. Manz, Ph.D.
Judith A. Silver, Ph.D.

The events that follow a report of suspected maltreatment to the child protective services (CPS) agency have a significant impact on the child and family. The report triggers an investigation to determine the report's precipitating circumstances and legitimacy. These determinations are followed by identifying services that need to be provided to the child and the family, including a variety of child protective services, as well as in-home and community-based services. The aims of this chapter are to enhance the mandated reporter's understanding of the range of possible outcomes after filing a report of suspected child abuse or neglect and to assist in defining his or her role in supporting children and families. It describes the investigation process and its outcomes, as well as the roles of CPS and child welfare professionals, child advocates, and foster parents. In addition, it concisely reviews out-of-home placements, such as foster care and kinship care; parent-centered programs; and community-based services, including early intervention programs, educational services, and community mental health centers. CPS laws and child welfare systems vary from state to state. This chapter presents general information, and readers are advised to consult the laws and regulations of the state(s) in which they practice for the specifics of their state's procedures.

Acknowledgement:
Preparation of this chapter was supported in part by a grant from The Pew Charitable Trusts to J. Silver. The authors gratefully acknowledge Eleanor Bush, Esq., and Raymond Meyers, D.S.W., for their careful review of the manuscript.

◆ THE INVESTIGATION PROCESS AND ITS OUTCOMES

The immediate response to a report of suspected maltreatment is to determine if the child has been intentionally harmed. This is done through an investigative process: a series of procedures to identify and respond to allegations of child abuse and neglect. This investigation is the responsibility of the county or state public child welfare agency, within its CPS section, and includes the following components and procedures:

- Notifying the parent/guardian or caregiver of the child that there is an allegation of maltreatment and describing the process of the investigation

- Examining the nature and circumstances of the injuries or event that led to the report of suspected maltreatment

- Interviewing and physically examining any child(ren) in the household

- Interviewing the parent(s) to obtain a brief social history regarding the family, personal situations, child care, discipline patterns, marital issues, drug or alcohol history, and employment history

- Interviewing any people alleged to have been involved in the maltreatment

- Possibly interviewing friends, relatives, neighbors, and others who know the child, family, or alleged perpetrator

- Seeking medical, psychological, or psychiatric evaluations of the child, depending on the characteristics of the case

- Considering any previous allegations of child maltreatment

- Determining whether the child is in immediate danger if he or she remains with his or her parent(s), guardian, or caregiver (Besharov, 1990)

In addition, the investigation may include interviews with other people who have had contact with the allegedly maltreated child and a review of pertinent records. For example, the CPS investigator may visit the child's school to interview teachers or other school personnel and review school records. In cases where a child is hospitalized due to injuries, the CPS investigator may interview hospital staff and review hospital records. The investigation might include visits to the child's home and other places where the child spends a lot of time, such as the homes of relatives, daycare providers, or babysitters.

The CPS investigation can result in one of two possible outcomes (see Figure 15-1 for an overview of the investigation process and possible outcomes). First, if the investigation yielded insufficient evidence to prove the allegation of abuse or neglect, the CPS worker will dismiss the complaint as *unsubstantiated*. This determination does not mean that no help can be offered to the family. The family may be eligible for services even if the case is unsubstantiated. For example, consider a case in which preschool personnel noticed bruises on Johnny's cheek and shoulder and contacted the child abuse hotline. The investigation indicated plausible explanations for Johnny's bruises, and there was no indication of abuse or neglect. However, during the course of the investigation, Johnny's mother commented that she was struggling with the management of Johnny's behavior and that of his siblings. The CPS worker provided a referral for the mother to enroll in a parent education and support program.

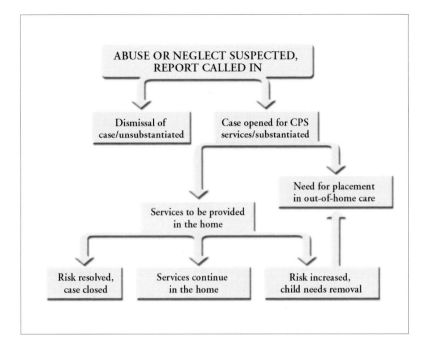

Figure 15-1. *Overview of the investigation process and possible outcomes.*

Alternatively, if the evaluation indicated that maltreatment occurred, the complaint is *substantiated*. In these cases, the immediate decision is to determine a safe placement for the child and to delineate needed support services for the child and family.

DETERMINATION OF SAFE PLACEMENT FOR SUBSTANTIATED CASES

The aims of the CPS or child welfare professional are to protect the child by attempting to strengthen the family while decreasing the risk of future abuse, and to prevent the unnecessary removal of the child from the parents' care. When there is a substantiated report of child maltreatment but removal of the child does not seem necessary, the CPS worker will recommend to the family or juvenile court judge that the conditions resulting in maltreatment can be addressed while the child remains in the home. Jones (as cited in Pecora, 1991a) describes the array of possible services to support family preservation as a "continuum of foster care prevention services" (p. 22). This continuum includes community-based education and support services that are available to any interested parent (i.e., there are no eligibility criteria to participate), and services for families at risk for continuing child maltreatment, such as in-home services, family-based services, and intensive family preservation services (Child Welfare League of America, 1988; Pecora, 1991a). The CPS worker makes specific recommendations or referrals or indicates the need for direct services to the family. If warranted, the CPS worker can take legal action to supervise the care of the child in the parents' home. Under this circumstance the family is legally required to accept services within the home.

At times, the CPS professional is faced with the difficult decision to remove the children from the parent's care. The CPS professional is compelled to ". . . balance the needs of children for protection with their need for family continuity . . . ," which can present " . . . a complex set of competing priorities . . . " (Berrick, Barth, & Gilbert, 1997, p. xi). As one expert on child welfare has noted:

> . . . Despite the proliferation of statutes, policies, and legal precedents, decision-making in this area is heavily influenced by a number of idiosyncratic factors. These include, among others, availability of prevention and placement resources; values and biases of service providers; presence of strong advocates for the parents or children; attitudes of juvenile court judges toward placement; rigor of the screening process (Pecora 1991c [Publisher's note: Pecora, 1991b]; Tracy, 1991); ambiguities in the definition of abuse, neglect and child protection; and the imprecise nature of information about human behavior and the impossibility of predicting the future (Pecora, Whittaker, Maluccio, Barth, & Plotnick, 1992, p. 327).

Out-of-home care may include placement in a variety of settings, including a non-relative family foster home, kinship care, a group home, or a children's shelter. For children with special needs, out-of-home care may involve residential care or inpatient treatment for drug and alcohol problems, psychiatric or behavioral problems, developmental disabilities, complex medical conditions, or any combination of these (Fig. 15-2).

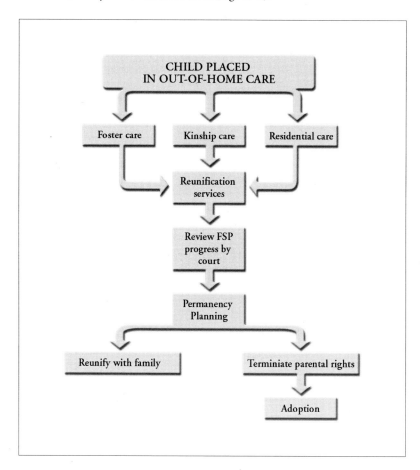

Figure 15-2. *Options for out-of-home care.*

LEGAL PROCEDURES TO REMOVE CHILDREN FROM THEIR HOMES

Despite all efforts by child welfare agencies and community-based service providers to provide supplemental and supportive services, some children are not going to be safe in their own homes and must be placed in out-of-home care. When children are removed from the home, there are well-defined legal steps that occur, depending upon the circumstances of the children's removal. The simplest situation occurs when the parents voluntarily agree to placement by CPS. An example is the case of a single parent who requires hospitalization and has no relatives or friends to care for the children. In this situation, no formal legal hearing needs to occur. The parent voluntarily places his or her children in foster care and the court is not involved. Hence, the court does not serve as an external monitor. In this arrangement, parents retain the right to terminate the placement at any time. It is a time-limited, written agreement that typically expires after an established number of days (e.g., in Pennsylvania it expires after 30 days; the amount of time varies widely among different states). There are other situations in which parents may be offered the option of voluntary placement, such as in cases where they have insufficient money to properly care for the children (e.g., the family has been cut off from welfare benefits), or if the parent is feeling despondent and unable to cope. These are conditions in which the children may have been experiencing neglect, and the CPS worker anticipates that over the period of time specified in the voluntary agreement, the parents will be able achieve whatever is necessary to properly care for the children. However, if the voluntary placement agreement expires and there have been insufficient changes in the home to protect the children, CPS will go to court to obtain a court order of temporary custody (OTC) and proceed to have the children maintained in out-of-home care through involuntary placement (Fig. 15-3).

Involuntary placement describes the situation in which the CPS worker will seek a court order to remove children from the home against the parents' wishes. In

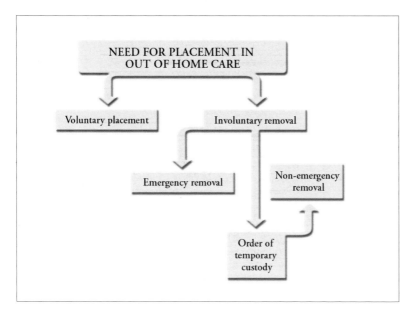

Figure 15-3. Process of involuntary placement.

extreme cases where the children are believed to be in immediate danger, an emergency involuntary placement may occur prior to the CPS investigation. Typically, this situation results in removal of all of the children in the home, not just the one whose alleged maltreatment prompted the investigation.

In the case of emergency involuntary placement, a detention hearing must be held within 24 to 72 hours to obtain an OTC. The OTC permits the CPS agency to maintain the children in emergency custody until a full court hearing with the parents can be held. The CPS worker can petition the court for an OTC without first having a custody hearing if the life or safety of a child is at risk, and the parents are refusing to allow removal from the home. The agency must submit an affidavit setting forth the facts that warrant immediate protection of the child or children. This detention hearing is the first involvement of the court.

Three additional formal hearings must be held within a brief period after the CPS agency has obtained the OTC. These hearings are conducted to formally evaluate and determine the custody of the children (Figure 15-4). First, a *preliminary hearing* (sometimes called a "detention" or "shelter" hearing) is held, in which parents either consent to or contest the petition by CPS for temporary custody of the children. The *adjudicatory hearing* determines whether abuse or neglect has occurred as defined by state law. The adjudicatory hearing is a fact-finding hearing in which evidence must be presented to prove that the children have been neglected or abused. This information is derived from the report of the CPS investigation. Professionals who are mandated reporters may be called as expert witnesses to present evidence and give opinions about the cause of a child's injuries. The emphasis is on the results of the parents' actions and not on the actions per se. Even if parental conduct is believed to be grossly inappropriate, unless the child has physical or demonstrable psychological damage or is in imminent peril of such damage, he or she is not a neglected or abused child. The third step is the *dispositional hearing*, which is conducted if

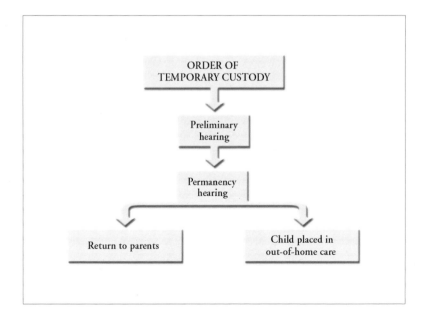

Figure 15-4. Legal process after obtaining a court order of temporary custody (OTC).

the evidence has proved that the child was neglected or abused. It is a decision-making hearing and represents the initial disposition of the case. At this time a child can be placed in a foster home or remain in his or her family's home under a program of protective supervision.

Under the Adoption Assistance and Child Welfare Act of 1980 (AACWA), the plan established in the dispositional hearing is reviewed every 6 months to monitor the continuing necessity for and appropriateness of the placement, the extent of the parents' compliance with the case plan, the degree of progress toward mitigating the causes of placement, and the projected date by which the child may be returned home or placed for adoption or legal guardianship. With the passage of the Adoption and Safe Families Act of 1997 (ASFA), the child's safety is also assessed in these biannual reviews. In other words, this review reassesses the parents' ability to care for the child and reviews the steps that have been taken by the child welfare agency to reunify the family (as outlined in the Family Service Plan developed by the child welfare professional; see below). If the initial disposition calls for reunification efforts to be made, a permanency hearing will occur later. Under ASFA, the first permanency hearing must occur no later than 12 months after placement in out-of-home care. Some states have legislation requiring a shorter time frame in which the first permanency hearing should be conducted. Thereafter the court must hold a permanency hearing every 12 months for as long as the child remains in placement. These hearings determine the actual permanency plan for the child (e.g., reunification or adoption), as opposed to simply reviewing compliance with the plan.

ASFA introduced certain circumstances under which an immediate permanency hearing must be held. These conditions are determined by state law. In general, if the court determines that the circumstances of the abuse, neglect, or other maltreatment were severe enough to warrant excusing the agency from making *any* reunification efforts, then a permanency hearing would have to be held fairly immediately to determine the permanent place for the child (such as adoption or placement in the legal custody of a relative).

Following a period of foster care placement, the court will re-evaluate the most suitable placement for the child. The court may permanently terminate parents' rights to their children if one of the three situations has occurred: (1) the parents have not complied with the objectives specified in the Family Service Plan, (2) the parents are not interested in having the children returned to their care, or (3) the parents have not made sufficient progress toward improving the home situation. Often, termination is not granted unless reasonable efforts to help the family have failed, and the parents have demonstrated no active efforts or ability to improve. The benefit of termination of parental rights is that it allows the children to be available for adoption (Fig. 15-2) and thus achieve permanency.

♦ PERTINENT LEGISTRATION DRIVING CHILD WELFARE POLICY AND PRACTICE

Two major pieces of legislation have shaped current policy and practice in CPS and child welfare activities: the Adoption Assistance and Child Welfare Act of 1980 (PL 96-272) and the Adoption and Safe Families Act of 1997 (PL 105-89). AACWA was passed by Congress to address concerns that too many children were placed in out-of-home care, including disproportionate numbers of minority children; that for many children, placement could have been prevented if supportive services had been provided to maintain them within their families; and that too many children lacked specific case plans and languished for years in out-of-home care without any efforts directed toward helping them achieve a permanent home (Pecora, 1991a). In response to these problems, AACWA directed states to increase efforts to prevent out-of-home placement by preserving families, reunifying families when possible, and proceeding to adoption (rather than long-term foster care) when reunification was not possible. State eligibility for federal funding for foster care was linked to these requirements. Specifically, these goals were addressed in the following steps:

- Mandating child welfare agencies to create and implement permanency plans with periodic reviews. These permanency plans, often called Family Service Plans (FSPs), were meant to move children towards either reunification or adoption more directly and eliminate "foster care drift" (i.e., children who become lost in the system without any genuine permanency plan year after year).

- Providing greater funding and attention to family preservation services (see below), both to prevent the placement of children and to give biological parents the supports they need to reunite with their children.

- Providing funding to subsidize adoptive placements for children who could not be returned to their families.

In 1997 Congress amended AACWA by passing ASFA. ASFA shifted the balance of efforts away from family preservation and reunification toward greater emphasis on the child's safety and swift achievement of permanency for the child. This legislation aims to accomplish these goals through the following:

- Clarifying that a child's health and safety are the paramount concerns in determining whether to remove a child from the home or to reunify the family. Therefore "reasonable efforts" at reunification or family preservation do not need to be taken under certain circumstances. Examples of such circumstances are if the child's parents have committed specific types of felonies, including murder or voluntary manslaughter of the child's sibling; had parental rights to a sibling involuntarily terminated; or subjected the child to abandonment, torture, chronic abuse, sexual abuse, or other "aggravated circumstances" (U.S. General Accounting Office [USGAO], 1999; Winterfield, 1998).

- Initiating the termination of parental rights proceeds when a child has been in foster care 15 out of the past 22 months and the parents have not made progress on the FSP (that is, the parents exerted minimal effort and/or demonstrated insufficient achievement of the objectives necessary for the child to be reunited with them).

In addition, to accomplish its goals, ASFA shortened the period to implement the child's permanency plan from 18 to 12 months. It authorizes concurrent planning for both reunification and adoption to occur after adjudication of a child as abused or neglected, rather than delaying adoption planning until after the termination of parental rights. Finally, ASFA provides financial incentives for states to increase the number of children adopted out of foster care (Children's Defense Fund (CDF), 1997; Winterfield, 1998).

◆ THE PLAYERS: ROLES AND RESPONSIBILITIES OF PROFESSIONALS, VOLUNTEERS, AND FOSTER PARENTS

CHILD WELFARE PROFESSIONALS

CHILD ABUSE HOTLINE WORKERS

At the core of child protection lies decision-making and judgments regarding individual cases. Those professionals who screen calls to the state or county child abuse hotline decide whether or not the report merits an investigation. They also determine the level of urgency given the case, which then affects the response time in initiating an investigation (Stein & Rzepnicki, 1983). The mandated reporter must be mindful that the hotline staff may be unfamiliar with certain medical, psychiatric, and other risk factors and with their adverse potentials. It is important for the mandated reporter to explain medical and other risks in terms laymen can understand rather than assume that they are familiar with the conditions and associated after-effects. This is especially true in cases of physical neglect and medical neglect. For example, a nurse observed that a toddler had an inflammation on her face that could spread rapidly to the eye, with the potential to cause blindness. She informed the toddler's foster mother of this danger and strongly urged her to have the child seen by a physician that day or within the next 24 hours. Follow-up calls to the foster family indicated that they did not comply with this urgent recommendation. In making the report to the child abuse hotline, the nurse presented her concern that the child may have been suffering from *cellulitis* and explained the imminent danger if the condition were not treated promptly.

CHILD PROTECTIVE SERVICE WORKERS

CPS workers play important roles in substantiating a report of suspected abuse and in connecting maltreating families to needed medical, psychological, and social services. As already stated, CPS workers investigate allegations of abuse and neglect. Based on their investigations, these individuals must determine whether or not a child has experienced maltreatment and what steps must be taken in protecting the child. Specific agency guidelines and policies, as well as supervisory direction, are critical factors in this decision-making process. The CPS worker must:

- Make a determination of immediate danger, that is, severe or life-threatening danger.

- Establish credible evidence of abuse or neglect. State laws define abuse and neglect. The CPS worker is mandated by state law to present clear and distinct evidence of maltreatment as defined by law. The subjective feelings of the CPS worker will not stand up in a court of law.

- Decide if the family is eligible for voluntary services. The CPS worker must determine if the family meets specific eligibility criteria as defined by individual programs.

- Define the specific problems to be addressed.

- Justify whether out-of-home placement is absolutely necessary and, if so, determine the most appropriate type of placement. This decision is made in direct response to the question of immediate danger and requires determination of a safe environment for the children if their home is not an option and there is no opportunity for placement with relatives. Often the CPS worker also must locate placement and secure necessary funding.

- Initiate appropriate court involvement. A judge will determine the necessity of out-of-home placement based on all of the evidence presented (Stein & Rzepnicki, 1983).

After the dispositional hearing is held, cases typically are transferred from the investigatory section of the public child welfare agency to the ongoing services section. Within the ongoing services section, a child welfare worker is assigned to work with the family to jointly establish the FSP, which specifies objectives for the family to achieve in order for the child welfare agency to close the case and, if the child has been removed from the home, for reunification to take place. This FSP also specifies the necessary medical, psychological, and social services to be offered to the family. The child welfare worker links the family to these services to support them in their efforts to achieve the FSP objectives (see section on alternatives to out-of-home care). This plan is reviewed semi-annually, within the context of a permanency hearing.

In many large urban communities, the public child welfare agency has contracts with private child welfare and social service agencies to provide the direct services to the child's family, the child, and, when children are in placement, the provider of out-of-home care. The public child welfare caseworker has ultimate responsibility for the case and provides oversight. The private contractual agency child welfare worker is responsible for working directly with the child's family to achieve the objectives of the FSP and working with the child and foster family to ensure that the child's needs are met. In less populated communities, this role may be fulfilled by the public child welfare agency caseworker.

CHILD ADVOCATES

After a report of child maltreatment is substantiated, the state or county may recommend interventions with the child's parents or caregivers, such as family support services or counseling. The court then authorizes implementation of the recommendations by the public child welfare agency. The parents may dispute these recommendations and resist the interventions. In such legal disputes, the child's interests may not be fully represented by the state or by the child's parents. Consequently, in most states the court appoints advocates specifically to represent the interests of the child. Assignment of a child advocate ensures that the child is recognized as an independent party, with distinct interests separate from those of the other litigants (that is, the state/public child welfare agency and the child's parents/caregivers). The presiding judge in a child abuse case may select a child advocate from a range of resources: public or private non-profit legal advocacy agencies, private law firms in which the attorney is providing pro bono services (working without financial compensation), "court-appointed" lawyers who are in private practice and receive a fee from the court for such cases, and court-appointed special advocates (CASAs). CASAs are volunteers (typically laypersons) who speak for and represent the interests of the child, and who often are paired with the court-appointed lawyer who represents the child in court (O'Grady & Birns, 1999).

The responsibilities of the child advocate may be determined by statute or by the nature of the judge's appointment. Among attorneys, the child advocate may be appointed as legal counsel for the child, or as a guardian ad litem. When the appointment is that of legal counsel, the child advocate functions in the same way that an attorney does for any adult client, by striving to advance the expressed interests and desires of the child. The attorney is essentially serving as a spokesperson for the child, regardless of whether the attorney agrees with the child-client that these desires are in the best interest of the child. This is the typical attorney-client relationship (O'Grady & Birns, 1999). In contrast, when serving as a guardian ad litem for a child, the attorney or other person appointed by the judge seeks information and then advocates in court regarding what, in the guardian ad litem's opinion, is in the best interest of the child.

Generally, child advocates are legally entitled to all information and records that concern a child. Consequently, it is not a breach of confidentiality for a healthcare or mental health professional or an educator to share information with the child's advocate. Professionals who interact with the child in various contexts (e.g., school, child care center) should contact the child's legal advocate if they believe that the child welfare agencies responsible for the child's care have failed to consider the professional's recommendations to the potential detriment of the child. Professionals can contact the legal advocates and CASAs by phone, fax, or mail. It is helpful to provide a succinct summary of the key issue(s) to the advocate in writing, with an offer to discuss the issue further. Professionals should maintain written documentation of their contacts with the child's caregivers and child welfare workers and be willing to testify in court when requested. It is important to keep in mind that both the lawyers and CASA volunteers working on behalf of the child typically are not trained in the healthcare professions, child development, or mental health. Therefore, unless the professional makes information available to the advocates, they very likely may overlook issues relevant to the child's health and well-being when in court. For example, in the case of a toddler who experienced a decline in her rate of weight gain over time, both the state CPS investigator and the legal advocate accepted the contention of the parent's attorney that the child had indeed gained several pounds between doctor's visits. However, a concerned pediatric nurse practitioner who was following the child noted that the small number of pounds gained was significantly (even dangerously) below the amount expected over the interval between clinic appointments. She explained that the *rate* of the child's weight gain was aberrant and that it indicated insufficient caloric intake and possible neglect. The nurse practitioner encouraged the child's advocate to seek an evaluation for failure to thrive by an experienced pediatrician in order to determine whether the child's poor growth was due to a medical problem or to neglect.

FOSTER PARENTS

The role of the foster parent is critical for the child's well-being: ". . . This person or couple has the responsibility to satisfy a child's basic needs for love, protection, food, shelter, clothing, education, exercise, health, and well-being . . . " (Ross & Crawford, 1999, p. 279). Foster parents are recruited by both public and private child welfare agencies to serve as surrogate parents for children who have experienced maltreatment or abandonment, or whose parents cannot care for them. Foster parents are charged with providing a nurturing family environment for the children under their supervision, yet this role contains inherent contradictions due to the unique legal context experienced by children in foster care. ". . . Foster parents repeatedly are caught in a double bind between assuming responsibility (including advocacy) for the child and not having the authority to accomplish what is needed in a given situation" (Ross & Crawford, 1999, p. 282). For example, the foster parent often cannot consent to medical interventions, which may include psychotherapy for a depressed child or early intervention services (such as physical therapy) for a developmentally delayed toddler. ASFA requires that foster parents receive notice of all administrative reviews and court hearings and be given the opportunity to speak. However, ASFA does not give foster parents legal standing to enforce their foster children's rights or to make requests for services on their behalf.

Prospective foster parents undergo an evaluation and pre-service training process before achieving a license or certificate that permits them to care for foster children, with requirements varying depending on the state of residence. Questions have been raised regarding the quality of the evaluation process, as well as preservice and continuing education programs, in relation to equipping foster parents to care for the complex behavioral, emotional, medical, and developmental needs of contemporary foster children (Ross & Crawford, 1999; Simms & Halfon, 1994; Zukoski, 1999). Foster parents typically do not receive payment for their efforts and legally are not considered employees of the child welfare agency that assigns foster children to their households and supervises the foster parents. They receive a small stipend for each foster child's expenses, which averaged far less than $20.00 per day at the time this chapter went to press (Ross & Crawford, 1999).

There is much confusion regarding issues of privacy and confidentiality, which often prevents child welfare professionals from communicating information important to the well-being of children in foster care to their foster parents (Ross & Crawford, 1999; Silver, Haecker, & Forkey, 1999). As a result, foster parents often are uninformed regarding children's social and medical histories, which can impede the children's timely access to needed health, mental health, developmental, and special education services, and can disrupt continuity of care. People often assume that information regarding a child's medical or psychosocial history cannot be shared, and this assumption may be wrong (although state and local statutes vary). For example, in Pennsylvania, confidentiality rules permit county child welfare agencies to share relevant information with service providers so that they can provide needed services. In Philadelphia, these rules have been interpreted to include providing pertinent health and psychosocial information to foster parents and health care providers to ensure that the child in foster care obtains appropriate health care. The reader is encouraged to consult with the National Center for Youth Law in Oakland California (www.youthlaw.org) to access information on laws and regulations of the state(s) in which they practice and to identify local legal advocacy organizations that may assist in discussing the interpretation of these statutes.

Mandated reporters who have had ongoing involvement with maltreated children should consider notifying the public child welfare authorities of the child's special needs, with the recommendation for measures that will ensure continuity of care after the child enters placement. A copy of this notification should be forwarded to the child's legal advocate to reinforce the likelihood that the recommendation will be considered.

With the dramatic rise in the numbers of children entering foster care since the mid-1980s, there has been an accompanying decrease in the pool of available foster homes as women have entered the workforce in large numbers. These demographic shifts have resulted in significant changes in the placement of children into foster care. On a positive note, there has been increasing reliance upon placing children with members of their extended families in kinship care (see below), which has been shown to decrease the number of placement changes and disruptions the child experiences (Berrick, Barth, & Needell, 1994). On the negative side, as many communities encounter a dearth of adequate foster homes, there has been a tendency toward overcrowding available homes with too many needy children or relying upon foster parents whose capabilities are known to be less than adequate (Kronstadt, 1999; Zuravin, Benedict, & Somerfield, 1993). Although all licensed or certified foster parents have undergone both criminal and child abuse background checks, children placed in foster care can be victims of neglect and abuse within these homes (Zuravin et al., 1993). Consequently, even if a child has an open case with the local child welfare agency, when the mandated reporter observes signs of suspected neglect or abuse, he or she is advised to follow the same procedures as with any child and to report the suspected maltreatment to the authorities.

♦ SERVICES RECEIVED BY CHILDREN AND FAMILIES AFTER THE CALL

FOSTER CARE

Children enter out-of-home care when the court orders their removal from the family home due to maltreatment, when the determination of immediate danger is made, or when voluntary arrangements are made with the child welfare system because of a parent's incapacity to care for the child. The public child welfare system is responsible for over 600,000 children placed in out-of-home care. The most prevalent type of placement is foster care, in which the child lives with a non-related caregiver in the caregiver's family home. The second most widely used placement option is kinship care, when the child is placed in the home of a related family member (Petit & Curtis, 1997). The reliance upon formal kinship care arrangements as placement options has increased dramatically since the late 1980s (Barth, Courtney, Berrick, & Albert, 1994; Gleeson & Craig, 1994; Needell & Gilbert, 1997; Wulczyn, Hardin, & Goerge, 1997).

Foster care and other forms of out-of-home care are meant to be temporary arrangements. Indeed, approximately half of all children entering placement are reunited with their parents after approximately 1 month (Halfon, Berkowitz, & Klee, 1992; Kutzler, 1997). For the mandated reporter, this information highlights the importance of a thoughtful approach in dealing with the child's family, even the perpetrator of maltreatment, at the time one is compelled to file a child abuse report. In a large number of cases, children who are removed from their parents' care will be returned to their homes. To decrease the likelihood that the family will subsequently avoid helping agencies or services represented by the mandated reporter, it is important to maintain a professional, nonjudgmental demeanor that is supportive of the family's dignity. The aim is to "keep the door open" so that the family will continue to seek healthcare or mental health services and support the child's school attendance. In most cases, it is suggested that the mandated reporter calmly inform the parent of the concern for the child's well-being and the legal requirement to report, rather than conceal this action. The parent can be informed that the alleged maltreatment suggests that the family may benefit from supports that can be made available through child welfare services.

Unfortunately, placement in foster care does not ensure that the best interests of the child are met. There are complex systemic problems, including lack of adequate funding, high worker turnover due to high case loads, stressful working conditions, limited training to cope with children and families' complex problems, and an insufficient number of experienced foster parents. Children often experience multiple placements, which are deeply disruptive for them. Multiple placements affect children's emotional functioning and development, as well as their education. If children have special needs, such as chronic medical conditions, developmental delays or disorders, or psychiatric and behavioral problems, changing placements disrupts the continuity of health care, early intervention, special education, and/or mental health services.

Ironically, children's health care needs tend to be underserved when they are in foster care. This is true for even routine, preventive health care (i.e., "check-ups" or "well child visits"). Many children in foster care are underimmunized and fail to visit a healthcare provider according to appropriate pediatric guidelines. Consequently, emerging medical problems may go unidentified and untreated (USGAO, 1995). Medical problems can result from physical abuse, neglect, or sexual abuse, or they may be related to medical conditions untreated prior to placement. Delays in immunizations and poor control of chronic diseases such as asthma, undernutrition, and growth deficiency are common. Many children suffer from a mother's inadequate prenatal care or from prenatal exposure to drugs or alcohol. The number of children in foster care with genetic malformation syndromes, central nervous system abnormalities, and isolated birth defects is unusually high. These needs have been well-documented (Chernoff, Combs-Orme, Risley-Curtiss, & Heisler, 1994; Halfon, Mendonca, & Berkowitz, 1995; Hochstadt, Jaudes, Zimo, & Schachter, 1987; Kavaler & Swire, 1983; Schor, 1988; Simms, 1989). Research conducted by the USGAO on 22,000 children, however, indicated that the medical needs of children under age 3 years in foster care were met in fewer than half the cases. One third were not adequately immunized and 12% had no medical care at all (USGAO, 1995).

State regulations vary regarding the time frame in which child welfare agencies must ensure that children who have recently entered out-of-home care receive a comprehensive pediatric evaluation. In many states this interval is 60 days for children in family foster care, despite the recommendations by the American Academy of Pediatrics (1994) and the Child Welfare League of America (1988) that comprehensive pediatric evaluations should be conducted within 14 days of the child entering foster care. The 14-day time frame is preferable, considering approximately half of all children entering foster care return to their parents within 1 month. In these cases, when a physical examination is not scheduled to be conducted before placement ends, the opportunity to address unrecognized healthcare needs is lost.

KINSHIP CARE

In the 1980s a number of demographic and policy changes resulted in an increased reliance on members of children's extended families to provide out-of-home care. Kinship care increased as a formal arrangement due to the increasing number of children in need of placements and the decreasing number of non-related foster families available to provide care. The passage of AACWA in 1980 supported this trend with the mandate that children should be placed in "the most family-like setting possible . . . " (Courtney & Needell, 1997, p. 131).

Historically, informal child care arrangements with relatives from the extended family have been a resource to many parents who are unable or unwilling to provide adequate care for their children. These arrangements, often sought by child welfare professionals, were unregulated, with no efforts to monitor children's well-being or to provide supports to the kin who cared for them (Needell & Gilbert, 1997; Takas, 1993). In the 1980s states began to formalize kinship care arrangements. These measures included a stipend for providing children's care and formal means of documenting and monitoring care, although there is broad variability among the states in terms of payment and supervision (Needell & Gilbert, 1997).

Research indicates that kinship care providers tend to have fewer financial resources and less education than foster parents. Many confront the challenges of poverty (Needell & Gilbert, 1997). Children placed with relatives often continue to have unidentified and unmet healthcare needs in levels similar to children placed in foster care (Dubowitz et al., 1994). On a positive note, several empirical studies have indicated that children placed in kinship care, when compared to those in foster care, are less likely to experience abuse, multiple placements, and placement in a group home. In addition, they are less likely to re-enter substitute care after reunification of their families (Barth, 1997; Courtney, 1995; Courtney & Needell, 1997).

ALTERNATIVES TO OUT-OF-HOME CARE

The problems associated with out-of-home care, including those that led to the passage of AACWA, resulted in the increasing reliance on a broad array of community-based and home-based prevention and intervention programs. Some aim to prevent maltreatment and/or out-of-home placement; others strive to strengthen families. The sad reality that parents are the perpetrators in the overwhelming majority (87%) of substantiated child maltreatment cases underscores the need to include them in preventive and treatment services (U.S. Department of Health and Human Services [USDHHS], 2000). Parents who abuse or neglect their children are often coping with numerous economic or personal difficulties, such as poverty, loss of employment, or other incidences of family or domestic violence (Egeland, Jacobvitz, & Sroufe, 1988; Zigler, Hopper, & Hall, 1993). In addition, many of these parents are socially isolated and do not have strong interpersonal connections with extended family members and neighbors or adequate resources for accessing health and human services in their communities (Zigler & Black, 1989).

PARENT- OR FAMILY-CENTERED PROGRAMS

Parent- or family-centered programs focus on supporting parents who are at risk to harm their children or who have previously harmed them (see Repucci, Britner, & Woolard, 1997, for a thorough review).

Parent Education Programs

Parent education programs are based on the assumption that maltreating parents have limited knowledge about the developmental capacities and limitations that affect child behavior, in addition to limited and harsh ways of directing and disciplining their children. As a result, these parents are likely to experience children's behavior as negative or defiant and respond harshly. Evidence for the relationship of parents' unrealistic or negative attributions about child behavior and child maltreatment is contradictory (Rosenberg & Repucci, 1983). Evaluations of parent education programs have demonstrated their effectiveness in teaching child development and positive parenting strategies (Wekerle & Wolfe, 1993). However, significant evidence for their effectiveness in reducing child abuse or neglect has not been documented.

Family Support Programs

Programs that support the family unit are strategically situated within communities. By integrating the program within the community, services are more easily accessed and can create a social network within the neighborhood. Family support programs strive to respond to the perceived needs of the families residing within the community and offer an array of services, including parent education, health and nutrition education, counseling, and child care (Andrews, Bishop, & Sussman, 1999; Wekerle & Wolfe, 1993). Evaluations of family support programs are favorable. These programs are associated with a reduction in child maltreatment, in addition to improvements in parent and child health, child development, and parent-child relationships (Andrews et al., 1982; Armstrong & Fraley, 1985; Olds & Kitzman, 1990).

Home-Visiting Programs

Home-visiting programs provide comprehensive services to families at risk for, or with a history of, child maltreatment. Similar to family support programs, home-visiting programs can include an array of educational, health, and child development services. A professional or paraprofessional delivers these services in the home. The effectiveness of this approach varies greatly according to the type of services offered and the method for delivering them. Components of effective home-visiting programs include the availability of multiple services, the delivery of services over an extended period of time, and the provision of services community-wide to avoid stigmatizing families in which maltreatment has been suspected or found (Olds & Kitzman, 1990). Research has indicated that among high-risk families, home visiting by a nurse initiated during the pregnancy up to the child's second birthday resulted in lower rates of child abuse and neglect, and fewer accidental injuries, ingestions, and trips to hospital emergency rooms than among matched controls (Olds, Henderson, Chamberlin, & Tatelbaum, 1986). Marcenko (1999) found that home visits by a paraprofessional resulted in more foster care placements, but that the children's length of stay in substitute care was significantly briefer. There was also a greater rate of reunification among home-visited families than among the matched controls.

INTENSIVE FAMILY PRESERVATION SERVICES

In contrast to the above alternatives to placement, Intensive Family Preservation Services (IFPS) are provided to families who are in significant crisis and who are at imminent risk of having their children placed in out-of-home care. These programs are characterized by an intensive provision of crisis-oriented services involving both clinical services and concrete supports on a time-limited (4 to 8 weeks) basis. Professionals providing IFPS typically work with the family in their home 5 to 8 direct contact hours per week and are available to the family on call 24 hours per day. IFPS workers have small caseloads to accommodate this intensive schedule (Fraser, Pecora, & Haapala, 1991). In some communities IFPS is followed up by a less intensive, more typical home-visiting program to reinforce any gains accomplished during the IFPS phase of services. Evaluation of the pioneering IFPS program, known as the Homebuilders Program, indicated favorable outcomes in improving child and parent interactions and in preventing foster placement (Kinney, Haapala, Booth, & Leavitt, 1990). This program provided a high degree of training and supervision for its providers. Research on other IFPS efforts has been inconsistent due to methodological difficulties inherent in field studies (Pecora, 1991a). Research suggests that IFPS is not effective with families in which the parents or children are struggling with alcoholism or drug abuse, or when the child is delinquent (Lewis, 1991). Fraser et al. (1991) and associates also present ". . . one serious implication. Because the provision of these services leads to a situation in which children who are thought to be at risk of child neglect and other social problems are not removed from the home, some children may be endangered by the decision to provide IFPS rather than substitute care services" (p. 10).

COMMUNITY RESOURCES FOR MALTREATED CHILDREN

There is an extensive body of research indicating that children who have been maltreated have elevated rates of emotional and behavioral problems, developmental delays, and poor school achievement (Aber, Allen, Carlson, & Cicchetti, 1989; Crittendon, 1985; George & Main, 1979; McIntyre, Lounsbury, Berntson, & Steel, 1988; Toth, Manly, & Cicchetti, 1992; Van der Kock & Fisler, 1994). It is not surprising that the high rates of these problems have also been documented among children who are placed in foster care and kinship care (Dubowitz, Zuravin, Starr, Feigelman, & Harrington, 1993; Halfon, Mendonca, & Berkowitz, 1995; Hochstadt et al., 1987; Silver et al., 1999). Due to these vulnerabilities, children with histories of neglect or abuse often need additional supports to improve their social, emotional, and cognitive outcomes. This section will discuss systems that can serve as resources for maltreated children: community-based mental health services, Head Start and Early Head Start programs, early intervention services, and public schools.

COMMUNITY-BASED MENTAL HEALTH SERVICES

Community-based mental health centers are subsidized programs for providing a variety of psychological services. These centers were designed to expand the availability of mental health services in low-income communities, where many families experience financial and logistical constraints in seeking appropriate healthcare programs. Community mental health centers are located within neighborhoods to ease accessibility and are structured to accommodate the financial circumstances of the families. The availability of mental health services for children and families varies among community-based mental health centers and can include psychiatric assessment, psychological evaluation, counseling, and partial hospitalization programs.

Although community mental health centers are advantageously located to enhance the accessibility of psychological services to economically disadvantaged families, there are limitations which impede the delivery of sufficient, quality services that the mandated reporter may be able to mitigate. Despite a proliferation of community mental health centers over the past three decades, the availability of centers is not proportional to the needs of many children and families across the United States (CDF, 1995). Given this reality, the mandated reporter can serve an important role in supporting and assisting families in connecting to community mental health centers. Families can benefit from assistance in locating the appropriate center, making the initial appointment, and preparing for the visit (i.e., making transportation arrangements, completing paperwork, organizing information and records).

Once connected to community mental health centers, families may need support in sustaining their participation. For example, families with economic and employment difficulties may find frequent intervention visits to be incompatible with parents' work schedules. In addition, some families may find intervention strategies to be inconsistent with their cultural values or perspectives of acceptable child-rearing practices (Fantuzzo, 1990). As a consequence of these or other obstacles, families may become discouraged and discontinue participation in these services (a response which is often perceived by professionals as resistant). The mandated reporter can encourage families to proactively manage their involvement in community mental health services. They can affirm the important role families play in children's development and mental health, prepare families for the possibility that treatment may seem unfitting at times, and guide them in discussing their needs and cultural values with therapists.

Children placed in foster care can benefit from a variety of services provided in the mental health context: psychiatric consultation, psychotherapy, counseling, partial hospitalization, or any combination of these. Initiating this treatment is contingent upon the foster child's biological parent providing informed consent, unless parental rights have been terminated or the child is old enough to legally consent to mental health services. The legal age varies among the states. For example, in Pennsylvania, a 14-year-old may legally consent to mental health services without the knowledge or consent of the parent or legal guardian. It is recommended that children in foster care receive a comprehensive psychological evaluation to identify their need for intervention.

HEAD START AND EARLY HEAD START PROGRAMS

Head Start preschool programs are federally funded enrichment programs for children, ages 3 to 5 years, from financially disadvantaged households. All children who are placed in foster care meet the eligibility requirements, regardless of the income of their foster families. Head Start programs are designed to compensate for early social and cognitive deprivation by offering comprehensive services, including early childhood education, as well as access to health care, nutrition, and social services (Kamerman & Kahn, 1995). Parent involvement in the classroom and on policy councils is an important component of the program and contributes to its success in improving the outcomes for disadvantaged children (Haskins, 1989).

For preschool children who have experienced neglect or abuse and for those placed in out-of-home care, this early childhood education program can provide an enriched, structured, and predictable environment on a daily basis. Head Start programs have health and mental health coordinators and consultants available to work with the teachers, children, and parents. The active support for parent involvement provides parents with good role models in caring for and disciplining preschool children, and offers them a meaningful way to participate in their children's program.

Over the years, Head Start personnel expressed concern that they were not intervening early enough in children's lives and that programming should be available to disadvantaged children who were younger than age 3 years. Research on infant development supported these observations. As a result, in 1995 the United States Department of Health and Human Services authorized support for Early Head Start Programs in many communities. These community-based programs serve pregnant women and mothers of infants and toddlers. Early Head Start focuses on the parent-child relationship as the most significant means of enhancing child development. Early Head Start programs aim to improve parenting skills to enhance infant health and development. They offer parents healthcare and nutrition supports. Early Head Start can be a helpful resource to parents, kinship care providers, and foster parents in enhancing their care of infants and toddlers.

EARLY INTERVENTION SERVICES

Early Intervention (EI) involves a variety of services to prevent and remediate developmental delays and disorders for infants, toddlers, and preschool children (ages birth to 5 years). This is a federal entitlement program originating from legislation passed in 1986 (The Education of the Handicapped Act Amendments of 1986, PL 99-457) and re-authorized as Part C of the Individuals with Disabilities Education Act (IDEA) Amendments of 1997 (PL 105-71). These services include multidisciplinary developmental assessments for children who are suspected of having developmental delays in the domains of communication, cognition, movement, physical growth, social-emotional functioning, or self-help skills. Children who have medical conditions that are highly associated with developmental delays or mental retardation also qualify (e.g., those with Down's syndrome, fetal alcohol syndrome, seizure disorders). Specific requirements for eligibility for EI services vary across states.

EI services for infants, toddlers, and preschool age children include a potentially wide range of interventions and supports provided by professionals and paraprofessionals. Depending on the individual child's needs, these services may include therapeutic interventions by speech-language pathologists, occupational therapists, physical therapists, psychologists, audiologists, special instructors, and others. Services are family-centered and can include transportation, family training or counseling, and service coordination supports. Each Individual Family Service Plan is tailored to the individual child's needs. The plan is developed by the multidisciplinary team that conducted the initial evaluation and the child's parent or legal guardian, and is reviewed semi-annually. Services are often provided to infants and toddlers within their homes, with a greater likelihood of center-based programs for preschool age children. (For a comprehensive discussion of early intervention services for children in foster care, see Spiker & Silver, 1999.)

There is an extensive body of research supporting the effectiveness of EI programs for infants and preschoolers with developmental disabilities and for those at risk for developing developmental problems (Casto & Mastropieri, 1986; Guralnick, 1997; Guralnick & Bennett, 1987; Ramey & Ramey, 1996; Simeonsson, Cooper, & Scheiner, 1982). These programs have been shown to improve children's functional abilities and, for some, their potential for school readiness (Infant Health and Development Program [IHDP], 1990; Ramey & Ramey, 1996). Children who have histories of premature birth and associated low birth weight; those who were born with prenatal drug and alcohol exposure; and those who experienced neglect, poor nutrition, or abuse should receive a multidisciplinary developmental assessment to evaluate whether they have developmental delays and to access EI services. These services are available in every state and county across the nation. Information on how to schedule an evaluation can be obtained by contacting the local county office of mental retardation services and/or the local school district's intermediate unit for special education services.

In order for a child to receive an evaluation and intervention services, informed consent must be obtained from the child's parent or legal guardian, even if the child has been removed from the parent's care and placed in out-of-home care. Sometimes the children's parents may be reluctant to agree to EI evaluations or services. They may be concerned that the evaluation will label their child and that the child will be stigmatized. They may resent the perceived intrusiveness of in-home child welfare interventions and see EI services (which are completely independent of child welfare services) as an additional intrusion. For whatever reason, the mandated reporter can encourage parents by explaining how the service plan will be developed with the parent's input, that there are concrete supports available to the parents (such as service coordination and transportation for appointments), and that early intervention has been shown to improve children's readiness for later elementary school. In cases in which parents cannot be located or parental rights have been terminated, the EI system has a program in which "educational surrogate parents" participate in the IFPS meetings and advocate EI programming in the best interests of the child. It is recommended that the child's foster parent receive the appointment as "educational surrogate parent" rather than the child welfare caseworker or legal advocate assigned to the child, to ensure attendance at IFSP meetings. It is also recommended that the child's early intervention services be family-centered, in the spirit of the IDEA legislation.

Schools as Resources for Maltreated Children

The prevalence of maltreatment among school and preschool age children underscores the important role schools can have in promoting competencies among those whose development has been compromised by abuse or neglect. Over half of the population of maltreated children is below age 12 years, with the highest incidence of abuse and neglect noted for children between ages 2 and 8 years (USDHHS, 2000). The experience of maltreatment during these formative years can adversely alter a healthy developmental trajectory and increase risks for lasting cognitive, emotional, and behavioral difficulties (Egeland, 1997).

Public schools are accessible to all children and can provide various educational support services for those who are experiencing cognitive, emotional, or behavioral difficulties as a consequence of maltreatment. Schools provide support services to children through the regular education or special education programs. Pre-referral intervention services are provided to children in regular education programs prior to involving more restrictive and costly special education services. Following are descriptions of pre-referral and special education procedures and services, with examples of how these services may apply to maltreated children.

Pre-referral Intervention Services

The scope of educational support services offered in schools has broadened from special education to include pre-referral interventions that aim to modify the instructional approach or classroom environment. The pre-referral intervention process is often initiated by the classroom teacher. Interventions are developed through a collaborative network of teachers and other school professionals, such as the counselor, nurse, social worker, or psychologist. This network is commonly referred to as the Instructional Support Team, Pupil/Teacher Assistance Committee, or Comprehensive Student Support Team. Parents or legal guardians can initiate the pre-referral process, or they may be invited to participate when the classroom teacher initiates the process. However, their consent or presence is not legally required. Features of a pre-referral intervention plan include clear identification of the child's needs, appropriate educational goals, specific intervention strategies, methods for monitoring progress, and review dates. At the time of review, the team may decide to continue or gradually eliminate the intervention plan if the educational goals for the child have been achieved. Alternately, the team may recommend proceeding to obtain special education services.

Pre-referral interventions can be helpful for maltreated children who experience academic, emotional, behavioral, or social difficulties that prohibit them from effectively participating in class and achieving in school. Some examples of difficulties that could be addressed through pre-referral interventions are poor completion of homework, inattention, aggression, social isolation, or difficulty mastering a mathematical concept. Possible pre-referral interventions for these difficulties could include strategies such as systematic reinforcements for increases in appropriate behaviors (e.g., homework completion, improved attention), repositioning the child's desk in the classroom, including the child in a social skills group conducted by the school counselor, alternative instructional strategies, or tutoring.

Special Education and Related Services

The Individuals with Disabilities Education Act of 1997 (IDEA) is a federal law that mandates that all children are entitled to a free and appropriate public education. IDEA sets forth guidelines for the provision of special education and related services to children who have cognitive, emotional, or behavioral difficulties that impede their academic achievement. Special education is an instructional program that is specifically designed to meet the learning needs of these children. There is a continuum of special education services in public school systems, ranging from the provision of alternate instructional strategies for students who remain in regular education classrooms to the placement of students in self-contained special education classes. Related services are provided to facilitate children with disabilities in their participation in school instruction and programs. Related services can include transportation, physical therapy, speech and language therapy, counseling, occupational therapy, and school health services.

A multidisciplinary team, including a school administrator, teacher, psychologist, counselor, and specialists in relevant areas of concern, determines a student's eligibility for special education and related services. Eligibility decisions are based on a psycho-educational evaluation of the student that is prepared by the school psychologist. The evaluation must involve multiple methods of assessment, such as (1) standardized testing of cognitive ability, academic achievement, speech and language skills, or motor skills; (2) vision and hearing assessments; (3) classroom observations; and (4) interviews with the child, teacher, and primary caregivers. Unlike the pre-referral process, consent from the student's parent or guardian is legally mandated before a psycho-educational evaluation can be conducted and eligibility for special education and related services determined.

Based on the results of the psycho-educational evaluation, the student must meet criteria for one of the 13 special education classifications specified in IDEA in order to receive special education services. These classifications include autism, deaf-blindness, deafness, hearing impairment, mental retardation, multiple disabilities, orthopedic impairment, other health impairment, serious emotional disturbance, specific learning disability, speech or language impairment, traumatic brain injury, and visual impairment. In some instances the student may have a diagnosis not represented by one of the special education categories. However, under section 504 of the Rehabilitation Act of 1973, the student can be eligible for special education services. Students diagnosed with attention deficit-hyperactivity disorder commonly receive services under this act.

Once a student is determined eligible for special education or related services, an Individualized Educational Plan (IEP) is developed. Based on the psycho-educational evaluation, the IEP specifies the educational goals, educational setting, instructional approach, related services, and process for evaluating the student's progress. Parents or legal guardians must be invited to participate in developing the IEP. Their approval of the IEP is required. The IEP is reviewed and updated annually by the multidisciplinary team and parent or guardian for the time that the student is receiving special education services.

Many maltreated children experience cognitive and/or socio-emotional difficulties that significantly impair their academic achievement and warrant special education services. Although all forms of maltreatment can adversely impact children's learning, neglect is most frequently associated with poor academic achievement (Egeland, 1997). For example, young children who are neglected often show significant delays in speech and language abilities and enter school with underdeveloped school readiness skills and behaviors (Egeland, 1988). The unfortunate consequence of these weaknesses during the crucial transition into school can be the onset of a perpetual cycle of learning difficulties, often in reading, and possible behavioral and emotional problems.

For this child, a psycho-educational evaluation may be conducted and could indicate that the child meets classification criteria for a specific learning disability. The IEP would reflect the multidisciplinary team's goal for the child in the upcoming year (i.e., specify expected reading level) and recommendation for educational placement, such as a self-contained, full-time learning support classroom or part-time resource room support. Based on what was learned about the child's learning style in the psycho-educational evaluation, instructional approaches could be specified. For example, the child may benefit from visual or tactile learning strategies. At the end of one year, the child's progress toward these educational goals and possible re-evaluation will guide the multidisciplinary team in making appropriate modifications to the IEP.

◆ CONCLUSION

The mandated reporter is a crucial player in identifying families at risk for child maltreatment and in preventing continued harm to children. The immediate period following a report of suspected child maltreatment involves many urgent activities, such as investigating the child's risk of being harmed, ensuring a safe place for the child, and connecting the family and child to medical, psychological, and social services. The reporting of maltreatment can serve as a valuable and compassionate act in helping families in need. However, the family may perceive the report as a threatening or unfair process unless it occurs in a supportive context. The mandated reporter can alter this perception by reporting in a supportive manner. The family should be informed about the need for and benefits of reporting and about the process that will follow. Moreover, to the best of their ability, mandated reporters should directly provide or utilize their institutional resources to offer ongoing support to families as they proceed through CPS investigation and intervention plans. For children placed in out-of-home care, the mandated reporter should strive to support continuity of special education, mental health, and medical or other on-going services, so that the child's needs are not overlooked.

This chapter was written with the intent of helping mandated reporters reflect on their contributions to directing this legally mandated act toward positive and helpful interventions for families whose level of distress may place them at risk for harming their children.

◆ REFERENCES

Aber, J.L., Allen, J.P., Carlson, V., & Cicchetti, D. (1989). The effects of maltreatment on development during early childhood: Recent studies and their theoretical, clinical, and policy implications. In D. Cicchetti and V. Carlson (Eds.), Child maltreatment: Theory and research on the causes and consequences of child abuse (pp. 579-619). Cambridge, England: Cambridge University Press.

American Academy of Pediatrics, Committee on Early Childhood, Adoption and Dependent Care. (1994). Health care of children in foster care. Pediatrics, 93, 335.

Adoption and Safe Families Act. (ASFA). (1997). PL 105-89.

Adoption Assistance and Child Welfare Act. (AACWA). (1980). PL 96-272.

Andrews, B., Bishop, A. R., & Sussman, M. S. (1999). Emergency child care and overnight respite for children from birth to 5 years of age: Development of a community-based crisis nursery. In J. Silver, B. Amster, and T. Haecker (Eds.), Young children and foster care: A guide for professionals (pp. 324-345). Baltimore: Paul H. Brookes Publishing Co.

Andrews, S. R., Blumenthal, J. B., Johnson, D. L., Kahn, A. J., Ferguson, C. J., Lasater, T. M., Malone, P. E., & Wallace, D. B. (1982). The skills of mothering: A study of parent-child development centers. Monographs of the Society for Research in Child Development, 47(6, Serial No. 198).

Armstrong, K. A., & Fraley, Y. L. (1985). What happens to families after they leave the program? Children Today, 14, 17-20.

Barth, R. P. (1997). Foster family care: Before, during, and beyond. In J. D. Berrick, R. P. Barth, and N. Gilbert (Eds.), Child welfare research review (Vol. 2) (pp.151-159). New York: Columbia University Press.

Barth, R. P., Courtney, M. E., Berrick, J. D., & Albert, B. (1994). From child abuse to permanency planning: Child welfare services, pathways, and placements. Hawthorne, NY: Aldine de Gruyter.

Berrick, J. D., Barth, R. P., & Needell, B. (1994). A comparison of kinship foster homes and foster family homes: Implications for kinship foster care as family preservation. Children and Youth Services Review, 16, 33-63.

Berrick, J. D., Barth, R. P., & Gilbert, N. (Eds.) (1997). Children welfare resarch review (Vol. 2) (p. xi). New York: Columbia University Press.

Besharov, D. J. (1990). Recognizing child abuse: A guide for the concerned. New York: The Free Press.

Casto, G., & Mastropieri, M. A. (1986). The efficacy of early intervention programs: A meta-analysis. Exceptional Children, 52, 417-424.

Chernoff, R., Combs-Orme, T., Risley-Curtiss, C., & Heisler, A. (1994). Assessing the health status of children entering foster care. Pediatrics, 93, 594-601.

Child Welfare League of America (CWLA). (1988). Standards for health care for children in out-of-home care. Washington, DC: Author.

Children's Defense Fund (CDF). (1995). The state of America's children. Washington, DC: Author.

Children's Defense Fund. (1997, November 20). Adoption and Safe Families Act (H.R. 867) protects children's safety and promotes permanent homes for children. Retrieved July 6, 2000 from the World Wide Web: hhtp://www.childrensdefense.org/ss_asfa_basics.htm

Courtney, M. E. (1995). Re-entry to foster care of children returned to their families. Social Service Review, 69, 226-241.

Courtney, M. E., & Needell, B. (1997). Outcomes of kinship care: Lessons from California. In J. D. Berrick, R. P. Barth, and N. Gilbert (Eds.), Child welfare research review (Vol. 2) (pp.130-149). New York: Columbia University Press.

Crittendon, P. M. (1985). Maltreated infants: Vulnerability and resilience. Journal of Child Psychology and Psychiatry, 26, 85-96.

Dubowitz, H., Feigelman, S., Harrington, D., Starr, R., Zuravin, S., & Sawyer, R. (1994). Children in kinship care: How do they fare? Children and Youth Services Review, 16, 85-106.

Dubowitz, H., Zuravin, S., Starr, R. H., Feigelman, S., & Harrington, D. (1993). Behavior problems of children in kinship care. Journal of Developmental and Behavioral Pediatrics, 14, 386-393.

Education of the Handicapped Act Amendments. (1986). PL 99-457.

Egeland, B. (1988). The consequences of physical abuse and emotional neglect on the development of young children. In A. Cowan (Ed.), Child neglect. Washington, DC: National Center on Child Abuse and Neglect.

Egeland, B. (1997). Mediators of the effects of child maltreatment on developmental adaptation in adolescence. In D. Cicchetti and S. Toth (Eds.), Developmental perspectives on trauma: Theory, research, and intervention (pp. 403-434). New York: University of Rochester Press.

Egeland, B., Jacobvitz, D., & Sroufe, L. A. (1988). Breaking the cycle of abuse. Child Development, 59, 1080-1088.

Fantuzzo, J. W. (1990). Behavioral treatment of the victims of child abuse and neglect. Behavior Modification, 14, 316-339.

Fraser, M. W., Pecora, P. J., & Haapala, D. A. (Eds.). (1991). Families in crisis: The impact of intensive family preservation services. New York: Aldine De Gruyter.

George, C., & Main, M. (1979). Social interactions of young abused children: Approach, avoidance, and aggression. Child Development, 50, 300-318.

Gleeson, J. P., & Craig, L. C. (1994). Kinship care in child welfare: An analysis of states policies. Children and Youth Services Review, 16, 7-31.

Guralnick, M. J. (Ed.). (1997). The effectiveness of early intervention. Baltimore: Paul H. Brookes Publishing Co.

Guralnick, J. J., & Bennett, F. C. (Eds.). (1987). The effectiveness of early intervention for at-risk and handicapped children. New York: Academic Press.

Halfon, N., Berkowitz, G., & Klee, L. (1992). Mental health service utilization by children in foster care in California. Pediatrics, 89, 1238-1244.

Halfon, N., Mendonca, A., & Berkowitz, G. (1995). Health status of children in foster care: The experience of the Center for the Vulnerable Child. Archives of Pediatric Adolescent Medicine, 149, 386-392.

Haskins, R. (1989). Beyond metaphor: The efficacy of early childhood intervention. American Psychologist, 44, 274-282.

Hochstadt, N. J., Jaudes, P. K., Zimo, D. A., & Schachter, J. (1987). The medical and psychosocial needs of children entering foster care. Child Abuse & Neglect, 11, 53-62,

Individuals with Disabilities Education Act (IDEA) Amendments. (1997). Part C. PL 105-71.

Infant Health and Development Program (IHDP). (1990). Enhancing the outcomes of low birth weight, premature infants: A multisite, randomized trial. JAMA: The Journal of the American Medial Association, 263, 3035-3042.

Kamerman, S. B., & Kahn, A. J. (1995). Starting right. New York: Oxford University Press.

Kavaler, F., & Swire, M. R. (1983). Foster child health care. Lexington, MA: D.C. Heath.

Kinney, J. M., Haapala, D. A., Booth, C., & Leavitt, S. (1990). The homebuilders model. In J. K. Whittaker, J. M. Kinney, E. Tracy, and C. Booth (Eds.), Reaching high risk families: Intensive family preservation services in human services (pp. 31-64). New York: Aldine De Gruyter.

Kronstadt, D. (1999). Providing positive, stable placements for infants and toddlers in foster care: A services research project. Zero to Three, 19, 19-23.

Kutzler, P. (1997). Unpublished raw data from the Family and Child Tracking System, Philadelphia Department of Human Services.

Lewis, R. E. (1991). What are the characteristics of intensive family preservation services? In M. W. Fraser, P. J. Pecora, and D. A. Haapala (Eds.), Families in crisis: The impact of intensive family preservation services (pp. 93-107). New York: Aldine De Gruyter.

Marcenko, M. O. (1999). Family-centered, home-based prevention strategies for vulnerable families of young children. In J. Silver, B. Amster, and T. Haecker (Eds.), Young children and foster care: A guide for professionals (pp. 309-324). Baltimore: Paul H. Brookes Publishing Co.

McIntyre, A., Lounsbury, K. R., Berntson, D., & Steel, H. (1988). The psychosocial charactieristics of foster children. Journal of Applied Developmental Psychology, 9, 125-137.

Needell, B., & Gilbert, N. (1997). Child welfare and the extended family. In J. D. Berrick, R. P. Barth, and N. Gilbert (Eds.), Child welfare research review (Vol. 2) (pp.63-83). New York: Columbia University Press.

O'Grady, S. P., & Birns, R. D. (1999). Collaboration with the child advocate. In J. Silver, B. Amster, and T. Haecker (Eds.), Young children and foster care: A guide for professionals (pp. 293-305). Baltimore: Paul H. Brookes Publishing Co.

Olds, D. L., Henderson, C. R., Chamberlin, R., & Tatelbaum, R. (1986). Preventing child abuse and neglect: A randomized trial of nurse home visitation. Pediatrics, 78, 65-78.

Olds, D. L., & Kitzman, H. (1990). Can home visitation improve health of women and children at environmental risk? Pediatrics, 86, 108-116.

Pecora, P. J. (1991a). Family-based and intensive family preservation services: A select literature review. In M. W. Fraser, P. J. Pecora, and D. A. Haapala (Eds.), Families in crisis: The impact of intensive family preservation services (pp. 17-47). New York: Aldine De Gruyter.

Pecora, P. J. (1991b). Using risk assessment technology and other screening methods for determining the need for child placement in family-based services. In V. Pina, D. Haapala, and C. Sudia (Eds.), Empowering families: Papers from the Fourth Annual Conference on Family-Based Services. Riverdale, IL: National Association for Family Based Services.

Pecora, P. J., Whittaker, J. K., Maluccio, A. N., Barth, R. P., & Plotnick, R. D. (1992). The child welfare challenge: Policy, practice, and research. New York: Aldine De Gruyter.

Petit, M. R., & Curtis, P. A. (1997). Child abuse and neglect: A look at the states 1997 CWLA stat book. Washington, DC: Child Welfare League of America.

Ramey, C. T., & Ramey, S. L. (1996). Early intervention: Optimizing development for children with disabilities and risk conditions. In M. L. Wolraich (Ed.), Disorders of development and learning: A practical guide to assessment and management (2nd ed.) (pp. 141-157). St. Louis, MO: C.V. Mosby.

Repucci, N. D., Britner, P. A., & Woolard, J. L. (1997). Preventing child abuse and neglect through parent education. Baltimore: Paul H. Brookes Publishing Co.

Rosenberg, M. S., & Repucci, N. D. (1983). Abusive mothers: Perceptions of their own and their children's behavior. <u>Journal of Consulting and Clinical Psychology, 51,</u> 674-682.

Ross, P. E., & Crawford, J. (1999). On the front lines: Foster parents' experiences in coordinating services. In J. Silver, B. Amster, and T. Haecker (Eds.), <u>Young children and foster care: A guide for professionals</u> (pp. 279-291). Baltimore: Paul H. Brookes Publishing Co.

Schor, E. L. (1988). Foster care. <u>Pediatric Clinics of North America, 35,</u> 1241-1252.

Silver, J., DiLorenzo, P., Zukoski, M., Ross, P. E., Amster, B., & Schlegel, D. (1999). Starting young: Improving the health and developmental outcomes of infants and toddlers in the child welfare system. <u>Child Welfare, 78,</u> 148-165.

Silver, J. A., Haecker, T., & Forkey, H. C. (1999). Health care for young children in foster care. In J. Silver, B. Amster, and T. Haecker (Eds.), <u>Young children and foster care: A guide for professionals</u> (pp. 161-193). Baltimore: Paul H. Brookes Publishing Co.

Simeonsson, R. J., Cooper, D. H., & Scheiner, A. P. (1982). A review and analysis of the effectiveness of early intervention. <u>Pediatrics, 69,</u> 635-641.

Simms, M. (1989). The foster care clinic: A community program to identify treatment needs of children in foster care. <u>Developmental and Behavioral Pediatrics, 10,</u> 121-128.

Simms, M. D., & Halfon, N. (1994). The health care needs of children in foster care: A research agenda. <u>Child Welfare, 73,</u> 505-524.

Spiker, D., & Silver, J. A. (1999). Early intervention services for infants and preschoolers in foster care. In J. Silver, B. Amster, and T. Haecker (Eds.), <u>Young children and foster care: A guide for professionals</u> (pp. 347-371). Baltimore: Paul H. Brookes Publishing Co.

Stein, T. J., & Rzepnicki, T. L. (1983). <u>Decision-making at child welfare intake: A guide for practitioners.</u> New York: Child Welfare League of America.

Takas, M. (1993). Kinship care: Developing a safe and effective framework for protective placement of children with relatives. <u>Zero to Three, 13</u>(3), 12-17.

Toth, S. K., Manly, J. T., & Cicchetti, D. (1992). Child maltreatment and vulnerability to depression. <u>Developmental Psychopathology, 4,</u> 97-112.

Tracy, E. M. (1991). Defining the target population for family preservation services. In K. Wells and D. E. Biegel (Eds.), <u>Family preservation services: Research and evaluation</u> (pp.138-158). Newbury Park, CA: Sage Publications.

U.S. Department of Health and Human Services (USDHHS), Administration on Children, Youth, and Families. (2000). <u>Child maltreatment 1998: Reports from the states to the National Child Abuse and Neglect Data System.</u> Washington, DC: U.S. Government Printing Office.

U.S. General Accounting Office (USGAO). (1995). <u>Foster care: Health needs of many young children are unknown and unmet </u>(GAO/HEHS-95-114). Washington, DC: Author.

U.S. General Accounting Office (USGAO). (1999). <u>Foster care: States' early experiences implementing the Adoption and Safe Famlies Act</u> (GAO/HEHS-00-1). Washington, DC: Author.

Van der Kock, B. A., & Fisler, R. E. (1994). Childhood abuse and neglect and loss of self-regulation. <u>Bulletin of the Menninger Clinic, 58,</u> 145-168.

Wekerle, C., & Wolfe, D. A. (1993). Prevention of child physical abuse and neglect: Promising new directions. <u>Clinical Psychology Review, 13,</u> 501-540.

Winterfield, A. P. (1998). An overview of the major provisions of the Adoption and Safe Families Act of 1997. <u>Protecting Children, 14</u>(3), 4-8.

Wulczyn, F. H., Hardin, A. W., & Goerge, R. M. (1997). <u>Foster care dynamics 1983-1994: An update for the multistate foster care data archive.</u> Chicago: Chapin Hall Center for Children at the University of Chicago.

Zigler, E., & Black, K. B. (1989). America's family support movement: Strengths and limitations. <u>American Journal of Orthopsychiatry, 59,</u> 6-19.

Zigler, E., Hopper, P., & Hall, N. W. (1993). Infant mental health and social policy. In C. H. Zeanah, Jr. (Ed.), <u>Handbook of infant mental health</u> (pp. 480-492). New York: Guilford Press.

Zukoski, M. (1999). Foster parent training. In J. Silver, B. Amster, and T. Haecker (Eds.), <u>Young children and foster care: A guide for professionals</u> (pp. 473-490). Baltimore: Paul H. Brookes Publishing Co.

Zuravin, S. J., Benedict, M., & Somerfield, M. (1993). Child maltreatment in family foster care. <u>American Journal of Orthopsychiatry, 63,</u> 589-596.

Chapter 16

PREVENTION EFFORTS: LOCAL

PEGGY S. PEARL, ED.D.

Child abuse prevention depends on neither a program nor a system of services. It must be founded on a society that values its children and provides resources to sufficiently support children and families. The more a society values its children, the less it will tolerate their victimization and the more effectively it will seek to protect them (Wurtele & Miller-Perrin, 1992). Within such a context, society will be willing to fund preventive services, programs, and policies rather than merely attempting to solve the crises caused by the lack of interest in the welfare of its children after they have occurred (Fortin & Chamberland, 1995; Giovannoni, 1991). Table 16-1 lists some of the characteristics that are apparent when a nation makes its children a high priority. A society must also place greater emphasis on tolerance, nonviolence, and respect for all its members regardless of race, gender, age, color, national origin, or religious beliefs. To prevent child maltreatment, our society must make many changes at the individual, family, community, and cultural levels.

A nation where children are valued is a composite of many communities where all citizens demonstrate a concern for all children.

- Citizens who expect for all children what they expect for their own children–the opportunity to achieve their maximum potential.

- Communities where each person accepts the responsibility to help and support his or her own family as well as neighbors.

- Neighborhoods where individuals are proactive in the support and praise of their fellow men and women.

- Communities where each person is valued and brought to the table to share in the country's resources.

The prevention of child abuse involves providing all parents with the necessary resources for successful parenting. The basic national commitment to children and the prevention of their maltreatment begins when the nation's leaders take the initiative to help families through policy and financial support. However, child abuse prevention is not a function of government alone. The leadership to create these changes must come from both the public and the private sectors, as well as the religious community. The private sector must support

> **Table 16-1. Characteristics of Communities with Children as a High Priority**
>
> - Individuals are informed about child abuse and neglect in their community.
>
> - Outraged citizens are motivated to action when they hear that children are being maltreated.
>
> - Parents expect for all children what they expect for their own children–the opportunity to achieve their maximum potential.
>
> - Citizens are tolerant of differences, and accept and respect diversity.
>
> - Adequate and affordable housing is available for all families.
>
> - Recreation, arts, sports, and esteem-building activities are available to all children and families.
>
> - Access to abuse treatment programs is included in insurance coverage.
>
> - Mental health, medical, and dental care are accessible to all families–insurance coverage for both mental and physical health.
>
> - Families in need of assistance access social service delivery systems before maltreatment occurs, rather than depending on systems that treat after abuse occurs or punish for maltreating.
>
> - Universal instruction in the care and guidance of children is found in the curriculum of all public and private schools (kindergarten to grade 12, as well as adult continuing education).
>
> - Instruction in interpersonal communications, nonviolent conflict resolution, and resource management is provided to all students (kindergarten to grade 12, as well as adult continuing education).
>
> - When families are separated by divorce, child support is awarded by the courts and paid by the noncustodial parent.
>
> - Job training and education programs provide all workers with access to jobs as an avenue out of poverty.

families through intervention and prevention programs offered in the workplace. Workplace policies that are supportive of families include job sharing; flextime; mental health, medical, and dental insurance; parental leave; employee assistance programs; and dependent care assistance programs. The business community must recognize the positive correlations between unemployment and child abuse and neglect, and between job training and full employment ("Balancing Work," 1996; Finkelhor, Asdigian & Dziuba-Leatherman, 1995; Fortin & Chamberland, 1995; Reppucci, Land, & Haugard, 1998; Wurtele & Miller-Perrin, 1992).

◆ PREVENTIVE SERVICES

To prevent child maltreatment, a wide range of services and resources must be available to *all* parents. These preventive strategies are commonly classified as primary, secondary, or tertiary:

> **Table 16-1. Characteristics of Communities with Children as a High Priority—***continued*
>
> • Workplaces have policies that support families, including parental leave; job sharing; flextime; employee assistance programs; dependent care assistance programs; mental health, medical, and dental insurance; career ladders; and employee wellness programs.
>
> • Nonviolent societal role models are highly visible.
>
> • All parents have access to self-help and support groups.
>
> • Adequate funding exists to research environments that facilitate optimal development of individuals throughout the life span and to monitor the effectiveness of prevention programs.
>
> • Policy decisions are grounded in research.
>
> • Legal systems–juvenile, criminal, and civil–are properly funded, staffed, and trained to promptly and fairly resolve child, spouse, and/or elder maltreatment cases.
>
> • Good supervision, peer support, and self-care are available for all workers in the child protective system, to access as needed.
>
> • Adequate salaries are provided for professionals who work in child-related professions to attract and retain the best and the brightest in jobs caring for the nation's priority–children and families.
>
> • Culturally and ethnically sensitive home-based parent education programs are available to all new parents.
>
> • Religious organizations are supportive–emotionally, socially, and financially–of all families and children.
>
> • Each individual is equally valued without regard for gender, race, ethnic background, ability, disability, or economic status.

Primary prevention: Training, resources, and policies are provided to all parents to enhance their parenting and to keep abuse from occurring. Examples include health care, adequate child care, supportive workplace policies, and life skills training.

Secondary prevention: Training, resources, and policies are provided to targeted high-risk populations to enhance their parenting skills. Secondary prevention programs commonly consist of training and services to victims to keep abuse from occurring in the next generation. Secondary prevention includes self-help groups for parents who consider themselves at risk for maltreating their children, home visitor programs for new parents, and parent education programs for adolescent parents.

Tertiary prevention: Therapy, assistance with resources, and home visitors are provided to enhance parenting and to keep abuse from recurring once it has been identified. Specific programs also included are respite day care for parents, treatment for abused and neglected children, crisis intervention services, and stress management training.

Within our society, primary prevention programs should be available to all parents before any maltreatment occurs. All parents benefit from access to parenting information, especially when they have their first child. Perinatal coaching, home visitor, and parent aide programs have proven effective for parents with young children. Additionally, all parents need access to health care both for themselves and for their children. All parents can benefit from stress and anger management training and from access to positive support services to help them cope with the stress of parenting. In our highly mobile society, many families lack the positive support of family and friends; consequently, this support must be supplied by other sources. For example, churches, recreational facilities, social organizations, or mental health agencies can assist these families. Accessible and affordable child care must be available to all working parents, especially to single parents and those with low incomes (Daro & McCurdy, 1994).

Treatment programs, including anger management, should be added within the penal systems for individuals of all ages to prevent them from abusing children after their release from incarceration. Juvenile offenders must have appropriate therapy to deal with their own problems and to learn more appropriate ways to handle stress, anger, and aggression. Most people in the penal system will return to the community and live in family units. They need assistance in learning how to not abuse and mistreat others within that family. All programs must be respectful of cultural issues to be effective.

In private, religious, and public schools, children need instruction regarding positive ways to interact and communicate with others as much as they need instruction in math, English, and science. Life skills education should be integrated into the curriculum beginning with kindergarten and continuing into adult education. Life skills education includes nonviolent conflict resolution, stress and anger management skills, resource management, effective decision-making, and effective interpersonal communication, as well as information regarding child development and guidance. Additionally, the basics of substance abuse prevention should be a component of education for parenting or life skills. Schools should provide the role model of positive discipline and not use corporal punishment (Daro & McCurdy, 1994; Helfer, Kempe & Krugman, 1997; National Clearinghouse, 1998; Wurtele & Miller-Perrin, 1992).

Every community should make parent education classes part of a comprehensive adult education program accessible to parents. Individuals and social institutions need to remove the current stigma against admitting one needs help with parenting. Topics suggested for these parent education classes include principles of child development, positive child guidance, and basics of child care, such as child nutrition and safety.

One vital area that should be addressed with parents of children at any age is techniques to improve the parent-child interaction. Learning to play with and enjoy their children enhances both this interaction and the parents' pleasure and pride in their parental role.

Corporal punishment can easily become abuse when administered by parents who are angry and under stress. Therefore, parents should be instructed in positive methods of child guidance. Additionally, parents need constructive methods of coping with stress. Self-help groups such as Parents Anonymous

(PA) give parents alternatives to abusing their children emotionally or physically and provide positive support networks when stress occurs. PA uses the Alcoholics Anonymous (AA) model of self-help, which has proven successful. Both primary and tertiary support groups should be developed to prevent and combat abuse (Cohn, 1987).

All new parents can benefit from various instruction and support services to enhance parenting skills and competence as well as prevent child abuse. The specific content and structure and the sponsoring agency or institution of these programs will vary. The goals for new parent programs include the following:

1. Increasing the parent's knowledge of both child development and the demands involved in parenting

2. Enhancing the parent's skill in coping with stress, including the specific stresses of infant and child care

3. Enhancing parent-child bonding, emotional ties, and communication skills

4. Increasing the parent's skill in coping with the stress of caring for children with special needs

5. Increasing the parent's knowledge about home and child management

6. Reducing the burden of child care

7. Increasing access to social and health services for all family members

8. Increasing parental knowledge of how to teach and model tolerance to their children

9. Increasing the quality and quantity of time spent playing with, talking with, and listening to their children (Daro, 1998; Daro & McCurdy, 1994)

Parent education offered as tertiary prevention for various types of maltreatment differs in informational need from primary or secondary programs. All programs should be culturally sensitive and targeted to the appropriate developmental level of the parents. Group parent education that emphasizes impulse control and alternative methods of discipline is particularly successful with physically abusive parents, whereas one-on-one, home-based services with individual counseling and problem-solving techniques are more effective with neglectful parents. Churches are very effective providers of culturally sensitive support services and positive parenting. Neglectful parents need instruction in practical child care tasks, such as diapering and feeding an infant, or distracting and communicating with a 2-year-old. Programs successful in preventing emotional abuse include group-based services that define nonphysical methods of discipline, emphasize the need for consistency in determining and implementing rules, and offer parents ways of demonstrating affection toward their children (Daro, 1998).

◆ PREVENTION PROGRAMS

Although different in form, child maltreatment practices share common causes and, therefore, the societal approaches to prevention have an impact on most types of maltreatment. However, mention should be made of the minor differences in prevention programs relating to each particular type of abuse (physical, neglect, emotional, sexual).

PREVENTION OF PHYSICAL ABUSE

There are multiple theories, with many overlapping variables, about the causes of physical abuse. Among the most common theories are previous exposure of the abuser to violence (abuse by partner or parent), exposure to stressors, and limited access to resources. The most commonly mentioned variable, and the most significant variable in many studies, is a mother's abuse by her mother in childhood. This risk factor increases when the mother is currently being battered or was formerly battered by a relationship partner. All families are exposed to stressors; however, physical abuse is more common when families experience either chronic stressors, such as poor living conditions and relationship problems, or acute stressors, such as a death in the family. The lack of access to resources may involve either internal or external resources. Internal resources include lack of parenting knowledge, self-esteem, and social skills. External resources include a positive support network of friends and family, child care professionals, teachers, and economic resources. When resources are severely limited, the appropriate management of the available resources and good problem-solving skills are very important (Erickson, Egeland & Pianta, 1989; Karr-Morse & Wiley, 1997; Fortin & Chamberland, 1995).

When mental health treatment is warranted, all members of the family should receive therapy. Whatever the cause and whoever is the victim or perpetrator (parent, spouse, or sibling), the whole family needs treatment. With therapy, family members learn new interpersonal communication skills and develop stronger self-esteem. The members of the family then need life skills and parenting classes to increase each individual's resources and reduce stressors. Because physical abuse is common in families where one or more adult(s) are substance abusers, substance abuse must be treated to stop the child abuse. The community must make substance abuse treatment available and accessible to all those in need of the service. Children from these homes must participate in support groups and substance abuse prevention services (Crittenden, 1992).

Reducing chronic stressors for many families would mean providing the resources for them to move out of poverty. Education and training for jobs that pay a living wage provide a beginning for many people. Communities are also responsible for making sure there is affordable housing, child care, health care, and transportation available for individuals at all income levels. Families that make a living wage may need training and assistance in financial management and problem-solving. Families at all income levels may be poor decision-makers who fail to recognize the relationship between their decisions and the life stressors they are experiencing. When individuals make the bad decision to purchase controlled substances, the results are often financially disastrous and chronically stressful for the family (Crittenden, 1992; Erickson, Egeland, & Pianta, 1989; Karr-Morse & Wiley, 1997; Krugman, 1995).

Corporal punishment can become abuse when parents are especially stressed or angry. Corporal punishment is correlated with a variety of behavorial problems in children, including aggression, delinquency, low self-esteem, depression, and emotional and behavioral problems (Strauss, 1994). Straus (1997) interviewed over 800 mothers of children aged 6 to 9 years and found that the greater the use of corporal punishment, the higher the level of antisocial behavior over the next 2 years. Parents must be aware of the short-term and long-term impact of using corporal punishment and have opportunities to learn alternative methods of discipline. Parents may fail to understand that children need guidance, supervision, and education to allow them to learn self-control instead of punishment for failing to follow rules. Children learn self-control more quickly with positive methods of guidance than with punishment. Children who experience corporal punishment are more aggressive, exhibit more behavior problems, and have less positive relationships with peers and adults. Adopting nonviolent forms of discipline has both short-term and long-term benefits. In the short term, more positive guidance improves the child's behavior and opinion of self and others. In the long term, positive guidance provides children with an appropriate role model of how to interact with others and how to parent their own children (Crittenden & Ainsworth, 1989). Child abuse prevention must include children learning appropriate alternatives to violence in their own homes and schools.

PREVENTION OF NEGLECT
To prevent child neglect, parents require the basic resources to provide proper care for their children. Parents with low incomes may not be able to provide the necessary food, shelter, clothing, or mental health, medical, and dental care for their children. Additionally, parents may also be experiencing stress or be without adequate support systems. Currently in our society, many individuals are employed full-time at jobs that do not pay enough to provide the basic needs for the family. Some parents lack the job skills necessary for entry-level jobs; even if they had these skills, many entry-level jobs fail to provide a living wage, medical insurance, and dental insurance.

When society makes adequate child care a national priority, it ensures, through various public and private sector means, that all parents have access to the basic resources to care for their families. To care for our nation's children, all parents must have access to decent and affordable housing; adequate mental health, medical, and dental care; nutritious food; developmentally appropriate child care; and recreational activities for youth of all ages. The cycle of poverty must be interrupted with culturally sensitive, multi-generational programs that work by addressing housing, jobs, substance abuse treatment, and family support (Claussen & Crittenden, 1991; Crittenden, 1988; Fortin & Chamberland, 1995; Giovannoni, 1991; U.S. Advisory Board, 1993; Wurtele & Miller-Perrin, 1992).

To prevent neglect, parents must function at optimal levels so that they can focus on their children's needs. Some parents are impaired in their ability to parent because of substance abuse or untreated psychopathologic disorders. To prevent child maltreatment, these adults and adolescents must have access to culturally sensitive, developmentally appropriate substance abuse prevention and treatment programs and mental health services. These services must be available to all parents at no cost, at fees based on ability to pay, along sliding scales, or under provisions of employee insurance or employee assistance programs. One solution used in many post-industrialized countries is to have insurance pay for mental health services equal to medical health care. Medicines for mental health care could be covered at the same reimbursement rate as other medications. Only when parents are functioning at their best can they appropriately care for dependent children.

One method of reducing the number of children living in poverty is to ensure that court orders following divorce or legal separation include child support payments from the non-custodial parent. Child support payments often make the difference between children having or not having their basic needs met. Government enforcement of child support orders is vital to ensure that child support payments are paid.

PREVENTION OF EMOTIONAL ABUSE

Improving conditions favorable to family well-being reduces the risk of family problems and child maltreatment. Since psychological abuse often occurs as a precursor to other forms of child maltreatment and continues along with other forms of maltreatment, societal emphasis needs to be on family support, education, and treatment to prevent the initial problems developing in a parent-child relationship. The support should be for both the individual and family unit. Parents need to be aware of the potential damage to children from psychological abuse.

To improve conditions for all age groups, citizen groups in Canada, England, Finland, and other countries are attempting to change societal approval of physical and verbal violence. These efforts begin with (a) educating the public to the potential for and great dangers of psychological abuse, and (b) decrying the impact of television on social norms and promoting more appropriate activities for everyone. The goals also include reducing the amount of violence on television and in music, and reducing the marketing of violent toys. These advocacy efforts are by professional and lay groups to educate parents and the general public in an attempt to change the attitudes of both the private and public sectors (Fortin & Chamberland, 1995).

Other family support efforts include reducing socio-environmental stress and the lack of educational and employment opportunities. These societal changes focus on reducing materialism and the emphasis on financial success. This change in values and priorities would shift societal emphasis from things to people and relationships. The emphasis on interpersonal relationships would place priority on parent-child attachment. The improved attachment would result in caregivers paying more attention to the child's ever-changing needs, developmental abilities, and unique personality, and would result in respect for the child as a person. Improving parent-child attachment and quality of parenting prepares the child to become a more effective parent of the next generation (Fortin & Chamberland, 1995; Olds et al., 1997; U.S. Advisory Board, 1993b). Parents need to be encouraged to participate in both informal and formal support systems that enhance their self-esteem, value their attachment to their children, and support the priority they place on effective parenting (Crittenden, 1992; Krugman, 1995).

Reducing socio-environmental stress is very different from the stress management often provided for individuals seeking relief from the pressures of everyday life (Fortin & Chamberland, 1995). The former is long-term and systemic while the latter is short-term and specific to one or more persons taking a class. As the U.S. Advisory Board on Child Abuse and Neglect (1993b) has consistently stated, people, as well as government and workplaces, must recognize their roles in changing the climate in which children grow up and the way people interact with each other in neighborhoods, places of worship, workplaces, schools, and places of recreation. They must extend to all members of society the same respect given to individuals who are valued for their own dignity as individuals. Each individual must embrace the dignity of children and the elderly (Wolfe & Jaffe, 1999).

Part of the reduction of socio-environmental stress is the increase of resources available to young parents. Stress from lack of resources can be alleviated through changes in workplace policies, salaries, and attitudes, as well as making resources available in the community. Community resources could include educational and leisure activities provided by parks and recreation departments or places of worship. Neighborhoods can provide important support by changing individual attitudes to become more family-friendly and concerned about the individuals with whom they live, work, and play (Daro, 1998).

PREVENTION OF SEXUAL ABUSE

In the 1980s and early 1990s many programs to prevent sexual abuse were developed and widely implemented. Generally, these sexual abuse prevention programs teach children how to protect themselves from sexual abuse (Wurtele, 1998). However, researchers, educators, and clinicians caution that the major responsibility for prevention of sexual abuse cannot be placed on the victims or potential victims because they are children (Finkelhor, Asdigian & Dziuba-Leatherman, 1995; Finkelhor & Dziuba-Leatherman, 1995). Sexual abuse prevention programs must focus on the perpetrator. Prevent Child Abuse America has developed a comprehensive strategy for preventing adults from becoming child sexual abusers (Daro, 1998). This prevention strategy includes the following:

1. Provision of quality sex education, including healthy sexuality, during the pre-teen and teenage years to enhance knowledge of what activity is normal and what should be reported.

2. Training for professionals and volunteers who work with children that teaches how to identify and help children who are being abused, how to teach children to protect themselves from abuse, and how to detect those who may be potential molesters.

3. Quality education for new parents that provides support to enhance early attachment and bonding when their first babies are born. This should include information about appropriate and inappropriate touch and what to do about it. Parents must know how to detect and handle the sexual abuse of their own children, specifically, how to interpret symptoms that may indicate that sexual abuse has occurred.

4. Institutional changes to ensure that all child-serving institutions and programs (e.g., schools, boys and girls clubs, Girl Scouts/Boy Scouts, day care) train children in self-awareness and self-protection.

5. Guidelines and regulations to screen, train, supervise, and monitor all volunteers and staff working with children and youth.

6. Availability of treatment services for all victims and perpetrators of sexual abuse. The treatment services must be accessible to the victims at repeated times in their lives as therapeutic needs change, i.e., at time of abuse, during adolescence, before marriage, at the time of the birth of their first child, and when their own child is the age they were at the time of their abuse.

7. Media messages that create an environment in which the prevention programs and concepts just outlined will be effective by communicating two messages:

First, for adolescents and adults, messages that say:

Child sexual abuse is a crime.

Help is available.

Abuse is a chronic problem unless you get help.

Children get hurt when you sexually abuse them.

Children cannot consent to sexual activity with adults or older youth.

Second, messages to children, including:

It's okay to say "No" and run away.

Sexual abuse is not your fault.

Reach out for help if this happens to you.

Help is available for you; ask someone you trust.

The comprehensive child sexual abuse prevention strategy just outlined, like all prevention programs, strengthens individuals and families by enhancing parenting skills.

Because some sexual abuse perpetrators are former victims, it is essential that all victims receive treatment. In addition, all convicted offenders must have treatment in prison or while on probation to prevent them from abusing again. Perpetrators who refuse to participate in prison treatment programs in a meaningful way should be denied their right to return to full community participation. Sixty percent of male sexual abuse perpetrators abuse their first victim in adolescence, and one half of the perpetrators were themselves maltreated as children; therefore, treatment programs for victims and young perpetrators must be expanded and funded to ensure therapy as needed over the life span of the individual. The treatment must include individual, group, and family therapy. It is not just the victim who needs to be helped, but rather the entire family needs help to improve their interpersonal relationships, to learn respect for the privacy of others, and to learn about each other's stress management techniques and communication skills (Finkelhor, Asdigian, & Dziuba-Leatherman, 1995; Finkelhor & Dziuba-Leatherman, 1995).

♦ CHANGES IN SOCIAL INSTITUTIONS
THE ROLE OF GOVERNMENT: THE COURTS AND LAW ENFORCEMENT

Because children lack the resources to protect themselves, they must turn to society for protection in the form of government and religious institutions. Comprehensive child abuse prevention, therefore, includes action taken within the judicial system. The judicial system—criminal, civil, and juvenile courts— must support laws and procedures both to ensure the protection of children and to support families. Laws and judicial procedures should be sensitive to the needs and special circumstances of children. Additionally, adequate numbers of well-trained judges, lawyers, and court support staff with manageable caseloads must be available to address the complex and demanding nature of child abuse and neglect litigation in a timely manner. The legal system must be sensitive to the needs of abuse victims to prevent additional maltreatment of these vulnerable individuals, both within the legal system and in abusive, dysfunctional families. In addition to the training and staffing of the judicial system, the criminal justice workforce must be trained to recognize and investigate what happens to children when family and community violence occurs. For example, in drug cases, there may be children who have been neglected or abused by caregivers addicted to drugs. Child and elder abuse are common in homes where domestic violence is reported. In situations where legal authorities are called because of the maltreatment of animals, investigation often reveals children or the elderly lacking proper care. Human services professionals, including those in the criminal justice and public health and safety systems, require education about the dynamics of violence within the family.

Each community should have active child advocacy groups to continually monitor the effectiveness of the legal and protective service systems. These groups continually work to ensure that the policies of the private and public sectors offer the most appropriate support for families and children. Where services are not offered, advocacy groups work to create the necessary services (Barnett, Miller-Perrin & Perrin, 1997; Krugman, 1995; National Clearinghouse, 1998; Thomas, 1998; Weberle & Wolfe, 1993).

The one variable that can most significantly reduce the number of children living in poverty is awarding and ensuring the payment of child support by non-custodial parents. Children living in poverty are often denied the basic necessities of life because family/divorce courts failed to include adequate child support from non-custodial parents or the child support enforcement system was not effective (Matthews, 1999). A society concerned about the well-being of children maintains a strong societal norm that says, "Be responsible and take care of your own children," and a legal system to enforce the law when the social norm is not followed.

The Role of the Workplace

Each individual is greatly impacted by his or her workplace. How he or she is treated as an individual is important to worker productivity as well as to home life. Is the workplace a place where the individual can never do enough to please the supervisors and feel good about himself or herself? Does the employee work in clean, well-lighted areas, free of excessive noise, heat, and environmental pollutants? Are there appropriate breaks and access to water for all workers? Are workers allowed time off when children and other family members are ill and need care? Can workers get off work to attend parent-teacher conferences? Are all workers respected as people? Is the workplace tolerant of diversity? The way parents are treated at work significantly affects how they feel about themselves and how they will treat members of their family at home. According to a *Business Week* survey in 1996, 42% of workers surveyed responded their home life was negatively impacted by their work experiences. This is compared to 26% who said it was neutral and 32% who said that work had a positive impact. The private and public sector workplaces should realize that family-friendly workplaces are actually more productive, and have less staff turnover, higher morale, and better financial success, resulting in a better community for everyone (U.S. Advisory Board, 1993a).

The Role of the Media

The media must play a key role in the prevention of child abuse. As a major force in shaping public opinion, the media can offer responsible programming and reporting to de-emphasize the current societal acceptance of violence.

Through responsible programming choices, the media can help reverse the current trend toward a desensitization of individuals to the horrors of violence. As the acceptance and glamorization of violence are removed, a new message can be sent: violence in all forms is inappropriate. The media can then replace the violence with programs that depict nonviolent methods of conflict resolution. The media have been involved in educating the public about the magnitude and consequences of violence in the lives of families. They also need to teach possible alternatives to domestic violence. The media may also advocate policies beneficial to children and families. One important step involves portraying parenting as an important and valued job in our society (Fortin & Chamberland, 1995; U.S. Advisory Board, 1993a).

◆ SUMMARY

The resources, education, and services needed to parent effectively should be available to all parents, as well as to friends, family, and neighbors committed to their support and assistance. A comprehensive multidisciplinary approach to prevention is needed. No specific program or plan is effective with all parents. A mix of family support programs is needed in both the private and public sectors to enhance parenting. Families need the informal support of extended family and friends in neighborhoods where people feel connected to each other. Neighbors must not accept others' abuse as "none of their business." Once abuse has occurred, various resources, educational programs, and services are needed to stop the cycle and prevent additional abuse. Each family needs a culturally sensitive and developmentally appropriate individualized approach, with some families requiring intensive and ongoing services to prevent maltreatment. Studies have shown specific gains in the following areas after parental participation in secondary and tertiary prevention programs: improved mother-infant bonding and maternal capacity to respond to the child's emotional needs; demonstrated ability to care for the child's physical and developmental needs; a decreased rate of subsequent pregnancies; increased consistent use of healthcare services and job training opportunities; decreased reliance on the public welfare system; higher school completion rates; and higher employment rates (Olds et al., 1997; U.S. Advisory Board, 1993a). Prevention requires society's commitment to the welfare of children and to individuals who take personal responsibility for all children, not just their biological children, and who value all individuals equally. Additionally, the commitment must be backed by both the public and the private sectors and must extend beyond mere rhetoric to include allocating resources and changing existing policies that do not conform to this commitment. Society must recognize the importance of parenting and commit resources to assist all parents in succeeding at this challenging and rewarding job.

◆ REFERENCES

Balancing work and family: Big returns for companies willing to give family strategies a chance. (1996). Business Week, 74-80.

Barnett, O. W., Miller-Perrin, C. L., & Perrin, R. (1997). Family violence across the lifespan. Thousand Oaks, CA: Sage Publications.

Claussen, A. H., & Crittenden, P. M. (1991). The physical and psychological maltreatment: Relations among types of maltreatment. Child Abuse and Neglect, 15(1-2), 5-18.

Cohn, A. H. (1987). Our national priorities for prevention. In R. E. Helfer and R. S. Kempe (Eds.), <u>The battered child.</u> Chicago: University of Chicago Press.

Crittenden, P. M. (1988). Distorted patterns of relationships in maltreating families: The role of internal representation models. <u>Journal of Reproductive and Infant Psychology, 6,</u> 183-199.

Crittenden, P. M. (1992). Children's strategies for coping with adverse home environments: An interpretation using attachment theory. <u>Child Abuse and Neglect, 16,</u> 329-343.

Crittenden, P. M., & Ainsworth, M. D. S. (1989). Child maltreatment and attachment theory. In D. Cicchetti and V. Carlson (Eds.), <u>Child maltreatment: Theory and research on the causes and consequences of child abuse and neglect</u> (pp. 432-463). New York: Cambridge University Press.

Daro, D. (1998). <u>Confronting child abuse: Research for effective program design.</u> New York: Free Press.

Daro, D., & McCurdy, K. (1994). Preventing child abuse and neglect: Programmatic interventions. <u>Child Welfare, 73,</u> 405-430.

Erickson, M. F., Egeland, B., & Pianta, R. (1989). The effects of maltreatment on the development of young children. In D. Cicchetti and V. Carlson (Eds.), <u>Child maltreatment: Theory and research on the causes and consequences of child abuse and neglect</u> (pp. 647-684). New York: Cambridge University Press.

Finkelhor, D., Asdigian, N., & Dziuba-Leatherman, J. (1995). The effectiveness of victimization prevention instruction: An evaluation of children's responses to actual threats and assaults. <u>Child Abuse and Neglect, 19,</u> 141-153.

Finkelhor, D., & Dziuba-Leatherman, J. (1995). Victimization prevention programs: A national survey of children's exposure and reactions. <u>Child Abuse and Neglect, 19,</u> 129-139.

Fortin, A., & Chamberland, C. (1995). Preventing the psychological maltreatment of children. <u>Journal of Interpersonal Violence, 10</u>(3), 275-295.

Giovannoni, J. (1991). Social policy considerations in defining psychological maltreatment. <u>Development and Psychopathology, 3,</u> 51-59.

Helfer, M. E., Kempe, R.S., & Krugman, R. D. (1997). <u>The battered child</u> (5th ed.). Chicago: University of Chicago Press.

Karr-Morse, R., & Wiley, M.S. (1997). <u>Ghosts from the nursery: Tracing the roots of violence.</u> Berkeley, CA: Atlantic Group West.

<u>Kid's Count 2001.</u> (2001). Summary. Washington, DC: Children's Defense Fund.

Krugman, R. D. (1995). Future directions in preventing child abuse. <u>Child Abuse & Neglect, 19,</u> 272-279.

Matthews, M. A. (1999). The impact of federal and state laws on children exposed to domestic violence. <u>The Future of Children, 9</u>(3), 50-66.

National Clearinghouse on Child Abuse and Neglect Information. (1998). <u>NCCAN lessons learned: The experience of nine child abuse and neglect prevention programs.</u> Retrieved October 1, 2001 from the World Wide Web: http://www.calib.com/nccancn/pubs/lessons/prevcomp.html

Olds, D., Eckenrode, J., Henderson, C. R., Kitzman, H., Cole, R., Sidora, K., Morries, P., & Pettit, L. M. (1997). Long-term effects of home visitation on maternal life course and child abuse and neglect: Fifteen-year follow-up on a randomized trial. JAMA, 278(8), 637-643.

Reppucci, N. D., Land, D., & Haugard, J. J. (1998). Child sexual abuse prevention programs that target young children. In P. K. Trickett and C. J. Schellenbach (Eds.), Violence against children in the family and the community (pp. 317-337). Washington, DC: American Psychological Association.

Straus, M. A. (1994). Beating the devil out of them: Corporal punishment in American families. New York: Lexington Books.

Straus, M. A. (1997). Physical child abuse. In W. Barnett, C. L. Miller-Perrin, and R. D. Perrin (Eds.), Family violence across the lifespan. Thousand Oaks, CA: Sage Publications.

Thomas, J. N. (1998). Community partnerships: A movement with a mission. The APSAC Advisor, 11, 2-3.

US Advisory Board on Child Abuse and Neglect. (1993a). Agenda for action. The continuing child protection emergency: A challenge to the nation. Washington, DC: US Government Printing Office.

US Advisory Board on Child Abuse and Neglect. (1993b). Neighbors helping neighbors: A new national strategy for the protection of children. Washington, DC: Government Printing Office.

Weberle, C., & Wolfe, D. A. (1993). Prevention of child abuse and neglect: Promising new directions. Clinical Psychology Review, 13, 501-540.

Wolfe, D. A., & Jaffe, P. (1999). Emerging strategies in the prevention of domestic violence. Futures of Children, 9(3), 133-144.

Wurtele, S. K., & Miller-Perrin, C. L. (1992). Preventing child sexual abuse: Sharing the responsibility. Lincoln, NE: University of Nebraska Press.

Wurtele, S. (1998). School-based child sexual abuse prevention programs: Questions, answers, and more questions. In J. Lutzger (Ed.), Handbook of child abuse research and treatment. New York: Plenum Press.

Chapter 17

PREVENTION EFFORTS: NATIONAL

KATHRYN HARDING, M.A.

Efforts to prevent child abuse and neglect include a wide range of activities, such as raising public awareness of the problem, educating parents and other caregivers about child-rearing, providing support to new parents or those who face greater challenges, and ensuring that families have access to health care, decent housing, and other community resources. Because of the pervasive impact of child maltreatment on society, *prevention efforts can be found throughout public systems of social service, justice, health, and education. In addition to government agencies, numerous national, state, and community organizations share the goal of preventing child abuse and neglect. This chapter reviews current efforts to prevent child maltreatment, highlighting a handful of programs working at various levels and employing various strategies.*

◆ THE FAMILY SUPPORT MOVEMENT

Prevention of child maltreatment requires an understanding of the causes of maltreatment. Research has illuminated a wide range of demographic and behavioral risk factors associated with child maltreatment, such as teen-aged child-bearing, poverty, community violence, parenting skills deficits, parental substance abuse, spousal abuse, social isolation, and mental illness, to name but a few (Daro, 1993; Sedlak & Broadhurst, 1996). Prevention efforts must address these and other significant risk factors in order to prevent child maltreatment.

In addition to risk reduction, the goals of prevention encompass the strengthening of families and communities to create healthier environments for raising children. To achieve these goals, prevention efforts must comprise a continuum of support for families and communities at all levels of risk. By strengthening families and communities, prevention programs not only reduce the risk of child maltreatment, but also offer improved well-being for children, families, and communities.

With the growth of the family support movement, child abuse prevention has broadened in its approach from a singular focus on parenting deficits to addressing a host of family needs and contextual issues from a strengths-based perspective. The family support movement emerged in the 1970s with the recognition of mounting social pressures on families, such as increased mobility and isolation, single-parenting, and demands of work outside the home (Weissbourd, 1990). Family support embodies all services that help families function better and has helped to shift prevention toward a strength-based orientation. To nurture their children, all parents need access to community resources designed to help meet the demands they face today. The family support movement has evolved into a national public-private partnership to promote state and federal policies that support all families. The goal of the family support movement is to build a seamless system of community-based resources to strengthen families.

◆ PREVENTION EFFORTS

Prevention efforts can be categorized as primary, secondary, and tertiary. These terms generally refer to breadth of the target audience and timing of the intervention (before or after maltreatment occurs) rather than the content of the intervention itself. With regard to preventing child abuse and neglect, primary prevention refers to activities directed at all members of a population or community to prevent abuse or neglect before it begins. Secondary prevention targets families at increased risk for child maltreatment to reduce risk and strengthen families before abuse or neglect occurs. Tertiary prevention refers to preventing the recurrence of maltreatment once it has begun. In practice, however, the boundaries between each level are blurred and many programs operate on multiple levels. This chapter focuses on primary and secondary prevention efforts.

PRIMARY PREVENTION PROGRAMS

Primary prevention of child maltreatment seeks to influence all members of a community or population to prevent abuse or neglect before it begins. Because of this broad scope, most primary prevention efforts use strategies that can reach a large audience simultaneously, such as television, classroom-based programs, and workplace programs. When individually focused strategies are employed, as with new parent support programs, strategies are typically limited in duration to a few months.

PUBLIC AWARENESS AND EDUCATION

Media campaigns to raise awareness and educate the public about the problem of child maltreatment and its prevention use information and emotional appeals to influence attitudes or behaviors. Public service announcements on television and radio broadcasts, combined with posters, billboards, and other print media, can reach millions of individuals at a time. However, crafting a message that can change individual attitudes or behaviors in 60 seconds or less is a daunting task. Media campaigns give parenting tips, raise public awareness about different types of maltreatment, inform the public about the harmful consequences of child maltreatment, encourage reporting of suspected abuse or neglect, and motivate people to take action to prevent maltreatment.

Organizations such as Prevent Child Abuse America and its network of state chapters work to engage the media proactively in promoting public awareness and education on various topics aimed at preventing child abuse and neglect before it starts. As new information emerges about specific issues, media campaigns convey this information to the public. For example, educating professionals, parents, and other caregivers about the dangers of shaking young children is the focus of a large media campaign to prevent shaken baby syndrome (SBS) led by the National Center on Shaken Baby Syndrome and the National Exchange Club Foundation.

Do media campaigns prevent child abuse and neglect? There is relatively little research that addresses this question directly. Anecdotally, Prevent Child Abuse America indicates that calls to its information line, 1-800-CHILDREN, increase notably after public service announcements air on television or radio, opening the door for providing additional information and linkages to support services. Similarly, following "Scared Silent," a 1992 television special on child abuse hosted by Oprah Winfrey, a toll-free number received over 200,000 calls, mostly requests for help from parents and children (Dombro, O'Donnell, Galinsky, Melcher, & Farber, 1996). Professionals credit media attention for broad changes in public perceptions of the issue of child abuse. A nationally representative survey found that 50% of adults believe child abuse and neglect is a more serious issue than other major public health issues, such as substance abuse and HIV/AIDS, and illnesses, such as heart disease and cancer (Harding & Fromm, in press). The same survey found that parenting practices have changed as well, with the percentage of parents who reported spanking or hitting their children in the past 12 months declining from 62% in 1988 to 43% in 2000, a decline of 31%. Overall, there is agreement among professionals that the media impact parenting (Simpson, 1997).

Organizations employ many additional strategies to increase community-wide public awareness and education on child abuse and its prevention. Since 1983, April has been designated by presidential proclamation as Child Abuse Prevention Month. Community activities include distributing blue ribbons signifying the problem of child abuse, special events for families and children, fundraisers for prevention services, and conferences to share information among professionals. Many national organizations provide resources and information to help local communities plan their efforts during Child Abuse Prevention Month, including Family Support America, the National Alliance of Children's Trust Funds, the National Clearinghouse for Child Abuse and Neglect Information, the National Indian Child Welfare Association, and Prevent Child Abuse America.

WORKPLACE PROGRAMS

Because 86% of young children in the United States have at least one parent working part- or full-time, the workplace plays a major role in parents' lives and has a major impact on children as well (Knitzer & Page, 1998). Access to quality child care, medical benefits, family leave, and flexible work hours help parents care for their children while earning a living. From the employer's perspective, the potential benefits of decreased parenting stress include improved productivity and staff retention. The Work and Family Connection is a national resource center that provides information on supporting families in the workplace through family-friendly policies. Galinsky (1999) heads the Families and Work Institute (FWI), a non-profit research center that seeks research-based solutions to current issues facing working families. FWI offers reports such as *The 1998 Business Work-Life Study,* which provides a comprehensive study of employers' responses to the needs of working families.

Employers may partner with organizations that offer support directly to parents in the workplace. An example of workplace parent support programs is *Louisiana I.N.C.* (Industry Nurturing Children), a program of Prevent Child Abuse Louisiana. This program reaches out to busy parents on the job, offering parenting information and support through help lines, print materials, parent education, and workshops designed for working parents.

SUPPORT FOR ALL NEW PARENTS

Nearly four million babies were born in the United States in 1998, with roughly 40% born to first-time parents (Ventura, Martin, Curtin, Matthews, & Park, 2000). Most parents having their first child want information and support to help them understand and respond effectively to their infant's needs, but many are isolated from extended family or do not know where to turn for information and support.

Programs that offer this information and support typically connect with new or expectant parents through hospitals and prenatal clinics. Trained volunteers are commonly used in such programs, both for economic reasons and because volunteers can be more like friends instead of "workers" in relating to parents in a supportive and nonjudgmental relationship. Services are voluntary, meaning that parents have the option of accepting the help or refusing to participate. Because these services reach out to all families systematically, they provide the added benefit of early identification of families in need of more intensive support.

First Steps, a perinatal primary prevention program of the Georgia Council on Child Abuse, Inc. (GCCA), has been implemented in 20 states and over 100 communities. The *First Step*s program provides emotional support, parent education, and linkages to community resources for expectant parents and new families. Services are provided by staff and volunteers extensively trained in communication techniques to help them relate to parents in a nonjudgmental, supportive manner. Goals of the program are to improve (1) social support; (2) knowledge of child development, health, safety issues, and parenting; (3) use of community resources; and (4) realistic expectations regarding children. Families receive follow-up phone contact, mailings, and/or home visits for a minimum of 3 to 6 months. Some *First Steps* sites include prenatal, home visiting, and neonatal intensive care service components. In addition to reaching out to all new parents, the *First Steps* program model is designed to be a gateway into a system of supports. Families who require more intensive services receive referrals for home visiting programs and appropriate community resources.

CHILD-FOCUSED PROGRAMS

While most child maltreatment prevention efforts target parents, the National Children's Advocacy Center (NCAC) based in Huntsville, Alabama, points out that the last line of defense against child abuse and neglect is often the children themselves. One of NCAC's programs, titled *SCAN* (Stop Child Abuse and Neglect), reaches over 17,000 children each year in kindergarten through seventh grade classrooms, helping them to avoid physical and sexual abuse, neglect, bullying, and other interpersonal conflicts. The program presents information through puppet shows with younger children and video dramas with older children, followed by group discussion about skills and strategies with regard to personal safety, disclosure, communication, and self-respect (National Children's Advocacy Center [NCAC], 2000).

Many child-focused programs seek to prevent violence in tomorrow's families by better preparing children for their roles as future parents and prosocial citizens. Prevention programs of this type generally include a broad focus on teaching children the life skills they will need to function well as adults. The Collaboration for Advancing Social and Emotional Learning (CASEL) connects model programs for children of all ages that promote the development of healthy relationships, coping and problem-solving abilities, and other life skills. Many programs also emphasize prevention of substance abuse, violence, and other risky behaviors. Many programs also involve parents to help them reinforce their children's prosocial behavior at home.

Children form their ideas about relationships early on, including their acceptance of violence in interpersonal relationships. Early adolescence is a particularly important stage for developing healthy relationship skills. The *Youth Relationships Program* (YRP) focuses on preventing dating violence as a step toward breaking the intergenerational cycle of child and spousal abuse (Pittman, Wolfe, & Wekerle, 1998). YRP targets youth aged 14 to 16 years, with a particular emphasis on those who have experienced violence in childhood. The goals of the 18-week program include helping youth develop the following:

1. An understanding of the foundations of abusive behavior

2. Skills to build healthy relationships

3. Understanding of social pressures that lead to violence

4. Increased social competence

A long-term evaluation of program impacts is currently in progress.

CHILD SEXUAL ABUSE PREVENTION

Child sexual abuse (CSA) prevention efforts usually focus on children, teaching self-protection skills and awareness of CSA. Group-based programs in school settings have been widely implemented. The majority of school districts and states offer CSA prevention programs (Wurtele, 1998). Most CSA prevention programs for children encompass four objectives:

- Teach children to recognize potentially abusive situations.

- Teach them skills to resist CSA.

- Encourage them to report any abuse to an adult they trust.

- Reassure them that victims are never to blame for sexual abuse.

CSA prevention programs educate parents and teachers as well. Increasing adult awareness of CSA helps with early identification and makes the home and school environments safer for children. While most teachers consider these programs effective, and some evidence exists of success in achieving these objectives in terms of children's skills and knowledge, not all children demonstrate competency in each area (Abrahams, Casey, & Daro, 1992). More importantly, research on whether such programs actually deter child sexual abuse is lacking (Wurtele, 1998). However, a recent article cites such prevention efforts as one of several factors that may have contributed to an overall national decline in the incidence of child sexual abuse in recent years (Jones & Finkelhor, 2001).

One example of a program that goes beyond child self-protection efforts is the Kempe Children's Center *Perpetration Prevention Program,* which includes primary, secondary, and tertiary CSA prevention strategies (http://www.kempecenter.org/about.htm). The primary prevention component of the program provides workshops for educators and caregivers on the topic of understanding and responding to sexual behavior in children, with the goal of reaching children in the general population to prevent development of sexually abusive behavior patterns. The program also trains people to conduct the workshop in their own communities (Ryan, 2000). Secondary prevention strategies are described later in this chapter.

Since child abuse and neglect often occur in the privacy of the home, hidden away from potential sources of assistance and support, there is no guaranteed method of detecting families at risk or those already experiencing child maltreatment. Primary prevention forms an essential component for reducing child abuse and neglect through the fundamental objective of reaching out to all children and families. Programs like those already described form the first segment in a continuum of support and can benefit all families. When faced with significant challenges, however, parents may need more assistance than these programs can provide. Secondary prevention efforts are designed to serve families at greater risk.

SECONDARY PREVENTION PROGRAMS

At the secondary prevention level, efforts share the primary prevention goal of short-circuiting maltreatment before it begins but narrow their focus to children and families at elevated risk for experiencing maltreatment. "Elevated risk" for child maltreatment encompasses a broad segment of the population. It is important to note that the majority of at-risk families do not experience maltreatment. Nonetheless, the factors that constitute risk for child maltreatment, such as social isolation, parental substance abuse, domestic violence, single-parenting, poverty, low educational attainment, unemployment, and community violence are in and of themselves undesirable to families and contribute to a variety of poor outcomes for children (Schorr, 1989).

CENTER-BASED PREVENTION EFFORTS

Building on theories and research regarding the causes of child maltreatment, many types of center-based services have been implemented in communities, providing parent education, support, and resources. Based on the theory that abuse results from parents' lack of information about how to best care for their children, parent education programs teach parents about child development, help them understand and respond appropriately to their child's behavior, and instruct them in alternatives to physical discipline. Parent support programs operate on the theory that abuse results from parents' lack of material and social support and offer both professional and mutual support from other parents. Many programs combine education and support. Over the past decade, programs have evolved from a "one-size-fits-all" approach to tailoring information for specific populations and enhancing the cultural relevance of parenting information.

Family resource and support programs typically offer a menu of support services to families, including resource centers, parenting education, support groups, parent aides, and referrals to community resources. Programs vary according to the specific needs of community residents, but at their core emphasize strengthening the family as the primary resource for a child. With the goal of creating a seamless system of support, family support programs can serve an important networking function among local community agencies to enhance service coordination. Family Support America (formerly the Family Resource Coalition of America) and the Federal Community-Based Family Resource and Support (CBFRS) Program support the development of comprehensive, statewide systems of community-based family resource services.

The *Nurturing Program* developed by Stephen Bavolek is a widely acclaimed and implemented set of programs that foster nurturing skills and attitudes for healthy family interaction. This group-based approach emphasizes parents' needs for nurturing and re-parenting, and teaches knowledge and skills in weekly sessions over several weeks. Variations of the program have been developed, tailored to the needs of parents of children from birth to age 5 years, children age 4 to 12 years, and adolescents, in addition to programs for parents who themselves possess special learning needs, and for foster and adoptive families (Bavolek, 1999; Family Development Resources, Inc., 2000).

Parent support groups provide an opportunity for parents to share experiences, both positive and negative, with other parents. Groups vary substantially, from those facilitated by professional therapists to those that use a self-help approach, but the mutual support provided by parents with common experiences is an important common element to reduce social isolation. Many groups blend parenting education and support.

Parents Anonymous, Inc., founded in 1970, is one of the nation's oldest child abuse prevention organizations. Parents Anonymous and similar programs employ the principles of mutual support and parent leadership to stop the cycle of abuse and to strengthen families. Group meetings provide the opportunity for parents to share experiences in a nonjudgmental atmosphere and to gain the support they need to adopt more effective parenting practices. Children's groups may be offered concurrently with parent meetings, to provide both child care and therapeutic support to children. Parents may join a group in recognition of their own need for parenting support or may be referred after child maltreatment issues have been identified (Pion-Berlin & Polinsky, 2000).

MELD, a national organization based in Minnesota, offers parent group curricula that combine education and support. The name MELD comes from the former acronym for "Minnesota Early Learning Design" and is used now to reflect the organization's goals of combining child-rearing information with parenting support as well as creating a sense of community among families to reduce social isolation. MELD's two-year parenting groups reduce risk for child maltreatment by helping parents adopt more realistic expectations of children, understand their child's needs and developmental stages, and learn alternatives to spanking and other types of physical discipline. MELD curricula have been specially designed for new parents, teen parents, young single moms, young dads, African-American families, Latino families, Hmong families, parents with hearing impairments, and parents of children with special needs, among others (http://www.meld.org).

Parent Aide programs provide individualized support to strengthen families and prevent abuse. Parent aides may work with high-risk parents to avoid abuse (secondary prevention) or those with identified child maltreatment issues (tertiary prevention). Parent aides are trained individuals, sometimes volunteers, who work with parents individually to teach and model caring and responsible parenting practices, provide genuine support, link families to needed resources, and stop abusive and neglectful behavior. A survey conducted in 1992 estimated the number of parent aide programs at 800 nationally (Bryan, 1992). The National Parent Aide Network (NPAN), a program of the National Exchange Club Foundation, links parent aides across the country to support and promote the development of parent aide programs nationwide.

Respite care provides a needed break to stressed-out parents. Crisis nurseries care for children who are at risk for or who have experienced abuse or neglect. Most programs offer free child care on a temporary basis, often available 24 hours a day, while helping parents get back on their feet with counseling, parenting classes, and various other services. Crisis nurseries encompass a variety of models, including in-home and out-of-home care. While many crisis nurseries work in tandem with child protective services after maltreatment has occurred, respite care also is a valuable secondary prevention service, providing emergency assistance for parents who cannot turn to extended family or friendly neighbors. ARCH National Resource Center for Respite Care and Crisis Care Services promotes the development of respite care centers and helps parents locate respite services in their own communities.

Accessibility is a notable limitation of most center-based programs. Families must either seek services on their own or rely on referrals from professional sources after parenting problems are already evident. Once enrolled in center-based services, families must have the capacity to travel to the center to receive services and be motivated enough to do so. Many families may be unaware of such services may not recognize how they can benefit from them, or may be unable to physically access center-based services. As a result, center-based programs may fail to reach many of the most vulnerable families in time for prevention to make a difference. Home-based services, described next, are designed to overcome this limitation.

HOME VISITATION

Neonatal home visitation was noted in a report by the U.S. General Accounting Office (1990) as a promising strategy for preventing child abuse and neglect. Since that time, home visitation has gained widespread use in the

United States as a strategy to prevent child maltreatment and support families. By bringing services to parents in their own homes, this strategy can reach parents who might not otherwise seek support services because of obstacles like distrust of public services, language and cultural barriers, and lack of information about community resources. Home visiting programs share a basic rationale: Home visitors can help decrease parental stress by providing support and resources. They also help parents adopt positive parenting practices in the primary environment where child rearing takes place—the home.

Home visitation programs vary in several dimensions, including the central goals of the program, characteristics of the home visitor, frequency and length of service, and target population. While the primary orientation of the program may be maternal and child health, child development and education, or the parent-child relationship, most programs include each of these goals in various rankings of importance. Accordingly, some models stipulate that home visitors be trained in nursing or education. Perhaps more important than the particular educational background, however, are the personal qualities of the home visitor that facilitate the building of a genuine and trusting relationship with mothers in the target population. Programs typically begin prenatally or at the birth of a child; some focus exclusively on first-time parents to promote positive parenting before dysfunctional patterns have a chance to develop. Two home visiting program models with evidence of child maltreatment prevention are described here.

The *Nurse Home Visitation Program* (NHVP), initiated in 1977 as a demonstration program in upstate New York, has shown significant ability to reduce rates of child maltreatment among high-risk families. A central feature of the model is the use of registered nurses to deliver home visits to new parents. The program targets low-income first-time mothers, particularly unmarried teen mothers. While the primary focus is on health issues, such as improved pregnancy outcomes and child health, additional goals include child development, family economic self-sufficiency, and prevention of child abuse and neglect. Services begin prenatally, typically during the second trimester, and continue for two years after the child's birth. Home visits focus on maternal and child health and parental life course. The visits also address the broader context of the family by improving social support, community resource utilization, and other issues as needed. Rigorous research has demonstrated many positive results of the NHVP among high-risk families, including the prevention of child abuse and neglect (Olds et al., 1999).

Healthy Families America® (HFA) was launched by Prevent Child Abuse America in 1992 with the support of Ronald McDonald House Charities and Freddie Mac. HFA's design is based on Hawaii's Healthy Start program, identified in 1991 as an example of the promising potential of home visitation in preventing child abuse (U.S. Advisory Board on Child Abuse and Neglect, 1991). The Healthy Families America approach built on the experience of Healthy Start and more than two decades of research on family support, identifying a series of best practice standards. In contrast to curriculum-based programs, HFA was designed to allow local tailoring of the program while replicating the essential elements of the model (Daro & Harding, 1999). National training, technical assistance, and quality assurance services have been established to ensure that local programs adhere to the critical elements of the model. Over 400 programs in 39 states and the District of Columbia are currently affiliated with the national HFA initiative.

The primary goal of HFA is to prevent child maltreatment and build family strengths by enhancing parent-child interaction, fostering child health and development, and improving family functioning. The program uses a strength-based approach, working with the family to support and empower caregivers, and to reduce risk for child abuse and neglect. HFA sites typically screen new parents to identify those facing significant challenges. Participation is voluntary. Weekly home visits begin prenatally or at birth; the frequency of visits tapers off gradually over a period of three to five years. Home visitors are selected based primarily on personal characteristics rather than a specific educational degree or specialization. A distinguishing characteristic of HFA is the focus on enhancing community support systems for new parents through collaboration and networking with other family support providers.

HFA sites are currently under evaluation in over 45 studies, including several randomized clinical trials. A national HFA Research Network established in 1994 has provided a forum for sharing results and improving research efforts. To date, evaluations of programs in Arizona, Hawaii, Virginia, and other states provide some evidence of reduced risk for child maltreatment by improving parent-child interaction, parenting attitudes and knowledge, home environment, maternal life course, and use of preventive health care. In general, most studies of HFA programs show low rates of child maltreatment among high-risk families, a promising beginning that requires further long-term research.

In practice, the similarities across many home visiting models may be greater than their differences. However, considering the relative strengths of each model and different target audiences, each may play an important role in meeting the varied needs of families in a particular community. Because families participate on a voluntary basis in these programs, offering an array of programs increases the chances that at least one program will appeal to a particular family.

CHILD-PERPETRATED SEXUAL ABUSE (CSA) PREVENTION

Programs at the secondary level targeted to prevent children from becoming sexually abusive are less common, perhaps in part because little is known about risk for CSA. One risk factor that has empirical support is prior victimization as a child. The secondary prevention component of the Kempe Children's Center's *Perpetration Prevention Program* mentioned previously targets children at risk of becoming sexually abusive due to their own victimization by training treatment providers and caregivers of these children. Similarly, the program's tertiary component serves children and adolescents who have already molested others to prevent them from becoming habitual child molesters. The Kempe program works through the National Adolescent Perpetration Network to provide information and support to more than 1,000 professionals working with sexually abusive youth.

◆ BUILDING CAPACITY FOR PREVENTION

Prevention efforts have grown considerably in the past decade, yet rates of child abuse and neglect remain high. National estimates indicate that close to one million children are victims of child maltreatment each year (U.S. Department of Health and Human Services [USDHHS], 2000; Wang & Harding, 1999). Despite the growth of prevention and family support programs in many states, comprehensive prevention efforts are available to only a fraction of families who need them (Knitzer & Page, 1998). In January, 1999, leaders in the field of child maltreatment proclaimed a national call to action in response to the continuing epidemic of child abuse and neglect (Sadler, Chadwick, & Hensler, 1999). This effort seeks to develop a national action plan for a new coordinated, comprehensive, and multidisciplinary approach to eliminate child maltreatment.

Moving from the current collection of independent and often uncoordinated efforts to a comprehensive system calls for more effective collaboration and for broadening existing efforts. There is general agreement among professionals that current resources to combat child maltreatment add up to a mere fraction of society's investment in other major health issues. Greater prevention capacity is required to address this need.

Building prevention capacity requires change from traditional approaches in responding to child maltreatment. Schorr (1997) writes that existing public systems are fundamentally incompatible with the attributes of successful prevention programs. Public agencies and funding streams often compartmentalize services and limit local flexibility. This is in stark contrast to the implementation of programs that take a comprehensive approach to families' needs and give front-line service providers the power to do what needs to be done to meet the diverse needs of individual families. As a result, scaling up effective programs from a demonstration site to a state-wide public service often dilutes or strips away the key elements of success, such as comprehensiveness and flexibility. Some leaders are beginning to tackle the challenge of system reform to create a climate more conducive to prevention. These new strategies in child protection emphasize collaboration and the creation or changing of systems to better support prevention efforts.

Changing the child protection system from an agency-based approach to a community-based approach is a goal of the Community Child Protection project, involving a variety of public and private organizations such as the Edna McConnell Clark Foundation and the Center for the Study of Social Policy. This effort represents a "whole new philosophy and approach to child protection" (Edna McConnell Clark Foundation, 1998, p. 4). While the child protection system plays the lead role in this new approach, all types of neighborhood resources are engaged in a partnership to identify and prevent abuse and neglect. This approach teaches key members of a community, from pediatricians to day-care providers to apartment managers to corner grocers, how to help when a child is at risk. Parents, extended families, and neighbors make up the center of this approach, helping to design strength-based solutions to build stronger families and safer communities for children.

Building effective collaborations among the many organizations engaged in family support and child welfare calls for the concerted efforts and even retraining of service providers in information sharing and working collaboratively with other agencies traditionally viewed as rivals. The Cornell Curriculum on Collaboration and Community Building focuses on in-depth strategies to foster collaboration, training front-line CPS staff together with workers from other agencies in the service community to overcome barriers to working together effectively. The training curriculum promotes a family-strengths approach and discusses the family's role as a collaborative partner in the service delivery process. The federally funded project seeks to strengthen families by improving service coordination and use of community resources.

Supporting local prevention programs at the state or system level is the work of many organizations, only a few of which have already been named. Training and technical assistance, quality assurance, research and evaluation, advocacy, and public relations form the infrastructure for successful prevention efforts. Building these resources at a state or national level is essential so that individual programs can focus on strengthening families. State and national organizations also support the work of local programs through partnerships that foster collaboration and coordination of services at the local level. As an example, Prevent Child Abuse America provides many resources to assist state leaders in building the infrastructure for prevention through its chapter network and Healthy Families America programs. These efforts "behind the scenes" provide the infrastructure and support that is essential for effective programs.

In addition to supporting efforts targeted specifically at preventing child maltreatment and strengthening families, a host of resources that either directly or indirectly support good parenting are fundamental to successful prevention. For example, access to adequate housing, educational opportunities, health care, and quality child care; freedom from neighborhood violence and crime; and livable employment opportunities all serve the basic needs of families and thereby decrease the potential for child maltreatment. The foundation of a caring community increases the likelihood that prevention and support efforts will be successful (Leventhal, 1997).

◆ CONCLUSIONS

The prevention efforts described come in all sizes and configurations. The vast majority have numerous inspiring stories of families and children whose lives have changed for the better as a result of their efforts. Although the incidence of child abuse and neglect in the United States has begun to slowly decline in recent years, it continues to affect nearly a million children every year (USDHHS, 2000). Prevention of child maltreatment has turned out to be much more complex than originally believed.

We now have considerable knowledge about child maltreatment and its causes. Prevention strategies that work are available, yet many efforts continue to be poorly funded and narrowly focused. In addition, the relationship between prevention efforts is often competitive rather than collaborative. "Turf" issues, competition for limited funding, and staff burnout impede efforts to integrate community services into a seamless continuum of family support. Practitioners need to help build bridges between existing services and fill in the gaps, rather than seeking a single program to address all needs. Given the complexity of child maltreatment and its prevention, research must address the question of "what works best for whom, and why?" Such efforts are beginning to take root and should foster the development of a coordinated continuum of services to support families of all types and at all levels of risk.

The prevention programs described in this chapter can serve as examples for those who work to end child abuse and neglect. Alone, however, none of these programs can end the abuse and neglect of our children. The complex needs of families and communities vary widely and require that communities be given the flexibility to address the needs of their own unique citizenry. By weaving together a variety of prevention efforts, communities can create a tapestry of support for families to prevent child abuse and neglect.

◆ REFERENCES

Abrahams, N., Casey, K., & Daro, D. (1992). Teachers' knowledge, attitudes, and beliefs about child abuse and its prevention. <u>Child Abuse and Neglect, 16,</u> 229-238.

Bavolek, S. (1999). Nurturing parent program. <u>Strengthening America's Families.</u> Retrieved November 3, 2000 from the World Wide Web: http://strengtheningfamilies.org/html/programs_1999/25_NPP.html

Bryan, G. (1992). <u>Parent aide programs in the U.S.: Preventing and treating child abuse.</u> Winston-Salem, NC: National Parent Aide Network.

Daro, D. (1993). Child maltreatment research: Implications for program design. In D. Cicchetti and S. Toth (Eds.), <u>Child abuse, child development, and social policy. Advances in applied developmental psychology</u> (Vol. 8) (pp. 331-367). Norwood, NJ: Ablex Publishing Corporation.

Daro, D., & Harding, K. (1999). Healthy Families America: Using research to enhance practice. <u>The Future of Children, 9</u>(1), 152-176.

Dombro, A., O'Donnell, N., Galinsky, E., Melcher, S., & Farber, A. (Eds.) (1996). Engaging the public. In <u>Community mobilization: Strategies to support young children and their families, Chapter 9.</u> New York: Families and Work Institute.

Edna McConnell Clark Foundation. (1998). <u>We are in this together.</u> New York: Author.

Family Development Resources, Inc. (2000). <u>Program description.</u> Retrieved November 3, 2000 from the World Wide Web: http://familydev.com

Galinsky, E. (1999). <u>Ask the children: What America's children really think about working parents.</u> New York: William Morrow and Company, Inc.

Harding, K., & Fromm, S. (in press). <u>Public opinion and behaviors regarding child abuse prevention: 2000 survey.</u> Chicago: Prevent Child Abuse America.

Jones, L. M., & Finkelhor, D. (2001). <u>The decline in child sexual abuse cases.</u> Washington, DC: Office of Juvenile Justice and Delinquency Prevention.

Knitzer, J., & Page, S. (1998). <u>Map and track: State initiatives for young children and families.</u> New York: National Center for Children in Poverty.

Leventhal, J. (1997). The prevention of child abuse and neglect: Pipe dreams or possibilities? <u>Clinical Child Psychology and Psychiatry, 2</u>(4), 489-500.

National Children's Advocacy Center. (NCAC). (2000). <u>SCAN program summary.</u> Huntsville, AL: Author.

Olds, D., Henderson, C., Kitzman, H., Eckenrode, J., Cole, R., & Tatelbaum, R. (1999). Prenatal and infancy home visitation by nurses: Recent findings. <u>The Future of Children, 9</u>(1), 44-65.

Pion-Berlin, L., & Polinsky, M. (2000). <u>Research profile.</u> Washington, DC: Parents Anonymous, Inc.

Pittman, A., Wolfe, D., & Wekerle, C. (1998). Prevention during adolescence: The youth relationships project. In J. Lutzger (Ed.), <u>Handbook of child abuse research and treatment.</u> New York: Plenum Press.

Ryan, G. (2000). Childhood sexuality: A decade of study. Part II—Dissemination and future directions. Child Abuse and Neglect, 24(1), 49-62.

Sadler, G. L., Chadwick, D. L., & Hensler, D. J. (1999). The summary chapter: The national call to action: Moving ahead. Child Abuse and Neglect, 23(10), 1011-1018.

Schorr, L. (1989). Within our reach: Breaking the cycle of disadvantage. New York: Anchor Books.

Schorr, L. (1997). Common purpose: Strengthening families and neighborhoods to rebuild America. New York: Anchor Books.

Sedlak, A., & Broadhurst, D. (1996). The third national incidence study of child abuse and neglect. Washington, DC: U.S. Department of Health and Human Services, Administration for Children, Youth, and Families.

Simpson, A. (1997). The role of the mass media in parenting education. Boston: Center for Health Communication, Harvard School of Public Health.

U.S. Advisory Board on Child Abuse and Neglect (1991). Creating caring communities: Blueprint for an effective federal policy on child abuse and neglect. Washington, DC: U.S. Government Printing Office.

U.S. Department of Health and Human Services, Administration on Children, Youth and Families. (2000). Child maltreatment 1998: Reports from the states to the national child abuse and neglect data system. Washington, DC: U.S. Government Printing Office.

U.S. General Accounting Office. (1990). Home visiting: A promising early intervention strategy for at-risk families. GAO/HRD-90-83. Washington, DC: U.S. Government Printing Office.

Ventura, S., Martin, J., Curtin, S. Matthews, T., & Park, M. (2000). Births: Final data for 1998. Washington, DC: National Center for Health Statistics, U.S. Department of Health and Human Services.

Wang, C., & Harding, K. (1999). Current trends in child abuse reporting and fatalities: The results of the 1998 annual fifty state survey. Chicago: Prevent Child Abuse America.

Weissbourd, B. (1990). A brief history of family support programs. In S. L. Kagan, D. R. Powell, B. Weissbourd, and E. F. Zigler (Eds.), America's family support programs: Perspectives and prospects (pp. 38-56). New Haven, CT: Yale University Press.

Wurtele, S. (1998). School-based child sexual abuse prevention programs: Questions, answers, and more questions. In J. Lutzger (Ed.), Handbook of child abuse research and treatment. New York: Plenum Press.

APPENDIX A: PROFESSIONAL RESOURCES

FEDERAL CLEARINGHOUSES WITH INFORMATION ON CHILDREN AND FAMILIES

(http://www.calib.com/nccanch/pubs/reslist/childandfam.htm)

National Center for Missing and Exploited Children
699 Prince Street
Alexandria, VA 22314
PHONE: (800) THE-LOST   (800) 843-5678
(703) 274-3900
FAX: (703) 274-2220
http://www.missingkids.com

National Clearinghouse on Child Abuse and Neglect Information
330 C St., SW
Washington, DC 20447
PHONE: (800) FYI-3366
(703) 385-7565
FAX: (703) 385-3206
nccanch@calib.com
http://www.calib.com/nccanch

National Sudden Infant Death Syndrome Research Center (NSRC)
2070 Chain Bridge Rd., Suite 450
Vienna, VA 22182
PHONE: (703) 821-8955 ext. 249 or 474
FAX: (703) 821-2098
sids@circsol.com
http://www.circsol.com/sids

Office for Victims of Crime Resource Center
Box 6000
Rockville, MD 20849-6000
PHONE: (800) 627-6872
FAX: (301) 519-5212
askncjrs@ncjrs.org
http://www.ncjrs.org

RESOURCES FOR HEALTH PROFESSIONALS
(http://www.calib.com/nccanch/pubs/reslist/healthpros.htm)

American Academy of Child and Adolescent Psychiatry (AACAP)
3615 Wisconsin Ave., NW
Washington, DC 20016
PHONE: (202) 966-7300
FAX: (202) 966-2891
http://www.aacap.org

American Academy of Pediatrics (AAP)
141 Northwest Point Blvd.
Elk Grove Village, IL 60007-1098
PHONE: (800) 433-9016
FAX: (847) 228-5097
kidsdocs@aap.org
http://www.aap.org

American Professional Society on the Abuse of Children (APSAC)
940 N.E. 13th St.
CHO 3B-3406
Oklahoma City, OK 73104
PHONE: (405) 271-8202
FAX: (405) 271-2931
http://www.apsac.org

Center for Child Protection
Children's Hospital and Health Center
3020 Children's Way MC 5016
San Diego, CA 92123
PHONE: (858) 966-5803
FAX: (858) 966-2365
http://www.chsd.org/ccp

Family Research Laboratory (FRL)
126 Horton Social Science Center
University of New Hampshire
Durham, NH 03824-3586
PHONE: (603) 862-2761
FAX: (603) 862-1122
mas2@christa.unh.edu
http://www.unh.edu/frl

Kempe Children's Center
1825 Marion St.
Denver, CO 80218
PHONE: (303) 864-5252
FAX: (303) 864-5302
Kempe@KempeCenter.org
http://kempecenter.org

Prevent Abuse and Neglect through Dental Awareness (P.A.N.D.A.)
Dr. Lynn Douglas Mouden
4815 W. Markham, Slot 41
Little Rock, AR 72205
PHONE: (501) 661-2595
FAX: (501) 661-2055

Shaken Baby Syndrome Prevention Plus (SBS Prevention Plus)
649 Main St., Suite B
Groveport, OH 43125
PHONE: (800) 858-5222
FAX: (614) 836-8359
sbspp@aol.com
http://www.sbsplus.com

Wisconsin Clearinghouse for Prevention Resources
PO Box 1468
Madison, WI 53701-1468
PHONE: (800) 248-9244
(608) 262-9157
FAX: (608) 262-6346
wchpr@www.uhs.wisc.edu
http://www.uhs.wisc.edu/wch

RESOURCES ON CHILD SEXUAL ABUSE
(http://www.calib.com/nccanch/pubs/reslist/chabuse.htm)

American Professional Society on the Abuse of Children (APSAC)
940 N.E. 13th St.
CHO 3B-3406
Oklahoma City, OK 73104
PHONE: (405) 271-8202
FAX: (405) 271-2931
apsacmems@aol.com
http://www.apsac.org

Association for the Treatment of Sexual Abusers (ATSA)
4900 SW Griffith Dr., Suite 274
Beaverton, OR 97005
PHONE: (503) 643-1023
FAX: (503) 643-5084
atsa@atsa.com
http://www.atsa.com

Center for the Prevention of Sexual and Domestic Violence (CPSDV)
2400 45th St. #10
Seattle, WA 98103
PHONE: (206) 634-1903
FAX: (206) 634-0115
cpsdv@cpsdv.org
http://www.cpsdv.org

Childhelp USA
15757 North 78th St.
Scottsdale, AZ 85260
PHONE: (800) 4-A-CHILD
(800) 2-A-CHILD (TDD line)
(480) 922-8212
FAX: (480) 922-7061
http://www.childhelpusa.org

Family Research Laboratory (FRL)
126 Horton Social Science Center
University of New Hampshire
Durham, NH 03824-3586
PHONE: (603) 862-2761
FAX: (603) 862-1122
mas2@christa.unh.edu
http://www.unh.edu/frl

Kempe Perpetration Prevention Program
Kempe Children's Center, UCHSC
1825 Marion St.
Denver, CO 80218
PHONE: (303) 864-5252
FAX: (303) 864-5302
Kempe@KempeCenter.org
http://kempecenter.org

Mothers Against Sexual Abuse (MASA)
PO Box 2966
Huntersville, NC 28070
PHONE: (704) 895-0489
FAX: (704) 895-5964
masa@againstsexualabuse.org
http://www.againstsexualabuse.org

National Center for Missing and Exploited Children
Exploited Child Unit
699 Prince St.
Alexandria, VA 22314-3175
PHONE: (800) 843-5678
(703) 274-3900
FAX: (703) 274-2220
http://www.missingkids.com
http://cybertipline.com

National Children's Advocacy Center (NCAC)
200 Westside Square, Suite 700
Huntsville, AL 35801
PHONE: (256) 533-0531
FAX: (256) 534-6883
webmaster@ncac-hsv.org
http://www.ncac-hsv.org

Parents United International, Inc.
615 15th St.
Modesto, CA 95354
PHONE: (209) 572-3446
FAX: (209) 524-7780
parents.united@usa.net
http://members.tripod.com/#Parents_United/Chapters/PUI.htm

The Safer Society Foundation, Inc.
PO Box 340
Brandon, VT 05733-0340
PHONE: (802) 247-3132
FAX: (802) 247-4233
http://www.safersociety.org

Stop It Now!
PO Box 495
Haydenville, MA 01039
PHONE: (888) PREVENT (Available Monday-Friday, 1:00 pm – 5:00 pm EST)
(413) 268-3096
FAX: (413) 268-3098
help@stopitnow.com
http://www.stopitnow.com

TOLL-FREE CRISIS HOTLINE NUMBERS
(http://www.calib.com/nccanch/pubs/reslist/tollfree.htm)

Crisis Type	Who to Call	Hotline	Hours	Who They Help
Child Abuse	Childhelp USA	800-4-A-CHILD (800-422-4453)	24 hr/7 days	Child abuse victims, offenders, parents
Child Abuse	Youth Crisis Hotline	800-HIT-HOME (800-448-4663)	24 hr/7 days	Individuals reporting child abuse
Family Violence	National Domestic Violence Hotline	800-799-SAFE (800-799-7233)	24 hr/7 days	Children, parents, friends, offenders
Missing/Abducted Children	Child Find of America	800-I-AM-LOST (800-426-5678)	9-5 EST, M-F; 24 hr answering machine	Parents reporting lost or abducted children
Missing/Abducted Children	Child Find of America-Mediation	800-A-WAY-OUT (800-292-9688)	9-5 EST, M-F; 24 hr answering machine	Parents (abduction, child custody)
Missing/Abducted Children	Child Quest International Sighting Line	800-248-8020	24 hr/7 days	Individuals with missing child emergencies and/or sighting information
Missing/Abducted Children	National Center for Missing and Exploited Children	800-843-5678	24 hr/7 days	Parents, law enforcement
Missing/Abducted Children	Operation Lookout National Center for Missing Youth	800-782-SEEK (800-782-7335)	9-6 PST, M-F	Individuals with missing child emergencies and/or sighting information

Crisis Type	Who to Call	Hotline	Hours	Who They Help
Rape/Incest	Rape Abuse and Incest National Network (RAINN)	800-656-HOPE (800-656-4673)	24 hr/7 days	Rape and incest victims
Relief for Caregivers	National Respite Locator Service	800-7-RELIEF (800-773-5433)	8:30-5 EST, M-F	Professionals caring for children with disabilities, terminal illness, or at risk of child abuse or neglect
Victims of Violent Crimes	National Center for Victims of Crime	800-FYI-CALL (800-394-2255)	8:30-5:30 EST, M-F	All victims of violent crimes
Youth in Trouble/ Runaways	Covenant House Hotline	800-999-9999	24 hr/7 days	Problem teens, runaways, family members
Youth in Trouble/ Runaways	Girls and Boys Town	800-448-3000	24 hr/7 days	Troubled children, parents, family members
Youth in Trouble/ Runaways	National Referral Network for Kids in Crisis	800-KID-SAVE (800-543-7283)	24 hr/7 days	Professionals, parents, adolescents
Youth in Trouble/ Runaways	National Runaway Switchboard (NRS)	800-621-4000	24 hr/7 days	Adolescents, families
Youth in Trouble/ Runaways	Youth Crisis Hotline	800-HIT-HOME (800-448-4663)	24 hr/7 days	Individuals wishing to obtain help for runaways

PREVENTION RESOURCE LISTING
(http://www.calib.com/nccanch/pubs/reslist/prevres.htm)

American Humane Association (AHA)
Children's Division
63 Inverness Dr., East
Englewood, CO 80112-5117
PHONE: (800) 227-4645
(303) 792-9900
FAX: (303) 792-5333
children@americanhumane.org
http://www.americanhumane.org

AVANCE Family Support and Education Program
301 South Frio St., Suite 380
San Antonio, TX 78207
PHONE: (210) 270-4630
FAX: (210) 270-4612
http://www.avance.org

412

Center for the Prevention of Sexual and Domestic Violence (CPSDV)
2400 45th St. #10
Seattle, WA 98103
PHONE: (206) 634-1903
FAX: (206) 634-0115
cpsdv@cpsdv.org
http://www.cpsdv.org

Child Abuse Prevention Network
Cornell University
MVR Hall
Ithaca, NY 14853-4401
PHONE: (607) 255-3888
FAX: (607) 255-8562
tph3@cornell.edu
http://child-abuse.com

Child Trauma Academy
childtrauma@bcm.tmc.edu
http://www.childtrauma.org

Child Trends
4301 Connecticut Ave., NW, Suite 100
Washington, DC 20008
PHONE: (202) 362-5580
FAX: (202) 362-5533
http://www.childtrends.org

Childhelp USA
15757 N. 78th St.
Scottsdale, AZ 85260
PHONE: (480) 922-8212 or 1-800-4-A-CHILD
http://www.childhelpusa.org

Children's Institute International (CII)
711 S. New Hampshire Ave.
Los Angeles, CA 90005
PHONE: (213) 385-5100
FAX: (213) 383-1820
http://www.childrensinstitute.org

Committee for Children (CFC)
2203 Airport Way South, Suite 500
Seattle, WA 98134
PHONE: (800) 634-4449 (8-4:30 PST)
or (206) 343-1223 (8-4:30 PST)
FAX: (206) 343-1445
info@cfchildren.org
http://www.cfchildren.org

Family Life Development Center
Cornell University
N202 Martha Van Rensselaer Hall
Ithaca, NY 14853-4401
PHONE: (607) 255-7794
FAX: (607) 255-8562
http://fldc.cornell.edu

Family Support America (formerly Family Resource Coalition of America)
20 N. Wacker Dr., Suite 1100
Chicago, IL 60606
PHONE: (312) 338-0900
FAX: (312) 338-1522
http://www.familysupportamerica.org

International Society for Prevention of Child Abuse and Neglect (ISPCAN)
200 N. Michigan Ave., Suite 500
Chicago, IL 60601
PHONE: (312) 578-1401
FAX: (312) 578-1405
ISPCAN@ispcan.org
http://www.ispcan.org

Kempe Children's Center
1825 Marion St.
Denver, CO 80218
PHONE: (303) 864-5252
FAX: (303) 864-5302
Kempe@KempeCenter.org
http://kempecenter.org

MELD: Programs to Strengthen Families
219 N. 2nd St., Suite 200
Minneapolis, MN 55401
PHONE: (612) 332-7563
FAX: (612) 344-1959
meldctrl@aol.com
http://meld.org

National Alliance of Children's Trust and Prevention Funds (ACT)
Department of Psychology
Michigan State University
East Lansing, MI 48824-1117
PHONE: (517) 432-5096
FAX: (517) 432-2476
millsda@msu.edu
http://www.msu.edu/user/millsda/index.html

National Center for Education in Maternal and Child Health (NCEMCH)
2000 15th St., North, Suite 701
Arlington, VA 22201-2617
PHONE: (703) 524-7802
FAX: (703) 524-9335
info@ncemch.org
http://www.ncemch.org

National Children's Advocacy Center (NCAC)
200 Westside Sq., Suite 700
Huntsville, AL 35801
PHONE: (256) 533-0531
FAX: (256) 534-6883
webmaster@ncac-hsv.org
http://www.ncac-hsv.org

National Exchange Club Foundation for the Prevention of Child Abuse
3050 Central Ave.
Toledo, OH 43606
PHONE: (800) 924-2643 or (419) 535-3232
FAX: (419) 535-1989
info@preventchildabuse.com
http://www.preventchildabuse.com

National Indian Child Welfare Association (NICWA)
5100 SW Macadam Ave., Suite 300
Portland, OR 97230
PHONE: (503) 222-4044
FAX: (503) 222-4007
info@nicwa.org
http://www.nicwa.org

National Maternal and Child Health Clearinghouse (NMCHC)
207 Chain Bridge Rd., Suite 450
Vienna, VA 22182-2536
PHONE: (888) 434-4MCH or (703) 356-1964
FAX: (703) 821-2098
http://www.nmchc.org

National Resource Center for Community-Based Family Resource and Support Programs (FRIENDS)
Chapel Hill Training Outreach Project
800 Eastowne Dr., Suite 105
Chapel Hill, NC 27514
PHONE: (800) 888-7970
FAX: (919) 968-8879
http://friendsnrc.org

Parents Anonymous, Inc.
675 W. Foothill Blvd., Suite 220
Claremont, CA 91711
PHONE: (909) 621-6184
FAX: (909) 625-6304
parentsanon@msn.com
http://www.parentsanonymous-natl.org

Prevent Child Abuse America
200 S. Michigan Ave., 17th Floor
Chicago, IL 60604-2404
PHONE: (800) CHILDREN or (312) 663-3520
FAX: (312) 939-8962
mailbox@preventchildabuse.org
http://www.preventchildabuse.org

Safer Society Foundation, Inc.
PO Box 340
Brandon, VT 05733-0340
PHONE: (802) 247-3132
FAX: (802) 247-4233
http://www.safersociety.org

Shaken Baby Syndrome Prevention Plus (SBS Prevention Plus)
649 Main St., Suite B
Groveport, OH 43125
PHONE: (800) 858-5222
FAX: (614) 836-8359
sbspp@aol.com
http://www.sbsplus.com

Society for Prevention Research (SPR)
Meeting Solutions (Melissa Greenhouse)
111 S. Calvert, Suite 2700
Baltimore, MD 21202
PHONE: (410) 385-5236
http://www.oslc.org/spr/sprhome.html

Zero to Three: National Center for Infants, Toddlers and Families
2000 M St. NW, Suite 200
Washington, DC 20036-3307
PHONE: (800) 899-4301 or (202) 638-1144
FAX: (202) 638-0851
0to3@zerotothree.org
http://www.zerotothree.org

APPENDIX B: STATE TOLL-FREE CHILD ABUSE REPORTING NUMBERS

For states not listed, or when the reporting party resides in a different state than the child, please call Childhelp USA, 800-4-A-CHILD (800-422-4453), or your local child protective services (CPS) agency.

Alaska (AK)
800-478-4444

Arizona (AZ)
888-SOS-CHILD
(888-767-2445)

Arkansas (AR)
800-482-5964

Connecticut (CT)
800-842-2288
800-624-5518 (TDD/hearing impaired)

Delaware (DE)
800-292-9582

Florida (FL)
800-96-ABUSE
(800-962-2873)

Illinois (IL)
800-252-2873

Indiana (IN)
800-562-2407

Iowa (IA)
800-362-2178

Kansas (KS)
800-922-5330

Kentucky (KY)
800-752-6200

Maine (ME)
800-452-1999

Maryland (MD)
800-332-6347

Massachusetts (MA)
800-792-5200

Michigan (MI)
800-942-4357

Mississippi (MS)
800-222-8000

Missouri (MO)
800-392-3738

Montana (MT)
800-332-6100

Nebraska (NE)
800-652-1999

Nevada (NV)
800-992-5757

New Hampshire (NH)
800-894-5533

New Jersey (NJ)
800-792-8610
800-835-5510 (TDD/hearing impaired)

New Mexico (NM)
800-797-3260

New York (NY)
800-342-3720

North Dakota (ND)
800-245-3736

Oklahoma (OK)
800-522-3511

Oregon (OR)
800-854-3508

Pennsylvania (PA)
800-932-0313

Rhode Island (RI)
800-RI-CHILD
(800-742-4453)

Texas (TX)
800-252-5400

Utah (UT)
(not toll free)
801-538-4377

417

Virginia (VA)
800-552-7096

Washington (WA)
800-562-5624

West Virginia (WV)
800-352-6513

Wyoming (WY)
800-457-3659

INDEX

A

AA; *see* Alcoholics Anonymous
AACAP; *see* American Academy of Child and
Adolescent Psychiatry
AACWA; *see* Adoption Assistance and Child Welfare
Act of 1980
AAP; *see* American Academy of Pediatrics
AATA; *see* American Art Therapy Association
Abandonment, 49–50
    and neglect; *see* Neglect
    physical, 50
Abnormal responses, psychological abuse of children
    and, 82
Abrogation of privileged communications, mandated
    report and, 316–317
Absolute immunity, 320, 322
Abuse
    alcohol, 42, 114, 117, 200
    allegations of, child custody disputes
        and, 338–340
    animal, child abuse and, 186
    child; *see* Child abuse
    of discretion, 340
    drug, 42, 114, 117
    multiple-victim/multiple-perpetrator, ritualistic
        abuse and, 70–71
    neglect versus, 50–51
    peer; *see* Peer abuse
    physical; *see* Physical abuse
    psychological; *see* Psychological abuse
    ritualistic, 68–69, 70–71
    sexual; *see* Sexual abuse
Abuse-related syndromes, evidentiary issues
    and, 347–348
Abusive contact burns, 10
Academic skills
    improving, 202–203
    in prevention of violence, 122
Accessibility, center-based prevention programs
    and, 400

Accidental disclosure, sexual abuse and, 25
Accountability, social work and, 159
Acquired mineral deficiencies, 15
Acquired vitamin deficiencies, 15
Acronyms, Internet, 273
ACT; *see* National Alliance of Children's Trust and
        Prevention Funds
Acting out sexually, 141, 144–145
AD dolls; *see* Anatomically detailed dolls
Adjudicatory hearing, 326–327, 356
Admissions by parties, evidentiary issues and, 343
Adolescent art, 236, 238
Adolescents; *see also* Child(ren)
    screening for violence in, 119–120
    violence prevention programs for, 125–126
Adoption and Safe Families Act of 1997 (ASFA), 312,
        327–328, 357, 358
Adoption Assistance and Child Welfare Act of 1980
        (AACWA), 312, 357, 358
Adult bites, 11
Adult pornographic material in suspected perpetrator's
        residence, 293
Adults Molested as Children, 194
Advocacy, role of law enforcement in investigation of
        child abuse and, 280
Advocates, child, 360–361
Affective symptoms, multiple personality disorder
        and, 147
Age-inappropriate sexualized behavior, 141, 144
Age-inappropriate toilet training, 75–76
Age-specific language, interviewing children during
        sexual abuse evaluations and, 26
Aggression, 116–117
AHA; *see* American Humane Association
Alateen, 200
Alcohol abuse, 42, 114, 117, 200
Alcoholics Anonymous (AA), 194, 383
Alexithymia, human maternal deprivation and, 63
Allegations
    child custody disputes and, 338–340

G

Gang violence, prevention of, 126
GCCA; *see* Georgia Council on Child Abuse, Inc.
Genital herpes, 33
Genital warts, 31, 33
Georgia Council on Child Abuse, Inc. (GCCA), 396
Germain, 168
Gibson, William, 273
Girls and Boys Town, 412
Glancing blows, burns and, 10
Glove burns, 9
Gluteal coitus, 30
Gonorrhea, 31, 33
Good faith, actions taken in, 320
Good faith immunity, 322
Good faith reporters, immunity for, mandated report
        and, 316
Google, 275
Government, role of, local prevention efforts
        and, 388–389
Graduate training programs in art therapy, 229
Grand jury in criminal court, 333
Grasp marks, 4, 6
Grief, psychological abuse and, 77
Group home, children with special needs and, 59
Growth plates, 12
Growth velocity, failure to thrive and, 44
Guardian ad litem
        child advocates and, 360–361
        child custody disputes and, 339
        in juvenile court, 325
Guilty pleas in criminal court, 334
Gun control, 111, 117, 120–121

H

Hair loss, physical abuse and, 11–12
Hallucinations, auditory, multiple personality disorder
        and, 148
Harm, demonstrable, 40
Harm standard, neglect and, 40
Hawaii's Healthy Start program, 401–402
Head circumference, failure to thrive and, 44
Head Start, 51, 122, 124, 368–369
Health and Human Services, Department of, 311, 369,
        402
Health care needs in foster care, 364
Health departments, 314
Health insurance for children, 43
Health maintenance visits, scheduled, neglect and, 52
Health Professionals, Resources for, 408–409
Healthcare organization policies and procedures
        requirements, mandated reporting and, 167
Healthcare providers, education by, in prevention of
        violence, 119–120
Healthcare social workers, reporting duties of, 159–160
Healthy Families America (HFA), 401–402, 404
Healthy Start, 401–402
Hearing
        adjudicatory, 326–327, 356
        bifurcated, in juvenile court, 323
        custody

        in juvenile court, 326
    detention, 356
    dispositional, 323, 327–328, 356–357
    preliminary, 332–333, 356
    protective custody, 316
    shelter, 356
Hearsay
    evidentiary issues and, 342–346
    sexual abuse, evidentiary issues and, 344
Heater, burns from, 8–9
Hemophilia, bruising and, 5
Hemorrhages
    intracranial, retinal hemorrhages and, 17
    retinal; *see* Retinal hemorrhages
    subdural, shaken baby syndrome and, 16–17
Henoch-Schönlein purpura (HSP), bruising and, 6
Herpes, 33
Herpes simplex virus, 31
HFA; *see* Healthy Families America
History folder, Internet and, 262, 264
History that raises suspicion of abuse, 2
Hit, definition of, 274
HIV; *see* Human immunodeficiency virus
Home
    group, children with special needs and, 59
    legal procedures to remove children from, 355–357
Home hot water heaters, temperature of, 7
Home page, definition of, 274
Home schooling, 56
Home visitation, 123–124, 400–402
Homebuilders Program, 367
Home-visiting programs, 366
Homicide, children who die by, 110–112, 113
Hopefulness, social work and, 159
Hot curling iron, burns from, 8
Hot water heaters, temperature of, 7
Hotline
    child abuse and neglect, 312–313
    state toll-free, 417–418
    toll-free crisis, 411–412
Hotline workers, child abuse, 359
HSP; *see* Henoch-Schönlein purpura
HTML; *see* HyperText Markup Language
HTTP; *see* HyperText Transfer Protocol
Human bites, 11
Human immunodeficiency virus (HIV), 33, 45
Human maternal deprivation, alexithymia and, 63
Human papillomavirus, 31
Husband–wife privileged communication, 316–317
Hymenal examination, 29
Hyperlink, definition of, 274
HyperText Markup Language (HTML), definition of,
        274
HyperText Transfer Protocol (HTTP), definition of, 274
Hypoglycemia, failure to thrive and, 46
Hyponatremia, failure to thrive and, 46

I

ICRA; *see* Internet Content Rating System
Idaho v. Wright, 346
IDEA Amendments of 1997; *see* Individuals with

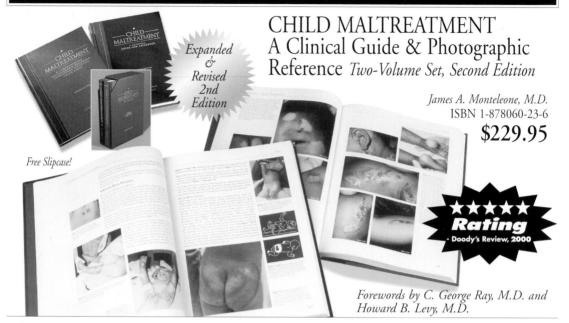

Child Maltreatment Order Form

✂ *Photocopy or detach this order form and mail or fax today.*

❏ **YES!** send me _____ set(s) of *Child Maltreatment* at $229.95* per set.

Please check payment option:

❏ Bill my credit card: ❏ MasterCard   ❏ VISA

Acct. No. _____

Signature _____

Exp. Date _____

❏ **Purchase order** _____

detach and mail to: **G.W. Medical Publishing, Inc.**
2601 Metro Boulevard • Maryland Heights, MO 63043 • 314-298-0330
Order Toll-Free 1-800-600-0330 or FAX orders 314-298-2820
* Tentative price

Shipping Information

Name _____

Title _____

Institution _____

Address _____

City _____

State _____ Zip _____

Daytime phone (_____) _____

*All orders are billed for postage, handling, and state sales tax where appropriate. All prices subject to change without notice. If using a purchase order, please attach to this form.

Money-back Guarantee: If you are not 100% pleased, simply return the book(s). Your money will be promptly refunded without question or comment, less a 15% restocking fee.

✂ *Photocopy or detach this order form and mail or fax today.*

❏ **YES!** send me _____ set(s) of *Child Maltreatment* at $229.95* per set.

Please check payment option:

❏ Bill my credit card: ❏ MasterCard   ❏ VISA

Acct. No. _____

Signature _____

Exp. Date _____

❏ **Purchase order** _____

detach and mail to: **G.W. Medical Publishing, Inc.**
2601 Metro Boulevard • Maryland Heights, MO 63043 • 314-298-0330
Order Toll-Free 1-800-600-0330 or FAX orders 314-298-2820
* Tentative price

Shipping Information

Name _____

Title _____

Institution _____

Address _____

City _____

State _____ Zip _____

Daytime phone (_____) _____

*All orders are billed for postage, handling, and state sales tax where appropriate. All prices subject to change without notice. If using a purchase order, please attach to this form.

Money-back Guarantee: If you are not 100% pleased, simply return the book(s). Your money will be promptly refunded without question or comment, less a 15% restocking fee.

✂ *Photocopy or detach this order form and mail or fax today.*

❏ **YES!** send me _____ set(s) of *Child Maltreatment* at $229.95* per set.

Please check payment option:

❏ Bill my credit card: ❏ MasterCard   ❏ VISA

Acct. No. _____

Signature _____

Exp. Date _____

❏ **Purchase order** _____

detach and mail to: **G.W. Medical Publishing, Inc.**
2601 Metro Boulevard • Maryland Heights, MO 63043 • 314-298-0330
Order Toll-Free 1-800-600-0330 or FAX orders 314-298-2820
* Tentative price

Shipping Information

Name _____

Title _____

Institution _____

Address _____

City _____

State _____ Zip _____

Daytime phone (_____) _____

*All orders are billed for postage, handling, and state sales tax where appropriate. All prices subject to change without notice. If using a purchase order, please attach to this form.

Money-back Guarantee: If you are not 100% pleased, simply return the book(s). Your money will be promptly refunded without question or comment, less a 15% restocking fee.

CHILD ABUSE QUICK-REFERENCE
for Healthcare Professionals, Social Services, and Law Enforcement

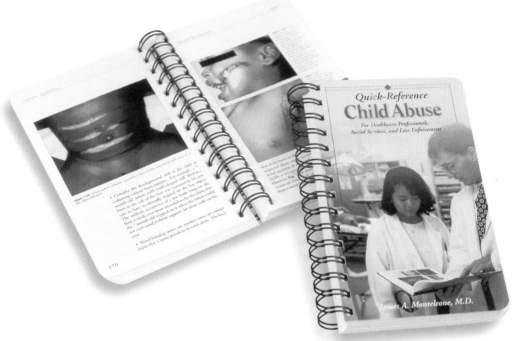

James A. Monteleone, M.D.
350 pages, 186 images, with 18 contributors;
ISBN 1-878060-28-7

$42.95

Foreword by Charles Wilson, M.S.S.W.

Sized for the on-the-go professional to carry in a pocket or a briefcase, *Child Abuse Quick-Reference* is the perfect comprehensive field guide for identifying child abuse and documenting an investigation. Now frontline professionals who must identify and report children who are at risk or have suffered abuse can get the information they need quickly with the pocket-sized *Child Abuse Quick-Reference*. _Law Enforcement Officers, Medical Professionals, Social Workers, Prosecuting Attorneys, Teachers,_ and others can all benefit from this easy-to-use reference that explains what to look for and what steps to take in identifying and reporting physical, sexual,

and emotional abuse. Lists are provided that describe indicators of the widest range of possible abuses.

Written by experts in various fields of child maltreatment, this practical guidebook walks you through each step involved in an intervention. Explicit instructions are provided for performing thorough examinations, assessing lab and radiologic studies, conducting effective interviews, and writing competent reports that will survive courtroom scrutiny. Every topic is designed to equip you in effectively handling the complexities of today's child abuse cases. **Order toll-free at 1-800-600-0330.**

Table of Contents

G W Medical Publishing, Inc.
2601 Metro Boulevard, Maryland Heights, MO 63043-2411
phone: 1-800-600-0330
e-mail: info@gwmedical.com
web site: http://www.gwmedical.com

Child Abuse Quick Reference Order Form

✂ *Photocopy or detach this order form and mail or fax today.*

❏ **YES!** send me _____ book(s) of *Child Abuse Quick-Reference* at $42.95 each.

Please check payment option:

❏ Bill my credit card: ❏ MasterCard ❏ VISA

Acct. No. _____

Signature _____

Exp. Date _____

❏ **Purchase order** _____

detach and mail to: **G.W. Medical Publishing, Inc.**
2601 Metro Boulevard • Maryland Heights, MO 63043 • 314-298-0330
Order Toll-Free 1-800-600-0330 or FAX orders 314-298-2820

Shipping Information

Name _____

Title _____

Institution _____

Address _____

City _____

State _____ Zip _____

Daytime phone (_____) _____

*All orders are billed for postage, handling, and state sales tax where appropriate. All prices subject to change without notice. If using a purchase order, please attach to this form.

Money-back Guarantee: If you are not 100% pleased, simply return the book(s). Your money will be promptly refunded without question or comment, less a 15% restocking fee.

✂ *Photocopy or detach this order form and mail or fax today.*

❏ **YES!** send me _____ book(s) of *Child Abuse Quick-Reference* at $42.95 each.

Please check payment option:

❏ Bill my credit card: ❏ MasterCard ❏ VISA

Acct. No. _____

Signature _____

Exp. Date _____

❏ **Purchase order** _____

detach and mail to: **G.W. Medical Publishing, Inc.**
2601 Metro Boulevard • Maryland Heights, MO 63043 • 314-298-0330
Order Toll-Free 1-800-600-0330 or FAX orders 314-298-2820

Shipping Information

Name _____

Title _____

Institution _____

Address _____

City _____

State _____ Zip _____

Daytime phone (_____) _____

*All orders are billed for postage, handling, and state sales tax where appropriate. All prices subject to change without notice. If using a purchase order, please attach to this form.

Money-back Guarantee: If you are not 100% pleased, simply return the book(s). Your money will be promptly refunded without question or comment, less a 15% restocking fee.

✂ *Photocopy or detach this order form and mail or fax today.*

❏ **YES!** send me _____ book(s) of *Child Abuse Quick-Reference* at $42.95 each.

Please check payment option:

❏ Bill my credit card: ❏ MasterCard ❏ VISA

Acct. No. _____

Signature _____

Exp. Date _____

❏ **Purchase order** _____

detach and mail to: **G.W. Medical Publishing, Inc.**
2601 Metro Boulevard • Maryland Heights, MO 63043 • 314-298-0330
Order Toll-Free 1-800-600-0330 or FAX orders 314-298-2820

Shipping Information

Name _____

Title _____

Institution _____

Address _____

City _____

State _____ Zip _____

Daytime phone (_____) _____

*All orders are billed for postage, handling, and state sales tax where appropriate. All prices subject to change without notice. If using a purchase order, please attach to this form.

Money-back Guarantee: If you are not 100% pleased, simply return the book(s). Your money will be promptly refunded without question or comment, less a 15% restocking fee.

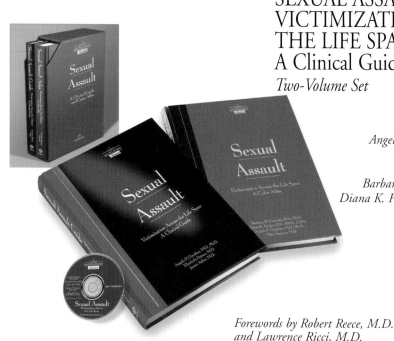

SEXUAL ASSAULT VICTIMIZATION ACROSS THE LIFE SPAN
A Clinical Guide and Color Atlas
Two-Volume Set

Angelo P. Giardino, M.D., Ph.D.
Elizabeth Datner, M.D.
Janice Asher, M.D.
Barbara W. Girardin, R.N., Ph.D.
Diana K. Faugno, R.N., B.S.N., C.P.N.
Mary J. Spencer, M.D.
*800 pages, 2,000 images,
with over 50 contributors*
ISBN 1-878060-62-7

$229.95*
*Tentative price.

*Forewords by Robert Reece, M.D.
and Lawrence Ricci, M.D.*

Sexual assault knows no boundaries. It crosses all gender, social, ethnic, religious, and cultural lines. As awareness of this problem grows, it has become evident that children, adolescents, adults, and the elderly are all vulnerable targets. This two-volume set is a comprehensive reference and color atlas for anyone who may come into contact with someone who has been sexually assaulted. Emergency room personnel, physicians, EMTs, social service agencies, judges, attorneys, and law enforcement personnel will find critical information on how to perform a physical examination, proper documentation, forensic evidence (including DNA analysis), and legal and prosecution issues. The special sections devoted to the unique problems of sexual victimization of each age group are invaluable, as well as chapters on male sexual assault, incarcerated rape, assault of the elderly and people with disabilities, and domestic violence and acquaintance rape.

This two-volume set debunks the myths surrounding sexual assault and presents specific findings related to behavior, affective functioning, cognitive ability, and physical conditions that can be observed in victims. Complete case studies are also present, including photos of the same injury in various stages of healing, to help determine the age of the injury, as well as whether or not it stems from assault. This reference is written by experts in various fields of assault—pediatricians, forensic nurses, psychologists, emergency room physicians, law enforcement personnel, social workers, and attorneys. Each contributor has dealt first-hand with sexual assault cases and has formulated the approaches presented here.

Table of Contents (tentative)

Each chapter contains sections on normal anatomy, findings in assault or abuse, and other variants.

G W Medical Publishing, Inc.
2601 Metro Boulevard, Maryland Heights, MO 63043-2411
phone: 1-800-600-0330
e-mail: info@gwmedical.com
web site: http://www.gwmedical.com

Sexual Assault Order Form

✂ *Photocopy or detach this order form and mail or fax today.*

❑ YES! send me _____ book(s) of *Sexual Assault Victimization Across The Life Span* at $229.95* per set.

Please check payment option:

❑ Bill my credit card: ❑ MasterCard   ❑ VISA

Acct. No. _____

Signature _____

Exp. Date _____

❑ **Purchase order** _____

detach and mail to: **G.W. Medical Publishing, Inc.**
2601 Metro Boulevard • Maryland Heights, MO 63043 • 314-298-0330
Order Toll-Free 1-800-600-0330 or FAX orders 314-298-2820
* Tentative price

Shipping Information

Name _____

Title _____

Institution _____

Address _____

City _____

State _____ Zip _____

Daytime phone (_____) _____

*All orders are billed for postage, handling, and state sales tax where appropriate. All prices subject to change without notice. If using a purchase order, please attach to this form.

Money-back Guarantee: If you are not 100% pleased, simply return the book(s). Your money will be promptly refunded without question or comment, less a 15% restocking fee.

✂ *Photocopy or detach this order form and mail or fax today.*

❑ YES! send me _____ book(s) of *Sexual Assault Victimization Across The Life Span* at $229.95* per set.

Please check payment option:

❑ Bill my credit card: ❑ MasterCard   ❑ VISA

Acct. No. _____

Signature _____

Exp. Date _____

❑ **Purchase order** _____

detach and mail to: **G.W. Medical Publishing, Inc.**
2601 Metro Boulevard • Maryland Heights, MO 63043 • 314-298-0330
Order Toll-Free 1-800-600-0330 or FAX orders 314-298-2820
* Tentative price

Shipping Information

Name _____

Title _____

Institution _____

Address _____

City _____

State _____ Zip _____

Daytime phone (_____) _____

*All orders are billed for postage, handling, and state sales tax where appropriate. All prices subject to change without notice. If using a purchase order, please attach to this form.

Money-back Guarantee: If you are not 100% pleased, simply return the book(s). Your money will be promptly refunded without question or comment, less a 15% restocking fee.

✂ *Photocopy or detach this order form and mail or fax today.*

❑ YES! send me _____ book(s) of *Sexual Assault Victimization Across The Life Span* at $229.95* per set.

Please check payment option:

❑ Bill my credit card: ❑ MasterCard   ❑ VISA

Acct. No. _____

Signature _____

Exp. Date _____

❑ **Purchase order** _____

detach and mail to: **G.W. Medical Publishing, Inc.**
2601 Metro Boulevard • Maryland Heights, MO 63043 • 314-298-0330
Order Toll-Free 1-800-600-0330 or FAX orders 314-298-2820
* Tentative price

Shipping Information

Name _____

Title _____

Institution _____

Address _____

City _____

State _____ Zip _____

Daytime phone (_____) _____

*All orders are billed for postage, handling, and state sales tax where appropriate. All prices subject to change without notice. If using a purchase order, please attach to this form.

Money-back Guarantee: If you are not 100% pleased, simply return the book(s). Your money will be promptly refunded without question or comment, less a 15% restocking fee.

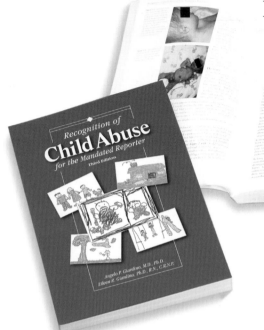

Recognition of Child Abuse for the Mandated Reporter Order Form

✂ *Photocopy or detach this order form and mail or fax today.*

❑ **YES!** send me _____ book(s) of *Recognition of Child Abuse for the Mandated Reporter* at $46.95* each.

Please check payment option:

❑ Bill my credit card: ❑ MasterCard ❑ VISA

Acct. No. _____

Signature _____

Exp. Date _____

❑ **Purchase order** _____

detach and mail to: **G.W. Medical Publishing, Inc.**
2601 Metro Boulevard • Maryland Heights, MO 63043 • 314-298-0330
Order Toll-Free 1-800-600-0330 or FAX orders 314-298-2820
* Tentative price

Shipping Information

Name_____

Title_____

Institution _____

Address _____

City _____

State _____ Zip_____

Daytime phone (   ) _____

*All orders are billed for postage, handling, and state sales tax where appropriate. All prices subject to change without notice. If using a purchase order, please attach to this form.

Money-back Guarantee: If you are not 100% pleased, simply return the book(s). Your money will be promptly refunded without question or comment, less a 15% restocking fee.

✂ *Photocopy or detach this order form and mail or fax today.*

❑ **YES!** send me _____ book(s) of *Recognition of Child Abuse for the Mandated Reporter* at $46.95* each.

Please check payment option:

❑ Bill my credit card: ❑ MasterCard ❑ VISA

Acct. No. _____

Signature _____

Exp. Date _____

❑ **Purchase order** _____

detach and mail to: **G.W. Medical Publishing, Inc.**
2601 Metro Boulevard • Maryland Heights, MO 63043 • 314-298-0330
Order Toll-Free 1-800-600-0330 or FAX orders 314-298-2820
* Tentative price

Shipping Information

Name_____

Title_____

Institution _____

Address _____

City _____

State _____ Zip_____

Daytime phone (   ) _____

*All orders are billed for postage, handling, and state sales tax where appropriate. All prices subject to change without notice. If using a purchase order, please attach to this form.

Money-back Guarantee: If you are not 100% pleased, simply return the book(s). Your money will be promptly refunded without question or comment, less a 15% restocking fee.

✂ *Photocopy or detach this order form and mail or fax today.*

❑ **YES!** send me _____ book(s) of *Recognition of Child Abuse for the Mandated Reporter* at $46.95* each.

Please check payment option:

❑ Bill my credit card: ❑ MasterCard ❑ VISA

Acct. No. _____

Signature _____

Exp. Date _____

❑ **Purchase order** _____

detach and mail to: **G.W. Medical Publishing, Inc.**
2601 Metro Boulevard • Maryland Heights, MO 63043 • 314-298-0330
Order Toll-Free 1-800-600-0330 or FAX orders 314-298-2820
* Tentative price

Shipping Information

Name_____

Title_____

Institution _____

Address _____

City _____

State _____ Zip_____

Daytime phone (   ) _____

*All orders are billed for postage, handling, and state sales tax where appropriate. All prices subject to change without notice. If using a purchase order, please attach to this form.

Money-back Guarantee: If you are not 100% pleased, simply return the book(s). Your money will be promptly refunded without question or comment, less a 15% restocking fee.

NURSING APPROACH TO THE EVALUATION OF CHILD MALTREATMENT

Eileen R. Giardino, Ph.D., R.N., C.R.N.P.
Angelo P. Giardino, M.D., Ph.D.
440 pages, 120 images, 18 contributors
ISBN 1-878060-51-1

$46.95*

*Tentative price.

Foreword by Anne Burgess, D.N.Sc.

Nurses and nurse practitioners are critical members of child abuse treatment teams. *Nursing Approach to the Evaluation of Child Maltreatment* provides the information nurses need to identify and accurately interpret the signs of maltreatment and then report it in a specific manner.

Presented in 16 chapters comprising three major sections—"The Problem," "Approaches to Patient Care," and "Special Issues"—the areas of physical abuse, sexual abuse, and neglect are extensively addressed. Each chapter is structured to give a general overview of the topic area, followed by a detailed treatment plan relevant to the specific types of abuse. In addition, each chapter includes easy-to-use checklists, examination hints, and flow charts for ready access to important information.

Edited by a nurse and a pediatrician, with chapter contributions by experts in the various fields of child maltreatment, this handy reference is a must-have for every nurse and nurse practitioner who may be confronted with possible child abuse. It clearly illustrates what is and what is not abuse and identifies the most common types of child abuse, as well as uncommon but possible causes. The steps to be taken when interviewing the child and the details to be addressed in performing a physical examination in a suspected abusive situation are also provided. This book is especially valuable for **nurse practitioners, school nurses, pediatric nurses, APNs, FNPs, social service and safety personnel, state and federal agencies, and allied health/emergency room technicians.**
Order toll-free at 1-800-600-0330.

Table of Contents

G W Medical Publishing, Inc.
2601 Metro Boulevard, Maryland Heights, MO 63043-2411
phone: 1-800-600-0330
e-mail: info@gwmedical.com
web site: http://www.gwmedical.com

Nursing Approach to the Evaluation of Child Maltreatment Order Form

❏ **YES!** send me _____ book(s) of *Nursing Approach to the Evaluation of Child Maltreatment* at $46.95* each.

Please check payment option:

❏ Bill my credit card: ❏ MasterCard   ❏ VISA

Acct. No. _____

Signature _____

Exp. Date _____

❏ **Purchase order** _____

detach and mail to: **G.W. Medical Publishing, Inc.**
2601 Metro Boulevard • Maryland Heights, MO 63043 • 314-298-0330
Order Toll-Free 1-800-600-0330 or FAX orders 314-298-2820
* Tentative price

Shipping Information

Name _____

Title _____

Institution _____

Address _____

City _____

State _____ Zip _____

Daytime phone ( ) _____

*All orders are billed for postage, handling, and state sales tax where appropriate. All prices subject to change without notice. If using a purchase order, please attach to this form.

Money-back Guarantee: If you are not 100% pleased, simply return the book(s). Your money will be promptly refunded without question or comment, less a 15% restocking fee.

❏ **YES!** send me _____ book(s) of *Nursing Approach to the Evaluation of Child Maltreatment* at $46.95* each.

Please check payment option:

❏ Bill my credit card: ❏ MasterCard   ❏ VISA

Acct. No. _____

Signature _____

Exp. Date _____

❏ **Purchase order** _____

detach and mail to: **G.W. Medical Publishing, Inc.**
2601 Metro Boulevard • Maryland Heights, MO 63043 • 314-298-0330
Order Toll-Free 1-800-600-0330 or FAX orders 314-298-2820
* Tentative price

Shipping Information

Name _____

Title _____

Institution _____

Address _____

City _____

State _____ Zip _____

Daytime phone ( ) _____

*All orders are billed for postage, handling, and state sales tax where appropriate. All prices subject to change without notice. If using a purchase order, please attach to this form.

Money-back Guarantee: If you are not 100% pleased, simply return the book(s). Your money will be promptly refunded without question or comment, less a 15% restocking fee.

❏ **YES!** send me _____ book(s) of *Nursing Approach to the Evaluation of Child Maltreatment* at $46.95* each.

Please check payment option:

❏ Bill my credit card: ❏ MasterCard   ❏ VISA

Acct. No. _____

Signature _____

Exp. Date _____

❏ **Purchase order** _____

detach and mail to: **G.W. Medical Publishing, Inc.**
2601 Metro Boulevard • Maryland Heights, MO 63043 • 314-298-0330
Order Toll-Free 1-800-600-0330 or FAX orders 314-298-2820
* Tentative price

Shipping Information

Name _____

Title _____

Institution _____

Address _____

City _____

State _____ Zip _____

Daytime phone ( ) _____

*All orders are billed for postage, handling, and state sales tax where appropriate. All prices subject to change without notice. If using a purchase order, please attach to this form.

Money-back Guarantee: If you are not 100% pleased, simply return the book(s). Your money will be promptly refunded without question or comment, less a 15% restocking fee.

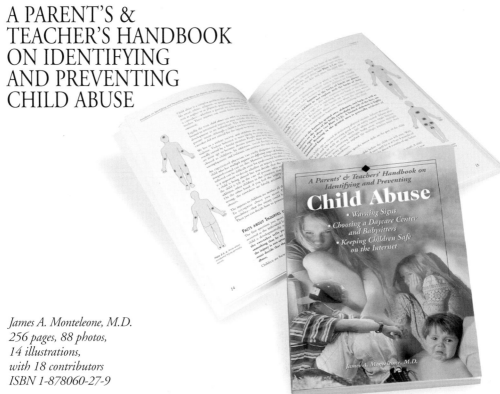

A Parent's & Teacher's Handbook on Identifying and Preventing Child Abuse Order Form

✂ *Photocopy or detach this order form and mail or fax today.*

❏ **YES!** send me _____ book(s) of *A Parent's and Teacher's Handbook on Identifying and Preventing Child Abuse* at $19.95 each.

Please check payment option:

❏ Bill my credit card: ❏ MasterCard ❏ VISA

Acct. No. _____

Signature _____

Exp. Date _____

❏ **Purchase order** _____

detach and mail to: **G.W. Medical Publishing, Inc.**
2601 Metro Boulevard • Maryland Heights, MO 63043 • 314-298-0330
Order Toll-Free 1-800-600-0330 or FAX orders 314-298-2820

Shipping Information

Name _____

Title _____

Institution _____

Address _____

City _____

State _____ Zip _____

Daytime phone (_____) _____

*All orders are billed for postage, handling, and state sales tax where appropriate. All prices subject to change without notice. If using a purchase order, please attach to this form.

Money-back Guarantee: If you are not 100% pleased, simply return the book(s). Your money will be promptly refunded without question or comment, less a 15% restocking fee.

✂ *Photocopy or detach this order form and mail or fax today.*

❏ **YES!** send me _____ book(s) of *A Parent's and Teacher's Handbook on Identifying and Preventing Child Abuse* at $19.95 each.

Please check payment option:

❏ Bill my credit card: ❏ MasterCard ❏ VISA

Acct. No. _____

Signature _____

Exp. Date _____

❏ **Purchase order** _____

detach and mail to: **G.W. Medical Publishing, Inc.**
2601 Metro Boulevard • Maryland Heights, MO 63043 • 314-298-0330
Order Toll-Free 1-800-600-0330 or FAX orders 314-298-2820

Shipping Information

Name _____

Title _____

Institution _____

Address _____

City _____

State _____ Zip _____

Daytime phone (_____) _____

*All orders are billed for postage, handling, and state sales tax where appropriate. All prices subject to change without notice. If using a purchase order, please attach to this form.

Money-back Guarantee: If you are not 100% pleased, simply return the book(s). Your money will be promptly refunded without question or comment, less a 15% restocking fee.

✂ *Photocopy or detach this order form and mail or fax today.*

❏ **YES!** send me _____ book(s) of *A Parent's and Teacher's Handbook on Identifying and Preventing Child Abuse* at $19.95 each.

Please check payment option:

❏ Bill my credit card: ❏ MasterCard ❏ VISA

Acct. No. _____

Signature _____

Exp. Date _____

❏ **Purchase order** _____

detach and mail to: **G.W. Medical Publishing, Inc.**
2601 Metro Boulevard • Maryland Heights, MO 63043 • 314-298-0330
Order Toll-Free 1-800-600-0330 or FAX orders 314-298-2820

Shipping Information

Name _____

Title _____

Institution _____

Address _____

City _____

State _____ Zip _____

Daytime phone (_____) _____

*All orders are billed for postage, handling, and state sales tax where appropriate. All prices subject to change without notice. If using a purchase order, please attach to this form.

Money-back Guarantee: If you are not 100% pleased, simply return the book(s). Your money will be promptly refunded without question or comment, less a 15% restocking fee.